# Oxford Specialist
# Handbooks in Surgery
# Surgical
# Oncology

### Edited by

### M. Asif Chaudry

Specialist Registrar in Surgery, London
& Surgical Research Fellow,
Division of Surgery & Interventional Science,
University College London,
London, UK

### Marc C. Winslet

Professor of Surgery, Head of Department & Chairman of
Division of Surgery & Interventional Science,
University College London,
London, UK

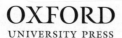

D1414225

# OXFORD
## UNIVERSITY PRESS

OXFORD
UNIVERSITY PRESS

Great Clarendon Street, Oxford OX2 6DP

Oxford University Press is a department of the University of Oxford.
It furthers the University's objective of excellence in research, scholarship,
and education by publishing worldwide in

Oxford New York

Auckland Cape Town Dar es Salaam Hong Kong Karachi
Kuala Lumpur Madrid Melbourne Mexico City Nairobi
New Delhi Shanghai Taipei Toronto

With offices in

Argentina Austria Brazil Chile Czech Republic France Greece
Guatemala Hungary Italy Japan Poland Portugal Singapore
South Korea Switzerland Thailand Turkey Ukraine Vietnam

Oxford is a registered trade mark of Oxford University Press
in the UK and in certain other countries

Published in the United States
by Oxford University Press Inc., New York

British Library Cataloguing in Publication Data
Data available

Library of Congress Cataloging-in-Publication Data
Chaudry, M. Asif.
  Surgical oncology / M. Asif Chaudry, Marc Winslet.
    p. ; cm. -- (Oxford specialist handbooks in surgery)
  Includes index.
  ISBN 978-0-19-923709-8 (alk. paper)
  1. Cancer--Surgery--Handbooks, manuals, etc. I. Winslet, M. C. (Marc
C.) II. Title. III. Series: Oxford specialist handbooks in oncology.
  [DNLM: 1. Neoplasms--surgery--Handbooks. QZ 39 C496s 2009]
  RD651.C43 2009
  616.99'4059--dc22
                                                     2009008905

Typeset by Cepha Imaging Private Ltd., Bangalore, India
Printed in China
on acid-free paper through
Asia Pacific Offset

ISBN 978-0-19-923709-8

10 9 8 7 6 5 4 3 2 1

Oxford University Press makes no representation, express or implied, that the drug dosages in
this book are correct. Readers must therefore always check the product information and clinical
procedures with the most up to date published product information and data sheets provided by
the manufacturers and the most recent codes of conduct and safety regulations. The authors and
publishers do not accept responsibility or legal liability for any errors in the text or for the misuse
or misapplication of material in this work.

Some of the medication discussed in this book may not be available through normal channels
and only available by special arrangements. Other examples used in research studies and recommended in international guidelines are unlicensed or may be subject to being used outside of their
licensed dosage ranges within the UK. We suggest consulting the BNF and local prescribing guide-
lines/protocols before using unfamiliar medication.

# Foreword

The editors and authors of this book are to be congratulated on the production of an excellent manuscript which will be of immense value both to specialist registrars in general surgery and to anyone who wants a contemporary reference text on their bookshelf.

Over the past decade especially, and in almost every sub-speciality of surgical oncology, there have been major changes in routine management as a result of improvement in technology and systemic therapies. Some of these changes have been dramatic and have taken many of us by surprise. The changes include staging techniques, neo– and adjuvant therapies and especially new surgical tools which have had a profound effect on our surgical practice. It is now more difficult then ever to keep abreast of changes in near-parallel sub-specialities which previously was not difficult.

This book will help to overcome some of these difficulties and will be of great value for life-long students of surgery. Throughout the book, the results of major trials which have brought about these changes are discussed and easy references provided. I have nothing but praise for this book which has been written by highly motivated members of our profession. The quality of the writing, its content, and presentation is exceptionally good and one is left with a sense of admiration for the authors and the reassurance that the future of surgery in this complex and challenging area is secure.

J Meirion Thomas MS FRCP FRCS
Professor of Surgical Oncology
Royal Marsden Hospital and Imperial College

# Foreword

# Preface

How should surgeons deal with cancer patients? The cornerstone of effective treatment is a multidisciplinary collaboration between many specialties in which surgeons are not only concerned about operative accessibility and technique, but rather have a deep understanding of the fundamental biology of the malignancy they are dealing with and appreciate the reach of multi-modal treatment.

Higher surgical trainees regularly moving to the variety of general surgical sub-specialties are required to rapidly assimilate updated clinical algorithms based on evidence-based guidelines that go beyond the basic level achieved at the MRCS. This is essential if we are to ensure that the clinical trajectory of our cancer patients is optimal. Clinical guidelines issued by national bodies usually run into hundreds of pages of dense text, as do the many textbooks of surgical oncology that often provide encyclopaedic reference material and conceptual information, but are not targeted at immediate practice.

In writing this handbook, our aim has been to provide a summarized yet reliable compendium of all of those books and resources online that both our colleagues and ourselves have quickly peered into on so many occasions: after reading a pathology report or CT scan in the outpatient's clinic; before presenting a case at a multidisciplinary team meeting at a regional cancer centre; or perhaps, before asking our seniors or colleagues for advice about surveillance for a complex case and before proceeding to the operating theatre. It is also the book that many were in search of when preparing for exams that contained the breadth of surgical oncology that had to be studied from an array of sub-specialty sources. It is an essential practical handbook that draws together all the varied guidelines and source materials that form the basis of this complex subject.

MAC
MCW

# Acknowledgements

We acknowledge all those who have helped in producing this book at OUP namely Susan Crowhurst and Suzy Armitage.

We gratefully acknowledge that many figures in this book have been reproduced from Operative Surgery, second edition, (2006) edited by Greg R. McLatchie and David J. Leaper (Oxford: Oxford University Press).

We are deeply thankful to and acknowledge the assistance of Dr Dhiren Shah, St Thomas's Hospital, London, who provided the radiological images used in this book.

We thank Christopher Liao for his invaluable input throughout.

We also thank Mr Don Menzies, ICENI Centre, Colchester, UK, for the laparoscopic images used—and Tino Solomon, ICENI Centre, Colchester, UK, for his assistance in the compilation of this book.

We gratefully acknowledge Mr Daren Francis, Chase Farm Hospital, Enfield, for his suggestions in the anal and colorectal chapters.

# Contents

Additional references including comprehensive trial references
can be found online at www.oup.com/uk/isbn/9780199237098

# Abbreviations

| | |
|---|---|
| $^{18}$FDG | $^{18}$fluorodeoxyglucose |
| 5-FU | 5-fluorouracil |
| 5-HT | 5-hydroxytryptamine |
| 5-HTP | 5-hydroxytryptophan |
| ♂ | male |
| ♀ | female |
| ↓ | decreased |
| ↑ | increased |
| ↑↑ | increased considerably |
| > | more than |
| < | less than |
| >> | much more than |
| AAT | alpha-1-antitrypsin |
| ABC–OAS | adjuvant breast cancer–ovarian ablation or suppression (trial) |
| AC | adriamycin, cyclophosphamide |
| ACC | adrenocortical carcinoma |
| ACS | American Cancer Society |
| ACTH | adrenocorticotrophic hormone |
| ADCC | antibody-dependent cellular cytotoxicity |
| ADH | anti-diuretic hormone |
| ADT | androgen deprivation therapy |
| AFP | alpha-1 foetoprotein |
| AGP | alpha-1-glycoprotein |
| AI | aromatase inhibitors |
| AIN | anal intra-epithelial neoplasia |
| AIDS | autoimmune deficiency syndrome |
| AJCC | American Joint Committee on Cancer |
| ALA | aminolaevulinic acid |
| AML | acute myeloid leukaemia |
| ANC | axillary nodal clearance |
| APC | adenomatous polyposis coli |
| APR | abdominoperineal resection |
| APTT | activated partial thromboplastin time |
| APUD | amine precursor uptake and decarboxylation |
| ASCO | American Society of Clinical Oncology |
| ATAC | anastrozole or tamoxifen alone or in combination (trial) |

| ATLAS | adjuvant tamoxifen longer against shorter |
|---|---|
| ATTOM | aTTom: adjuvant tamoxifen-to offer more? |
| AXR | abdominal X-ray |
| B | biopsy |
| BCC | basal cell carcinoma |
| BCG | bacillus Calmette–Guerin |
| BCS | breast conserving surgery |
| BEP | bleomycin-etoposide-cisplatin |
| BILCAP | biliary tract cancer capecitabine RCT |
| BMI | Body Mass Index |
| BRCA | breast cancer gene |
| BRCA-1 | breast cancer gene 1 |
| BRCAPRO | breast cancer pro statistical model and software |
| BV | bevacizumab |
| bx | biopsy |
| C | cytology |
| CA | 19-9: carbohydrate antigen 19-9 |
| Ca | cancer, carcinoma |
| CBD | common bile duct |
| CC | cranial-caudal |
| CCA | cholangiocarcinoma |
| CDDP | cisplatin |
| CEA | carcinoembryonic antigen |
| CFTR | cystic fibrosis transmembrane conductance regulator |
| CHOP | cyclophosphamide, hydroxydaunorubicin, vincristine, prednisolone |
| CHRPE | congenital hypertrophic retinal pigmentation |
| CHT | chemotherapy |
| CHT/RT | chemoradiotherapy |
| CIS | carcinoma *in situ* |
| CLOCC | chemotherapy and local ablation vs. chemotherapy |
| CMF | cyclophosphamide-methotrexate-5-fluorouracil |
| CNBCS | Canadian National Breast Cancer Screening Study |
| CNS | central nervous system |
| CORE | continuing outcomes relevant to evista |
| CPA | cyproterone acetate |
| CR | complete response rate or complete remission |
| CRC | colorectal cancer |
| CRP | C reactive protein |
| CSF | colony-stimulating factor |
| CT | computed tomography |
| CTZ | cyclophosphamide |

| CVA | cerebrovascular accident |
|---|---|
| CX | cetuximab |
| CXR | chest radiograph |
| DCBE | double-contrast barium enema |
| DCC | deleted in colorectal cancer |
| DCF | docetaxel, cisplatin and 5-FU |
| DCIS | ductal carcinoma *in situ* |
| DDFS | distant disease-free survival |
| DEXA | dual energy X-ray absorptiometry |
| DFS | disease-free survival |
| DFSP | dermatofibrosarcoma protuberans |
| DGE | delayed gastric emptying |
| DHT | dihydrotestosterone |
| DIEA | deep inferior epigastric artery |
| DIEP | deep inferior epigastric perforator |
| DJ | duodeno-jejunal |
| DM | diabetes mellitus |
| DRE | digital rectal examination |
| DTC | differentiated thyroid cancer |
| DVT | deep vein thrombosis |
| DXT | radiotherapy |
| EBCTG | Early Breast Cancer Trialists' Group |
| EBRT | external beam radiotherapy |
| EBV | Epstein–Barr virus |
| ECF | epirubicin, cisplatin, fluorouracil |
| ECOG | Eastern Cooperative Oncology Group |
| ECX | epirubicin, cisplatin, capecitabine |
| EGFR | epidermal growth factor receptor |
| EMR | endoscopic mucosal resection |
| EOF | epirubicin, oxaliplatin, 5-FU |
| EORTC | European Organization for Research and Treatment of Cancer |
| EOX | epirubicin, oxaliplatin, capecitabine |
| ER | oestrogen receptor |
| ERCP | endoscopic retrograde cholangiopancreatography |
| ES | endoscopic sonography |
| ESPAC | European Study Group for Pancreatic Cancer |
| ET | endotracheal |
| ETOH | ethanol |
| EUA | examination under anaesthetic |
| EUS | endoscopic ultrasound |
| FA | folinic acid |

| FAC | fluorouracil, adriamycin, cyclophosphamide (cytoxan) |
|---|---|
| FACS | Follow up after colorectal surgery |
| FAM | 5-FU, doxorubicin, and mitomycin |
| FAP | familial adenomatous polyposis |
| FBC | full blood count |
| FDG | fluorodeoxyglucose |
| FDR | 1st degree relative |
| FDR | fixed dose rate |
| FFP | fresh frozen plasma |
| FHx | family history |
| FISH | fluorescent *in situ* hybridization |
| FL-HCC | fibrolamellar hepatocellular carcinoma |
| FNA | fine needle aspiration |
| FNAC | fine needle aspiration cytology |
| FNH | focal nodular hyperplasia |
| FNNAC | fine needle non-aspiration cytology |
| FOB | faecal occult bloods |
| FOLFIRI | 5FU + leucovorin + irinotecan |
| FOLFOX | 5-fluorouracil + leucovorin + oxaliplatin |
| FPC | familial polyposis coli |
| FSH | follicle stimulating hormone |
| FTC | follicular thyroid cancer |
| FUDR | floxuridine |
| G&S | group and save |
| GA | general anaesthetic |
| GAP | gluteal artery perforator |
| GCT | germ-cell tumour |
| GDA | gastroduodenal artery |
| GFR | glomerular filtration rate |
| GI | gastrointestinal |
| GIA | gastrointestinal anastomosis |
| GIST | gastrointestinal stromal tumour |
| GIT | gastrointestinal tract |
| GITSG | Gastrointestinal Tumour Study Group |
| GM | granulocyte/macrophage |
| GnRH | gonadotrophin-releasing hormone |
| GORD | gastro-oesophageal reflux disease |
| GRE | gradient echo |
| GS | Gardeners' syndrome |
| GSA | galactosyl-human serum albumin-diethylenetriamine-pentaacetic acid |

| h | hours |
|---|---|
| HAI | hepatic artery infusion |
| HAL | (hexi)-aminolaevulinic acid |
| HASTE | Half fourier Acquisition Single shot Turbo spin Echo |
| HBV | hepatitis B virus |
| HCC | hepatocellular carcinoma |
| HCG | human chorionic gonadotropin |
| HD | haemodialysis |
| HDU | high dependency unit |
| HIAA | 5-hydroxyindoleacetic acid |
| HIF | hypoxia inducible factor |
| HIFU | high intensity focused ultrasound |
| HIP | health insurance plan |
| HIV | human immunodeficiency virus |
| HNPCC | hereditary non-polyposis colorectal cancer |
| HPF | high power field |
| HPV | human papillomavirus |
| HRPC | hormone-refractory prostate cancer |
| HRT | hormone replacement therapy |
| IBD | inflammatory bowel disease |
| ICS | intercostal space |
| IES | Inter-Group Exemestane Study |
| IGCCCG | International Germ Cell Cancer Collaborative Group |
| IGCNU | intratubular germ-cell neoplasia unclassified |
| IHC | immunohistochemistry |
| IJV | internal jugular vein |
| IM | intramuscular |
| IMA | inferior mesenteric artery |
| IMN | internal mammary node |
| IMPACT | immediate preoperative arimidex compared to tamoxifen |
| IMRT | intensity modulated radiotherapy |
| IMV | inferior mesenteric vein |
| INR | International Normalized Ratio |
| IPMN | intraductal papillary mucinous neoplasm |
| IPSS | International Prognostic Scoring System |
| ISUP | International Society of Urological Pathology |
| ITA | Italian Tamoxifen Anastrozole (study) |
| ITU | intensive care unit |

| | |
|---|---|
| IV | intravenous |
| IVAC | ifosfamide, mesna, etoposide, and cytarabine |
| IVC | inferior vena cava |
| IVU | intravenous urography |
| c-KIT | CD117 |
| LA | left atrial |
| LA | local anaesthetic |
| LCIS | lobular carcinoma *in situ* |
| LD | latissimus dorsi |
| LDH | lactate dehydrogenase |
| LFT | liver function test |
| LH | luteinizing hormone |
| LMS | leimoyosarcoma |
| LN | lymph node |
| LOH | loss of heterozygosity |
| LHRH | luteinizing hormone-releasing hormone |
| M | metastases |
| MAGIC | Medical Research Council Adjuvant Gastric Infusional Chemotherapy |
| MALT | mucosa-associated lymphoid tissue |
| MC&S | microscopy, culture & sensitivity |
| MCN | mucinous cystic neoplasm |
| MDCT | multi-detector computed tomography |
| MDT | multidisciplinary team |
| MEGX | monoethylglycinexylidide |
| MEN | multiple endocrine neoplasia |
| MFH | malignant fibrous histiocytomas |
| MI | myocardial infarction |
| MIBG | meta-iodobenzylguanidine$^{131}$I |
| MIBI | methoxyisobutylisonitrile |
| min | minutes |
| MLO | medio-lateral-oblique |
| MMC | mitomycin C |
| MMP | matrix metalloproteinases |
| MMR | mismatch repair |
| MMS | Mohs micrographic surgery |
| MORE | Multiple Outcomes for Raloxifene Evaluation (trial) |
| MPNST | malignant peripheral nerve sheath tumours |
| MRA | magnetic resonance arteriography |
| MRCP | magnetic resonance cholangiopancreatography |
| MRCS | member of the Royal College of Surgeons |

| MRI | magnetic resonance imaging |
| MRS | magnetic resonance spectroscopy |
| MRSA | methicillin-resistant *Staphylococcus aureus* |
| MSI | microsatellite instability |
| MTC | medullary thyroid carcinoma |
| MTD | malignant teratoma differentiated |
| MTI | malignant teratoma intermediate |
| MTU | malignant teratoma undifferentiated |
| MVAC | methotrexate, vinblastine, adriamycin, and cisplatin |
| MVD | microvessel density |
| MYH | MUTYH: mutY Homolog (gene) |
| N | nodes |
| NBM | nil by mouth |
| NCCN | National Comprehensive Cancer Network |
| Nd:YAG | neodynium: yttrium-aluminium-garnet |
| NG | nasogastric |
| NGT | nasogastric tube |
| NHL | non-Hodgkins lymphoma |
| NHSBSP | National Health Service Breast Screening Programme |
| NICE | National Institute for Health and Clinical Excellence |
| NO | nitric oxide |
| NPI | Nottingham Prognostic Index |
| NPV | negative predictive value |
| NSGCT | non-seminomatous germ cell tumour |
| OCP | oral contraceptive pill |
| O-G | oesophagogastric |
| OGD | oesophagogastro-duodenoscopy |
| OS | overall survival |
| PanIN | pancreatic intra-epithelial neoplasia |
| PD | pancreatico-duodenal |
| PDS | polydioxanone |
| PDT | photodynamic therapy |
| PE | pulmonary embolus |
| PEB | cisplatin, etoposide, and bleomycin |
| PEG | percutaneous endoscopic gastrostomy |
| PEI | percutaneous ethanol injection |
| PET | positron emission tomography |
| PFS | progression-free survival |
| PG | prostaglandin |
| PgR | progesterone receptor |
| PHex | protein-bound hexose |

| | |
|---|---|
| PICC | peripherally inserted central catheters |
| PJ | Peutz–Jeughers |
| po | orally by mouth |
| PPPD | pylorus preserving pancreatico-duodenectomy |
| PPV | positive predictive value |
| PR | progesterone receptor |
| PRLV | percentage remnant liver volume |
| PSA | prostate-specific antigen |
| PSC | primary sclerosing cholangitis |
| PTC | papillary thyroid cancer |
| PTEN | phosphatase and tensin homolog |
| PTH | parathyroid hormone |
| PUNLMP | papillary urothelial neoplasms of low malignant potential |
| PV | per vaginum |
| PVE | portal vein embolization |
| qds | four times daily |
| QUART | quadrantectomy + ANC + RT |
| RAS | a signal transduction protein |
| RBA | retinol-binding protein |
| RCC | renal cell carcinoma |
| RCT | randomized control trial |
| RF | radiofrequency |
| RFA | radiofrequency ablation |
| RH | rhenium |
| ROLL | radioisotope-guided occult lesion localization |
| RPLND | retroperitoneal lymph node dissection |
| RR | response rate |
| RT | radiotherapy |
| RTOG | Radiation Therapy Oncology Group |
| RT-PCR | reverse transcriptase polymerase chain reaction |
| Rx | treatment |
| s | seconds |
| SBFT | small bowel follow through |
| SCA | senile cardiac amyloidosis |
| SC | subcutaneous |
| SCC | squamous cell carcinoma |
| SCLN | supraclavicular lymph node |
| SCM | sternocleidomastoid |
| SCPRT | short course pre-operative radiotherapy |
| SCV | subclavian vein |

| SDR | 2nd degree relative |
|---|---|
| SERM | selective oestrogen receptor blocker |
| SHARP | Sorafenib HCC Assessment Randomized Protocol (trial) |
| SIEA | superficial inferior epigastric artery |
| SLE | systemic lupus erythematosus |
| SLN | sentinel lymph node |
| SLNB | sentinel lymph node biopsy |
| SMA | superior mesenteric artery |
| SMV | superior mesenteric vein |
| SNB | sentinel node biopsy |
| SOFEA | Study of Faslodex, Exemestane, and Arimidex |
| SPECT | single photon emission computerized tomography |
| SPIO | supermagnetic iron oxide particles |
| SRS | somatostatin receptor scintigraphy |
| SSFSE | single shot fast spin echo |
| STIR | short tau inversion recovery (MRI sequence) |
| STZ | streptozotocin |
| SVC | superior vena cava |
| T | tumour |
| TAC | taxotere, adriamycin, and cyclophosphamide |
| TAP | thoracodorsal artery perforator |
| TB | tuberculosis |
| TBG | thyroxine-binding globulin |
| TBPA | thyroxine-binding pre-albumin |
| TCC | transitional cell carcinoma |
| tds | three times daily |
| TE | echo time |
| TEAM | Tamoxifen Exemestane Adjuvant Multinational Trial |
| TEM | transanal endoscopic microsurgery |
| TFT | thyroid function test |
| Tg | thyroglobulin |
| TIN | testicular intra-epithelial neoplasia |
| TME | total mesenteric excision |
| TNM | tumour, nodes, metastases |
| TPA | tissue polypeptide |
| TPN | total parenteral nutrition |
| TRAM | transverse rectus abdominis myocutaneous |
| TRH | thyrotrophin-releasing hormone |
| TRUS | trans-rectal ultrasound |
| TS | thymidine synthase |

| | |
|---|---|
| TSE | turbo spin echo |
| TSH | thyroid stimulating hormone |
| TTP | time to tumour progression |
| TUG | transverse upper gracilis (flap) |
| TURBT | treatment of non-invasive bladder cancer |
| TURP | transurethral resection of the prostate |
| TVUS | trans-vaginal ultrasound |
| U&E | urea & electrolytes |
| UC | ulcerative colitis |
| UICC | International Union Against Cancer |
| UKCCCR | UK Coordinating Committee on Cancer Research |
| ULN | upper limit of normal range |
| US | ultrasound |
| USPIO | ultrasmall particle iron oxide |
| USS | ultrasound scan |
| UW | University of Wisconsin solution |
| VEGF | vascular endothelial growth factor |
| VIP | etopside-ifosfamide-cisplatin |
| VNPI | Van Nuys Prognostic Index |
| WLE | wide local excision |
| WHI | Women's Health Initiative |
| X | Xeloda |
| YSR | 5-year survival rate |
| ZEBRA | Zoladex Early Breast Cancer Research Association |

# Contributors

**Irfan Ahmed**
Department of Interventional Radiology,
St Thomas's Hospital, London

*Cancer Radiology*

**Manit Arya**
The Institute of Urology,
University College London

*Renal Cancer, Bladder Cancer,
Prostate Cancer, Testicular Cancer*

**Hennah Bashir**
Chelsea & Westminster Hospital,
London

*Palliative Care Topics*

**M. Asif Chaudry**
Division of Surgery & Interventional
Science, University College
London

*Editor and Author*

**Gemma Conn**
University Department of Surgery,
Royal Free Hospital, London

*Liver and Biliary Cancer*

**Jason Constantinou**
Department of Surgery,
Whittington Hospital, London

*Anal Cancer*

**Harleen Kaur Deol**
Department of Surgery,
The Royal London Hospital,
London

*Thyroid Cancer*

**Mark Emberton**
Institute of Urology,
University College London
and
Clinical Director,
Clinical Effectiveness Unit,
The Royal College of Surgeons
of England

*Renal Cancer, Bladder Cancer,
Prostate Cancer, Testicular Cancer*

**Asma Fikree**
Department of Gastroenterology
Barnet & Chase Farm Hospital
London

*Small Bowel Cancer*

**Said A. Mohamed**
Epsom & St Helier University
Hospital, Epsom

*Gastric Cancer*

**Borzoueh Mohammadi**
Department of HPB Surgery,
Royal Free Hospital, London

*Pancreatic Cancer*

**Antony Pittathankal**
Department of Surgery,
St Bartholomew's Hospital, London

*Breast Cancer*

**Shahnawaz Rasheed**
St Mark's Hospital & Academic
Institute, London

*Colorectal Cancer*

**James R. A. Skipworth**
Department of Upper
Gastrointestinal Cancer,
Division of Surgical & Interventional
Sciences,
University College London

*Oesophageal Cancer*

**Simon G. T. Smith**
Department of Breast and
Oncoplastic Surgery,
Broomfield Hospital, Chelmsford

*Thyroid Cancer, Breast Cancer*

**Ben Stubbs**
Princess Alexandra Hospital,
Harlow

*Soft Tissue Sarcoma*

**Hashim Uddin Ahmed**
The Institute of Urology,
University College London

*Renal Cancer, Bladder Cancer,
Prostate Cancer, Testicular Cancer*

**Marc C. Winslet**
Division of Surgery & Interventional
Science, University College
London

*Editor*

# Detailed contents

**3  Thyroid and parathyroid tumours**                                    **175**

**4  Oesophageal cancer**                                                 **221**

# Chapter 1

# Cancer radiology

# 1. Common imaging modalities

Imaging techniques for diagnosis, staging, surveillance, and treatment of cancer are rapidly improving. Advances in technology and development of novel techniques have meant that 'best practice' is constantly evolving. Radiologists are at the forefront of deciding which test is appropriate.

# Plain film 'X-rays' and barium studies

• In 1895 William Conrad Rontgen produced and detected electromagnetic radiation known today as X-rays.
• Since then X-ray use has developed as a useful diagnostic tool in the detection of cancer.
• Oral and IV contrast agents may be used in conjunction with plain film radiography to detect specific pathologies.
• X-rays are used therapeutically in radiotherapy.

Common indications for plain film and barium examinations in cancer diagnosis include:

• CXR – initial imaging for lung Ca or metastases.
• Barium enema for colorectal Ca.
• Barium swallow/meal/follow-through for upper GI malignancies.

## Oral contrast media

### Barium sulphate

Different preparations are used for different parts of the GI tract – e.g. E-Z HD® 250% 100mL for barium swallow. Advantages over water soluble contrast include cost and better coating, allowing better demonstration of mucosal pattern. The main risk is high morbidity associated with barium in the peritoneal cavity. CT and US must be done prior to barium studies if they are needed due to artefacts or difficulty in interpretation subsequent to barium ingestion.

### Water soluble contrast media

E.g. Gastromiro®, Gastrografin®. Used in cases of meconium ileus, suspected perforation, and as oral contrast for CT examinations. The main risks are allergic reactions, ileus, hypovolaemia, and pulmonary oedema if aspirated (the latter two are unlikely if low osmolar contrast media is used).

## Contraindications

• All barium studies are contraindicated in suspected perforation, where water-soluble contrast, e.g. Gastrografin®, may be used instead.
• Barium follow-through and meal is contraindicated in cases of complete large bowel obstruction.
• Barium enema is also contraindicated in cases of toxic megacolon, pseudomembranous colitis and recent rectal biopsy (via rigid endoscope within the previous 5 days or flexible endoscope within the previous 24 h).
• Gastrografin® may be used with care to diagnose SBO; as it is hyperosmolar it may increase intraluminal pressure. Paradoxically it may therefore have a therapeutic effect.

# Ultrasound

- Utilizes cyclic high frequency sound waves to produce images of the body. Most diagnostic procedures use frequencies between 2 and 20MHz.
- Internal organs, muscle, tendons, etc., are seen in real-time image. Doppler mode enables patterns of blood flow to be examined.
- Contrast agents are available, e.g. microbubbles. The most important application of this in US imaging is in the detection and differentiation of focal liver lesions.
- US in diagnostic imaging for cancer can be performed via a transcutaneous, transabdominal, transvaginal, transrectal endoscopic, and intraoperative approach.
- Endoscopic US utilizes a small US probe at the tip of an endoscope. It is useful in the staging of cancers of the oesophagus, stomach, pancreas, and rectum. It aids visualization of radial penetration of the tumour, as well as circumferential extent in viscous organs.
- Intraoperative US is used occasionally as an adjunctive tool to more conventional imaging for staging tumours and guiding segmental resection. It is of particular benefit in cases of non-palpable breast tumour surgery, as well as for hepatic tumours.
- The use of US as an imaging medium is limited because of the means by which US penetrates tissue. US does not readily cross tissue–bone and tissue–gas boundaries. Structures lying deep to gas-containing and bony structures are not visible. Hence, the use in imaging of lung and brain is limited (except in neonates with open fontanelles). The inspection of the bowel transabdominally is restricted for the same reason.
- It is highly useful in assessing tubular structures, such as the biliary ducts that may contain a small focal lesion that may be missed between sequential slices on CT. As a dynamic imaging modality it is highly useful to guide biopsies of relatively superficially lying lesions. Cystic structures are well visualized and can be aspirated, e.g. thyroid and breast cysts.
- Heat generated by US can be used therapeutically – high intensity focused US (HIFU) treatment is available for the treatment of early prostate cancer or as 'salvage treatment' if recurrence following other treatments (approved by NICE, March 2005). There may be a larger role for HIFU in the future for other tumours – clinical trials are ongoing.

# Computed tomography

- First introduced in the 1970s at Northwick Park Hospital, London.
- Tomographic images are produced from a large 2-D series of X-ray images taken around a single axis of rotation.
- Data produced is digitally reconstructed to demonstrate various organs based on differential radio-opacity.
- Most centres now use multi-detector CT (MDCT) scanners – longer scanning range and shorter scanning times due to multiple rows of detectors.
- Slice thicknesses of less than 1mm can be obtained using MDCT.
- Images from MDCT can be reconstructed in any plane without significant loss of image quality.
- Computed tomography is essential for the localization and staging of various malignancies. Its use as the gold standard for staging has been challenged by MRI and PET-CT for regional cancers such as the rectum.
- CT is also important in radiotherapy planning in the case of most tumours and for radiofrequency (RF) ablation (see 'Radiofrequency ablation', p. 74).

## IV water soluble contrast media

- First report of use in 1923 by Osborne et al. to opacify urinary tract.
- Newer non-ionic low osmolar contrast agents have fewer toxic effects.
- Risks include contrast extravasation leading to pain, skin erythema, and sloughing, contrast-induced nephropathy (incidence of 5%), cardiovascular and neurotoxicity with intracardiac and intracerebral arteriography, respectively, haematological changes (e.g. haemolysis, thrombus formation, etc.), thyrotoxicosis, and idiosyncratic reactions (ranging from mild to severe and even death).
- Use of N-acetylcysteine to prevent contrast-induced nephropathy is not agreed upon.
- Similarly, steroid prophylaxis for patients considered at risk of adverse reactions remains controversial. Lasser et al. recommend two oral doses of 32mg methylprednisolone, 12 and 2 h before high osmolar contrast media injection. They believe this may also prevent adverse reactions where newer non-ionic low osmolar contrast agents are used.

## Contraindications to CT scanning

- Pregnancy (relative contraindication).
- Allergies to iodine or contrast agents.
- Diabetic patients cannot take metformin for 48 h following IV contrast injections.
- Extremely overweight patients might have difficulties accessing the scanner.

## Further reading

Lasser EC, Lang J, Sovak M, Kolb W, Lyon S, Hamlin AE. Steroids: theoretical and experimental basis for utilization in prevention of contrast media reactions. *Radiology* 1977; **125(1)**:1–9.

Osborne ED, Sutherland CG, Scholl AJ, Jr., Rowntree LG. Landmark article Feb 10, 1923: Roentgenography of urinary tract during excretion of sodium iodid. By Earl D. Osborne, Charles G. Sutherland, Albert J. Scholl, Jr. and Leonard G. Rowntree. *JAMA* 1983; **250(20)**:2848–53.

# Magnetic resonance imaging

- Does not use ionizing radiation to obtain images.
- A magnetic field is employed to align the magnetization of hydrogen atoms in the body. Radio waves then alter the alignment of this magnetization causing the hydrogen atoms to produce a rotating magnetic field detectable by the scanner, from which an image can reconstructed.
- The spatial resolution of the image is not as good as CT, but there is superior contrast resolution and no radiation dose to patient.
- MRI use is central in the localization and staging of various malignancies.
- Gadolinium containing contrast agents often used to look for enhancement but risk of nephrogenic systemic fibrosis in chronic severe renal insufficiency (glomerular filtration rate <30 mL/min/1.73 m2), or acute renal insufficiency of any severity caused by hepato-renal syndrome or in the perioperative liver transplantation period.

## Magnetic resonance spectroscopy

- Magnetic resonance spectroscopy (MRS) is an application of MRI.
- MRS provides chemical information about tissue metabolites.
- Detects the resonance spectra of chemical compounds other than hydrogen, e.g. carbon 13, fluorine 19, etc.
- Primary clinical use is for brain cancer, but also has a role as an adjunct to conventional imaging in prostate, colon, breast, cervix, oesophageal, and pancreatic cancer.

## Absolute contraindications to MRI

- Electronically, magnetically, and mechanically activated implants, such as:
  - cardiac pacemakers;
  - defibrillators;
  - ferromagnetic or electronically-operated stapedial implants.
- CNS aneurysm clips.
- Ocular foreign body, e.g. metal shavings.

## Relative contraindications

- Other pacemakers, e.g. carotid sinus.
- Insulin pumps and nerve stimulators.
- Lead wires or similar wires.
- Non-ferromagnetic stapedial implants.
- Cochlear implants.
- Claustrophobia.
- Pregnancy (although there is no evidence that MRI is harmful to the foetus during any trimester).
- Prosthetic heart valves (if dehiscence is suspected).

# Positron emission tomography (PET) – CT

- PET-CT is a technique by which a 3-D image map of functional processes within the body is produced through the use of a positron emitting radioisotope introduced into the body on a metabolically active molecule. Images from a simultaneously taken CT scan (or MRI scan) are then reconstructed to provide metabolic and anatomical information.
- In current oncology imaging practice PET-CT is performed using the radioactive tracer isotope $^{18}$fluoro deoxyglucose ($^{18}$FDG) to localize cancer cells that have a higher rate of glucose metabolism and, therefore, concentrate the molecule within them (*Fig. 1.1*).
- FDG is not a tumour specific agent.
- Occasionally, PET-CT can detect functional abnormalities in structures that look normal on conventional CT and MR.
- PET-CT is now considered a key investigation in the management of several malignancies, particularly in primary tumour staging, assessment of treatment response, and as a prognostic indicator for detecting disease recurrence.
- Tumour specific radiotracers detected by PET-CT scanners are in development, e.g. radiotracers linked to oestrogen receptor/HER-2 in breast cancer.

## Common pitfalls

### False positives

Skin contamination (tracer or urine), normal uptake in skeletal muscle, brown fat and urinary tract, respiratory motion, inflammatory conditions (e.g. sarcoid, tuberculosis, abscesses, fungal infections), certain physiological states (e.g. lactating breast, thymus, growth plates in children, etc.), trauma, and recent surgery.

### False negatives

Small lesions size (less than 1cm), type of neoplasm (see 'Regional cancer imaging', p. 14), tumour grade, and lesion location, e.g. adjacent to urinary tract or bladder, respiratory motion, etc.

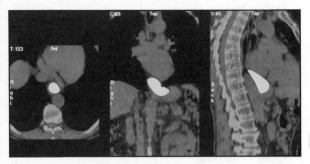

**Fig. 1.1** PET-CT demonstrating increased $^{18}$FDG uptake in the distal oesophagus, where there is increased mucosal thickening secondary to oesophageal malignancy.

# Radionuclide imaging

- Provides physiological or metabolic images by using tracer studies employing various radiopharmaceuticals, which are administered to patients.
- The radiation emitted is detected with a gamma camera and an image is formed.

Radionuclides in common use for cancer imaging and their clinical application

- *$^{131}$Iodine and $^{123}$Iodine:* thyroid malignancy.
- *$^{67}$Ga – gallium citrate:* lymphoma, used with variable success in a variety of other tumours, e.g. hepatoma, bronchial carcinoma, multiple myeloma, and sarcoma.
- *$^{99m}$Tc -sulphur colloid:* liver/spleen imaging.
- *$^{201}$Thallous chloride:* brain neoplasia and lung tumours. It may also be used to detect lymphomas, and thyroid and breast cancers.
- *$^{99m}$Technetium:* bone scans, diagnosis of breast cancer.
- *$^{99m}$Tc-MIBI:* parathyroid adenomas and carcinoma.
- *$^{111}$In-pentetreotide:* somatostatin receptor positive tumours.
- *$^{123}$I-MIBG:* neuroblastoma, phaeochromocytoma, carcinoid tumours, medullary thyroid carcinoma, other neuroendocrine tumours.

# 2. Regional cancer imaging
# Head and neck cancer

**Paranasal sinus neoplasms**
- Least common of all head and neck malignancies.
- Usually advanced at presentation (60% at stage T3 or T4) and poor prognosis.
- Imaging required for identification of the neoplasm, staging, determining suitability for surgery, planning radiotherapy treatment, and as baseline for assessment of recurrence.

### Imaging
*Plain radiography:*
- Used as a screening tool.
- Will identify ~80% of cases of bone destruction.

*CT*
- CT and MRI can both be used to identify and stage paranasal sinus neoplasms.
- 2–3mm axial sections if using spiral technique following IV contrast thought skull base and primary tumour. (MDCT slice thickness will depend on scanner capability). 5mm axial sections through whole neck for lymph node assessment and coronal reformats for pre-surgical planning.
- CT is better at identifying bony erosion than MRI.
- Aggressive bony destruction is observed in SCC, lymphoma, and metastases.
- Bone remodelling in inverted papillomas, olfactory neuroblastomas, most sarcomas, haemangiopericytomas, minor salivary gland tumours.
- Sclerotic bony changes not usually seen with tumours.
- CT accurately assesses nodal disease.
- CT is not accurate in identifying tumour margins, differentiating tumour from secretions and detecting early intracranial extension.

*MRI*
- MRI provides multiplanar imaging and superior soft tissue contrast allowing for better differentiation of tumour from surrounding tissue and fluid.
- Recommended sequences: coronal 3mm STIR, T1W, T1W + Gadolinium Fat Sat, axial 5mm T1W + Gad Fat Sat, T1W and 3mm axial T2W Fat Sat., sagittal 3mm T1W + Gad Fat Sat
- Patients with intracranial and perineural extension can be more accurately identified by MRI as they are excluded from surgery.
- Use of IV supermagnetic iron oxide particles (SPIOs) as MR lymphangiographic agents may increase specificity in nodal disease (metastatic nodes do not show signal drop on T2* sequences).
- Overall, MRI is considered more accurate in staging sinonasal tumours (MRI 94% accurate or 98% accurate if post-contrast images as opposed to CT accuracy of 78–85%).

*Ultrasound*
- Used in node staging – involved nodes are usually hypoechoic or inhomogenously echogenic with loss of echogenic hilum.
- Outlines may be indistinct and the node may show central necrosis.
- US sensitivity in diagnosis of nodal metastases is 75–90% with specificity of 63–91% or 100% if used with US guided FNA.

*FDG-PET*
- Most sensitive method for detection of cervical nodal metastases (US is most specific).
- FDG-PET is best imaging method for assessing recurrent tumour, but there can be false positives due to inflammation.

**Follow-up**
- Routine follow up 3–4 months post-treatment to establish baseline for future comparison. MRI is preferred to CT in the post-surgical patient.
- Where available $^{18}$FDG PET-CT can be used to accurately re-stage disease recurrence.

## Tumours of the pharynx, tongue, and mouth
- The pharynx is divided into three sections – nasopharynx, oropharynx, hypopharynx.
- Most primary tumours of the head and neck are best evaluated clinically.
- Role of imaging is in identifying extent of local tumour, including submucosal spread, bone and cartilage invasion, and evaluating areas such as base of skull, orbits, and brain that cannot be examined clinically.
- Imaging is also important to identify extent of lymph node metastases, and to identify organs at risk of radiotherapy-related damage and also monitor tumour response to treatment.

*Imaging*
*Conventional radiography*
Limited use. Barium swallow can be used to evaluate mucosal extent of hypopharyngeal cancer.

*CT*
- 3mm axial sections. If using a spiral CT following injection of IV contrast through the skull base with 5mm axial sections through the neck.
- If using MDCT slick thickness will depend on scanner capability.
- CT and MRI are considered complementary to each other and patients tend to have both.
- CT has a short acquisition time, reduced motion artefact, and accurate bone analysis.
- Supplementary dynamic images may be used, e.g. Valsalva manoeuvre for better distension of the hypopharynx in hypopharyngeal tumours.

*MRI*
- Considered superior to CT for assessing soft tissue extent of tumours.
- T-staging is best achieved with imaging in multiple planes. Combination of axial, coronal and sagittal STIR, T1W, T1W + Gad Fat Sat, T2W Fat Sat sequences are obtained.

- Disadvantages are related to motion artefacts from swallowing, breathing, pulsating carotid arteries, etc., due to patient symptoms from their pathology.

*Ultrasound*

Limited role in imaging of pharynx due to bone and air interfaces, but is valuable in staging of metastatic lymph node metastases, particularly when combined with FNAC.

*Nuclear imaging*

$^{18}$FDG PET is useful in initial diagnosis, staging of recurrent disease, and assessment of treatment response.

## Laryngeal tumours

- Commonest head and neck cancer site.
- Diagnosis is made at laryngoscopy.
- Imaging is complementary to endoscopic evaluation allowing for assessment of cartilage, subglottic space, tongue base, ventricle, lymph nodes, vascular invasion, perineural spread, extralaryngeal spread .
- Cross-sectional imaging is advised for all stage T2 lesions or above.
- Imaging is only indicated in lower stages where clinical assessment is difficult or subglottic disease is suspected.

### Imaging

*Fluoroscopy*

- Used in cases where patients cannot tolerate endoscopy.
- Cord mobility can be assessed fluoroscopically using various phonation manoeuvres.

*Barium swallow*

- Used to assess oesophageal reflux induced vocal cord inflammation, evaluation of pyriform sinuses, areas difficult to assess clinically, and to exclude synchronous oesophageal tumours.
- Also used post-laryngectomy to exclude anastomotic leaks.

*CT*

- Multidetector CT imaging is the preferred imaging modality due to speed of acquisition, reduced motion artefact from breathing and swallowing, and patient tolerance.
- CT and MRI have similar accuracy in diagnosis of cartilage invasion. Both modalities also have a similar accuracy of clinical staging.

*MRI*

- Generally used as adjunct to CT to clarify issues, such as early cartilage invasion or possible pre-epiglottic space and tongue base invasion.
- Axial, sagittal, and coronal T1W and T2W sequences, as well as contrast enhancement with spectral fat suppression are usually used to assess the larynx and soft tissue involvement.
- Pitfalls include swallowing motion artefact in patients whose airway is compromised by tumour.

*PET-CT*

- A silence protocol of 1 h is necessary prior to performing the study due to physiological uptake of $^{18}$FDG in the larynx as a result of vocal cord activity.

- $^{18}$FDG-Pet-CT can be used to detect and define extent of submucosal spread of disease.

*Follow-up imaging*
- 3–4 months following radiotherapy.
- The same modality used in the pretreatment stage should be utilized.

# Thyroid cancer

- Imaging role is determined by tumour histology because different types behave differently in terms of metastases and regional lymph node involvement.
- Initial role is to distinguish between benign and malignant lesions by radionuclide imaging and US with FNAC.
- For low volume and early stage disease further pre-operative imaging is rarely needed as surgery is primary treatment.
- MRI or CT are indicated where there is suspicion of tumour extension into larynx, trachea, or retrosternally into the mediastinum.

## Imaging

### Radionuclide imaging

*Purpose*
- Evaluation of a thyroid nodule.
- Detection of distant metastases.
- Follow-up following surgery or radioiodine treatment.

### Technetium-$^{99m}$-pertechnetate imaging
- Most widely used imaging agent.
- Used as a baseline study to evaluate anatomical location and trapping function of thyroid nodules.
- Low radiation dose to patient.
- Half-life of 6 h and emits gamma radiation.
- Also concentrates in choroid plexus, salivary glands, and gastric mucosa.
- Radioactive markers are placed on palpable abnormalities.
- Uptake of $^{99m}$Tc provides map of function of thyroid tissue.
- High sensitivity for detection of nodules >2cm, but not as sensitive for smaller lesions.
- Difficult to evaluate retrosternal extension.
- No role in detection of metastases or recurrent disease; poor uptake by metastatic cervical nodes.

### Radioiodine imaging
- Two important radioisotopes – $^{131}$I and $^{123}$I.
- Provide a physiological map of iodine metabolic pathway.
- $^{123}$I is preferred for imaging due to lower radiation dose and shorter half-life, but more costly as it requires a cyclotron.
- $^{131}$I is used for therapeutic irradiation of the thyroid and can be used for follow-up after treatment.
- Patient must stop thyroxine and liothyronine or carbimazole treatment prior to imaging or treatment with radioiodine.
- Most papillary and follicular carcinoma metastases are iodine avid.
- Anaplastic and medullary carcinomas are not iodine avid.

### Key points in diagnosis of cancer with Tc$^{99m}$ and radioiodine
- 10–20% of 'Cold' nodules are malignant; the remainder due to cysts, adenomas, degenerative nodules, colloid nodules, and thyroiditis.
- 10% of 'Warm' nodules on $^{99m}$Tc will be malignant. These need further imaging with $^{123}$I that usually shows them to be cold.

- 'Hot' nodules rarely malignant.
- Non-visualization of palpable nodule is due to normal function, and can be due to and adenoma or hyperplasia.
- Multinodular goitres are rarely associated with malignancy except in cases of a dominant nodule, where the risk is similar to that of a solitary nodule.

### Key points in follow-up of thyroid cancer with radioiodine

- Some thyroid tissue is left at thryoidectomy to spare parathyroid glands.
- $^{131}$I is given 1–4 weeks after surgery to ablate remaining thyroid tissue.
- Patient is imaged 4 days after ablation therapy.
- A series of follow-up studies are then carried out for up to 6 months.
- $^{123}$I is replacing $^{131}$I tracer imaging in follow-up of differentiated thyroid cancer. Other less commonly used radionuclide agents.
- **Thallium 201:** excellent for detecting local metasteaes, cervico-mediastinal nodes, and lung and bone metastases. Useful in differentiation of recurrent tumour from fibrosis.
- **Technetium-$^{99m}$methoxyisobutylisonitrile (MIBI):** does not require withdrawal of thyroid suppressive treatment when looking for recurrent disease.
- **Technetium-$^{99m}$-tetrofosmin:** promising agent for detection of metastatic foci and for follow-up. Also does not require thyroid hormone withdrawal.
- **Gallium-67 citrate:** not sensitive or specific in making diagnosis of thyroid cancer.

### Imaging agents for medullary thyroid carcinoma

- Pentavalent technetium dimercaptosuccinic acid. Sensitivity 77% and specificity 100% for primary. Sensitivity 66% and specificity 100% for metastatic disease. Agent is not taken up by normal thyroid tissue.
- Somatostatin receptor imaging using $^{111}$In-labelled octreotide (pentetreotide) visualizes MTC in 88% of cases. Sensitive to pulmonary metastases, but not liver or lymph node metastases. False positive uptake in areas of inflammation and granulomatous disease.
- Metaiodobenzylguanidine : $^{123}$I/$^{131}$I-MIBG used in imaging of tumour that store catecholamines. Not ideal agent to image MTC (positive uptake in 30% and negative rate of 52%), but allows for simultaneous imaging of phaeochromocytoma in MEN patients. If MTC is $^{123}$I-MIBG avid then treatment with $^{131}$I-MIBG is possible.
- $^{111}$In labelled anti-CEA antibody fragments.

### PET-CT

- $^{18}$FDG uptake not usually seen in normal thyroid.
- Low uptake in well differentiated thyroid cancers, but increased uptake in moderately and poorly differentiated types.
- Poorly differentiated types show loss of iodine uptake.
- Observation of low iodine/high $^{18}$FDG uptake and vice versa is called 'flip-flop' phenomenon.
- $^{18}$FDG-PET-CT indicated in thyroid cancer patients with negative radioiodine scans with elevated thyroglobulin levels, as PET-CT allows detection and localization of non-iodine avid metastases.

*Conventional radiology*
CXR to assess for tracheal deviation or pulmonary metastases.

*Ultrasound*
- Used for the evaluation of the morphology of the gland.
- Is nodule solitary or is it a multinodular gland?
- Measurement and characterization of nodule. ?Cystic.
- Search for non-palpable thyroid cancer in patients presenting with cervical lymphadenopathy.
- Guide FNA biopsy.
- Detect local recurrence following surgery.
- Specificity in differentiating benign from malignant lesions is poor unless direct invasion of adjacent tissues.
- Combination of imaging appearances of absent halo sign, microcalcification, and intranodular arterial Doppler flow increases specificity for malignancy.
- US-guided FNAC is the most accurate means of distinguishing benign and malignant lesions.

*CT*
- Not used routinely.
- Iodine-containing contrast can prevent or delay radioiodine scanning and therapy.

*Indications*
- To determine degree and location of invasive thyroid carcinoma.
- To demonstrate retrosternal or retrotracheal tumour extension.
- To detect regional metastatic disease, cervical and mediastinal lymphadenopathy, and lung metastases when strongly suspected.
- To identify local recurrence following surgery.

*MRI*
- Preferred to CT for determining local extent of thyroid cancer.
- Indications same as for CT.
- Protocol for imaging thyroid tumours: 3mm slice thickness; coronal STIR, T1W, T1W +Gad Fat Sat images, Axial 3mm T2W Fat Sat, 5mm T1W and 5mm T1W + Gad Fat Sat images as well as sagittal 3mm T1W + Gad Fat Sat images
- Unlike CT contrast enhanced MRI does not interfere with radioiodine imaging and therapy for differentiated thyroid cancer.

# Breast cancer

Screening

- Mammography is preferred technique.
- Screening reduces mortality by 25–30% in screened groups.
- Screening results in diagnosis of smaller tumours and at earlier stages.
- Age of commencing screening and interval not agreed upon.
- In the UK women aged 50–70 are offered two-view mammography at intervals of 3 years.

*Mammography*

- Usually at least two views in diagnostic mammography – mediolateral oblique and craniocaudal – with supplemental views tailored to specific problem, e.g. mediolateral and lateromedial views.
- Tends to over-estimate tumour size.
- Characteristic appearance of malignancy is stellate mass.
- *Other features of malignancy:* calcifications with features of clustering, polymorphisms, and multiplicity; parenchymal distortion, new opacities, lymphadenopathy.
- Malignancy can be mimicked by fat necrosis, radial scar, sclerosing adenosis, fibromatosis.
- Well-defined masses likely to represent fibroadenoma, cyst, intramammary lymph nodes, lipid cysts, galactocoeles.
- False-negative rate of at least 10% with mammography.
- *UK mammograms scored on Bi-Rads scale from 1–5:* (1) no abnormalities; (2) benign finding; (3) probably benign finding; (4) malignancy suspected; and (5) malignant finding.
- Computer-aided detection may increase cancer detection rate by 20%.
- Mammographic (stereotactic) guidance for biopsy (see 'Breast intervention, p. 84)

Ultrasound

- A diagnostic and not a screening procedure.
- Usually targeted to specific mammographic finding.
- Tends to underestimate tumour size.
- US may avoid need for biopsy, e.g. if lesion is cyst or normal fibroglandular tissue.
- Appearances suggesting malignancy include speculation, larger AP than transverse diameter, angular margins, hypoechoic lesion, shadowing, calcifications, branch pattern, microlobulation, disruption of tissue planes, duct extension.
- US findings scored on Bi-Rads scale – see 'Breast cancer: mammography'.
- US guidance used for biopsy of masses.

## MRI

- Indicated in suspected multifocal/multicentric cancer (Fig. 1.2) where treatment strategy may be altered (e.g. when breast conservation would be preferred) especially for large tumours in radiographically dense breast and for lobular cancers.
- Also indicated when trying to identify extent of residual cancer if positive surgical margin following breast conservation surgery.
- Most accurate technique for tumour size measurement.
- Low (40%) sensitivity for detecting DCIS, but high sensitivity for invasive carcinoma.
- TSE T2W transverse imaging of both breasts with a slice thickness of 4mm, as well as TSE T2W, dynamic contrast-enhanced T1 gradient echo + Fat Sat images, and delayed T1 gradient echo + Fat Sat post-contrast sagittal 4mm slice images of the affected breast are recommended.

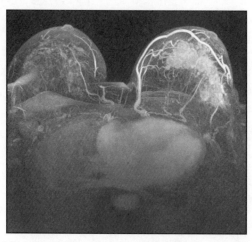

**Fig. 1.2**  T1 Fat Sat MIP MRI showing multifocal invasive ductal cancer left breast.

## CT

- Not indicated for early stage disease in asymptomatic disease.
- Even in cases of advanced disease (T3/T4) or symptomatic disease, routine CT is not generally done as a first line of investigation – the patient will have appropriate investigation, e.g. bone scan for bone pain, CXR initially for breathlessness.

## [18]FDG PET/CT

- Not routinely indicated for primary tumour/axillary staging due to low accuracy (64% sensitivity).
- Most accurate imaging modality for detecting metastatic disease recurrence.
- Currently only used in cases with equivocal imaging to provide definitive answer regarding the presence or absence of active recurrent metastatic disease.

# Oesophageal cancer

Responsible for 7% of all GI tract malignancies and 1% of all cancer in USA, with a poor survival rate – only 10% have a survival rate of 5 years.

## Radiological diagnosis

### Barium studies

- Double contrast studies have high sensitivity.
- Accurately predicts lesion length in 59% of patients.
- Polypoid and stenotic tumours are easier to visualize than flat lesions.

### Staging:

- Diagnosis is usually by barium studies or endoscopy with endoscopic biopsy for confirmation.
- Accurate staging is a prerequisite for selection of appropriate therapy.
- CT is more accurate than EUS in detecting metastases.
- EUS is more accurate than CT in local staging.

### CT

- Wall thickening greater than 5mm is abnormal.
- Intraluminal air, fluid, or contrast facilitates measurement of wall thickness.
- Generally, CT is poor for early T stage tumours.
- Accurate in demonstration of tracheobronchial, pericardial, aortic, and diaphragmatic invasion.
- Accurate in the detection of metastases to adrenals, omentum, para-aortic lymph nodes.
- Inaccurate in detecting subtle nodal disease.

### EUS

- Tumour stenosis can prevent adequate assessment in 30% patients.
- Very accurate in assessment of tumour depth invasion (T stage).
- Accurate in demonstration of para-oesophageal and gastric adenopathy.
- Poor demonstration of distant metastases.

### MRI

- May be used in staging advanced malignancies to help determine regional resectability.
- Superior to CT, US, and EUS in detection of liver metastases.

### [18]FDG PET-CT

- Malignant cells show avid uptake of [18]FDG.
- Used for delineating craniocaudal extent of disease.
- Also used to detect regional and distant lymphadenopathy and metastases.
- Useful in monitoring tumour response to therapy.

## Follow-up

- CT is primary imaging modality for follow-up.
- CT at 3 months following surgery advised.
- Subsequent imaging depends on disease status and patient symptoms.

# Gastric cancer

### Diagnosis
Endoscopy has largely replaced barium meals for diagnosis.

### Staging aims
- To identify metastatic disease.
- To identify peritoneal nodules and nodal enlargement.
- To determine proportion of stomach involved by tumour to assist with decision with regard to extent of surgery.
- To determine degree of outflow obstruction to guide clinical management of obstructive symptoms.

### CT
- CT of thorax, abdomen, and pelvis is primary imaging investigation.
- Performed with oral administration of 1L of water as contrast agent and IV contrast, preferably with patient fasted for 6 h prior to scan.
- CT accurately identifies spread to mesocolon/colon (76%) and peritoneal deposits (71%).
- High specificity in advanced disease with few false positives.
- Accuracy in assessment of depth of tumour invasion less in early than advanced tumour.
- Overall T stage accuracy is 69% because CT cannot resolve individual layers of gastric wall and, therefore, cannot discriminate early T stages.
- Accuracy of assessment of degree of serosal invasion 80%.

### EUS
- T staging accuracy is superior to CT at 89–92%.
- Particularly good in T staging of stage I and II disease.
- Reliable in predicting complete resectablity with sensitivity of 94% and specificity of 83%.
- Limited field of view; therefore, only useful to visualize peri-gastric nodes.

### MRI
Limited use due to motion artefact, lack of suitable contrast agents, time of examination, etc.

### [18]FDG-PET-CT
- Less useful than in oesophageal carcinoma as stomach often shows low/moderate physiological [18]FDG uptake.
- Local small lymph nodes may not demonstrate significant [18]FDG uptake.

# Primary tumours of liver and biliary tract

## Hepatocellular carcinoma

- Most common primary liver neoplasm.
- Fifth commonest malignancy worldwide.
- 90% have underlying cirrhosis or chronic viral infection.
- Screening of high risk patients with cirrhosis using US and serum alpha protein estimation undertaken in UK.

### Imaging appearances

- Often has non-specific appearance like other liver neoplasms.
- Cirrhosis causes difficulty in detection of small tumours.
- Contrast-enhanced CT and MR detect only approximately 50% of tumours in screening population and US is even less.
- Imaging appearances may be differentiated due to characteristic pathological features, such as presence of surrounding fibrous capsule, heterogenous nature of larger lesions, vascular nature of tumour leading to marked contrast enhancement, and vascular invasion with portal or hepatic thrombosis (indicating advanced stage).

### Ultrasound

- Internal echo pattern is variable, depending on fibrous and fat content.
- Smaller tumours more homogenous, larger tumours heterogeneous.
- Hypoechoic surrounding fibrous capsule.
- Procedure of choice for biopsy.

### CT

- Performed unenhanced, and then in arterial and portal venous phase post-IV contrast.
- Appearance depends on size.
- Small tumours are often homogenous, larger lesions heterogenous with mosaic appearance due to necrosis, haemorrhage, fatty metamorphosis, and fibrosis.
- Lesions are hypo- or iso-intense precontrast. Calcification in seen in 5–10%.
- Small lesions usually show homogenous enhancement in arterial phase.
- Usually, iso-intense in portal venous phase due to early washout. Larger lesions may be iso-intense in this phase.

### MRI

- Better than CT in depicting changes of cirrhosis.
- Appearances are variable.
- Larger lesions hypointense on T1- and hyperintense on T2- weighted images with heterogenous or mosaic appearance.
- Smaller lesions often iso-attenuate on T1- and T2-weighted images.
- Hypointense peripheral capsule on T1- and T2-weighted images is more commonly seen than on CT.
- Fatty metamorphosis is seen more frequently than in CT – high T1 signal foci.

- Enhancement characteristics similar to that with CT. Optimal MR detection requires use of arterial phase gadolinium contrast-enhanced imaging.

### [18]FDG PET-CT

- Limited use.
- Sensitivity for detection of HCC is 50–70%.

## Fibrolamellar hepatocellular carcinoma

- Occurs in young adults with non-cirrhotic livers.
- Pathologically fibrous central scar present in 70–80% cases, which has common imaging appearances.

### Imaging features

- Same technique as with HCC for CT and MR scanning with arterial phase imaging mandatory.
- Central scar is hypointense on T1- and T2-weighted MR in contrast to focal nodular hyperplasia, where fibrous central scar is usually low signal on T1 and high signal on T2.
- **CT:** calcification in central scar in two-thirds of FL-HCC (very uncommon with FNH). Well-defined vascular tumour is shown best during arterial phase imaging. Usually, heterogenous enhancement in comparison to FNH, which is very homogenous except for central scar.

## Cholangiocarcinoma

- Uncommon tumour arising from epithelial lining of bile ducts. 90% are extrahepatic.
- Most common location for CCA is at hilum – Klatskin tumour.
- Occur in 10–15% of patients with primary sclerosing cholangitis.

### Imaging findings

Usually lack characteristic findings.

### Ultrasound

Non-specific findings of dilated biliary tree, homo/heterogenous mass, which is usually hyperechoic, but can be iso- or hypoechoic.

### CT

- No capsule.
- Hypo or isodense on unenhanced imaging.
- Show early minimal/moderate rim enhancement with progressive concentric filling.
- Characteristic CT feature is marked homogenous delayed enhancement (in 74%).

### MR

- Non-specific findings.
- Typical lesions hypointense on T1- and mildly hyperintense on T2-weighted images.
- May show low central signal intensity on T2 if fibrous or high signal if high mucin content or necrosis present.
- Following contrast, enhancement pattern similar to that of CT.

## Biliary cystadenocarcinoma

- Rare malignant uni- or multilocular cystic mass originating from biliary cystadenoma.
- Cannot be differentiated from benign biliary cystadenoma on imaging.
- Other differentials include complicated hepatic cysts, liver abscess, cystic metastases, and hydatid cysts.

### Ultrasound

- Unilocular or mulitiloculated hypoechoic mass.
- Echogenic septations/papillary growths.
- May contain fluid/fluid levels.

### CT

- Multiloculated fluid density mass.
- Peripheral soft tissue nodularity and traversing septations, which show contrast enhancement.

### MR

Locules with variable signal intensity on T1W or T2W imaging dependent on protein content

## Angiosarcoma

- Rare tumour derived from endothelial cells.
- Associated with carcinogens like thorotrast, arsenic, polyvinyl chloride, and also haemochromatosis and von Recklinghausen disease.

### Plain film

May show circumferential displacement of residual thorotrast.

### Ultrasound

Solid/mixed echogenicity mass(es) with hypoechoic areas of haemorrhage and necrosis.

### CT

- Non-specific appearance.
- Can be confused with haemangiomas due to marked peripheral enhancement on dynamic contrast-enhanced CT.
- Usually presents when there are multiple masses.

### MRI

- Hypointense on T1 and hyperintense on T2WI.
- Peripheral gadolinium enhancement as with CT.

## Epitheloid haemangioendothelioma

Uncommon primary malignant vascular tumour.

### Ultrasound

Usually hypoechoic lesions due to central core of myxoid stroma.

### CT and MR

Non-specific findings that mimic other tumours.

## Gallbladder carcinoma
- Most common malignancy in biliary tract.
- Associated with choletlithiasis, precleain gallbladder, chronic cholecystitis, gallbladder polyp, PSC, congenital biliary anomalous, inflammatory bowel disease, familial polyposis coli.

### Plain film
May show gallstone or porcelain gallbladder.

### Ultrasound
- Gallbladder replaced by irregular walled mass.
- Heterogenous exotexture relating to degree of tumour necrosis.
- Echogenic foci with acoustic shadowing related to gallstones, calcification, porcelain bladder.
- Mass may be inseparable from liver (Fig.1.4).

### CT
- Hypoattenuating mass with direct invasion of liver with protrusion of anterior surface of medial segment of left lobe.
- Variable enhancement post-IV contrast.

### MRI
- Hypointense mass on T1WI.
- Ill-defined irregular areas of enhancement.

### Cholangiography
- GB filling defect (non-specific).
- Obstruction/stricture of extrahepatic bile duct, or confluence of right and left ducts.

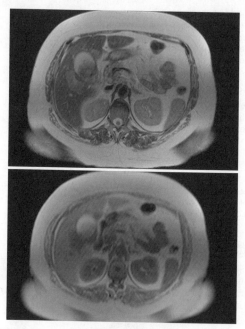

**Fig. 1.3** Gall bladder carcinoma in a 50-year-old woman. Extension into liver, irregular mass centred on gall bladder. Best seen on T2 axial, and in and out of phase sequences.

# Cancers of the pancreas

- 5-year survival for pancreatic malignancy is only 10%.
- Various pathological types arising from:
  - ductal epithelium (e.g. adenocarcinoma (most common);
  - cystadenocarcinoma, mucinous, etc.);
  - acinar cell carcinoma;
  - islet cells (e.g. malignant insulinoma, glucanoma, etc.);
  - non-epithelial tissue (very rare, e.g. lymphoma, fibrosarcoma, etc.).

## Imaging

### CT

- Non-contrast scans, late (40s delay) arterial phase, portal-venous phase images obtained.
- Pancreatic carcinoma hypoattenuating in 90% relative to surrounding enhancing pancreas on later arterial phase. Iso-attenuating in 10% – difficult to identify if small and no secondary signs of pancreatic/common bile duct obstruction.
- Liver metastases, portal venous occlusion, and venous collateral more easily detected on venous phase.
- *Important considerations:* arterial encasement (contraindicates surgery) and portal venous system involvement, gastric invasion, liver and peritoneal metastases, lymph node enlargement, bile duct and duodenal obstruction (Fig.1.5)

### MRI

- Equivalent to CT in diagnosis and staging accuracy.
- Generally reserved for problem-solving, particularly for small lesions and where IV CT contrast is contraindicated.
- MRCP is useful to visualize obstruction of CBD or pancreatic duct.
- Negative oral contrast is helpful.
- Sequences used include Fast T2W imaging (10mm axial slices for planning), 6mm axial GRE T1W (in and opposed phase to characterize lesions and eliminate effects of intrahepatic fat), 4mm axial T2W short and long TE or HASTE (for identifying neuroendocrine lesions and liver lesions), 5cm coronal MRCP SSFSE (for ductal anatomy), 5mm axial T1W with fat saturation (identify small tumours), 2.5mm axial/oblique coronal dynamic contrast medium-enhanced study T1W GRE with or without fat saturation (delineate primary tumour which shows diminished enhancement, vascular invasion, and liver metastases).

### Endoscopic ultrasound

- Used for local staging when no evidences of distant metastases.
- Hypoechoic pancreatic mass, focal, or diffuse gland enlargement, pancreatic/biliary duct dilatation.
- FNA biopsy.
- Not good at detecting tumour infiltration of coeliac and splenic arteries.
- Not used to detect distant metastases.

## ¹⁸FDG PET-CT

- Does not distinguish between acute pancreatitis and pancreatic carcinoma as both show increased uptake.
- Can distinguish between chronic pancreatitis and carcinoma.
- Not routinely indicated in pancreatic cancer, but used to a limited extent to exclude distant metastases.

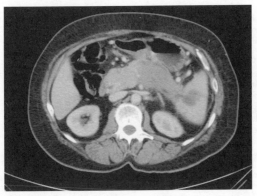

**Fig. 1.4** Post-IV contrast CT scan of a 5.5 × 4cm pancreatic mass of body and tail with invasion into the spleen.

# Colon and rectal cancer

Colorectal cancer is second commonest cause of cancer death in West.

## Screening

More effective than mammographic screening. Advised after age 50 by American Cancer Society.

High risk categories screening to start earlier:

- Strong family history.
- Hereditary colorectal cancer syndromes, e.g. FPC.
- Previous history of polyps or colorectal cancer.
- History of chronic inflammatory bowel disease.

## Methods

Screening by one of following options is advised by American Cancer Society:

- Yearly faecal occult bloods (FOB) with five yearly flexible sigmoidoscopy.
- Flexible sigmoidoscopy 5-yearly.
- Yearly FOB.
- Colonoscopy every 10 years.
- Double contrast barium enema every 5 years.
- CT colonography.

Positive results from anything other than colonoscopy should be followed by colonoscopy – considered the 'gold standard'

## Imaging and staging

### Barium enema

- Double contrast barium enema 82–97% sensitivity for detection polyps >1cm and 61–83% < 1cm.
- Various possible appearances: fungating polypoid, annular ulcerating, saddle lesion, scirrhous (signet-ring type).
- Calcifications (rare) in mucinous adenocarcinoma.

### CT

- Limited use in local staging due to insufficient spatial resolution to accurately detect tumour spread external to muscularis propria.
- Sensitivity for local invasions 48–55%.
- Use of size in detection of lymph node metastases means CT not accurate for detecting involved nodes (62%).
- More accurate for detecting metastases.
- Can identify complications including obstruction, tumour perforation, fistulas, pericolic abscess, intussusceptions, etc.
- Psammomatous calcifications, low density mass, and low density lymph nodes may be seen in mucinous adenocarcinoma.

### CT colonography and virtual colonoscopy

- Enables the internal contours of the bowel to be visualized in 2D or 3D.
- The empty bowel is distended by insufflation of air or carbon dioxide.
- Scan can demonstrate polyps and cancers that project into the bowel.

- CT colonography for the detection of colorectal cancer is a reliable alternative to barium enema where colonoscopy is incomplete and in the frail elderly or young unfit patient group, it is a valuable additional diagnostic tool (see Fig. 1.6).

## MR
- Disappointing for staging of colon cancer.
- Used to stage rectal carcinoma (see Fig. 1.7).
- Abdomino-pelvic surface coil is preferred by most to endorectal coil due to stenosis, pain, discomfort, bowel wall motion, difficulties in coil placement, coil migration, and inability to assess lesion in upper rectum.
- T2W sagittal and axial 5mm slice thickness, and 3mm oblique axial/coronal images advised.
- Reported 92% positive predictive value for prediction of histological status of the circumferential resection margin.

## $^{18}$FDG PET-CT
- Accurate for detection of local recurrence and hepatic and extrahepatic recurrence.
- Major role in patients with hepatic recurrence considered for surgical resection to exclude extrahepatic disease.

### Endoscopic ultrasound
- Intraluminal EUS can be used to assess rectal tumours.
- Rectal tumours are hypoechoic.
- Poor accuracy in assessing deep penetrating tumours.
- Highly accurate for staging early T stage rectal cancers.
- Unreliable for distinguishing malignant from benign nodes and nodes smaller than 5mm in diameter.

## Follow-up and imaging for recurrence
- Recurrence is difficult to detect clinically
- Recommended baseline CT 3 months post-surgery, 6-monthly CT examination for 3 years, and then yearly CT scans.
- Dynamic MR scanning helps distinguish post-surgical/radiotherapy fibrosis from tumour recurrence.
- $^{18}$FDG-PET-CT demonstrates uptake in tumour and not scar tissue and is, therefore, also very useful in detecting recurrence.

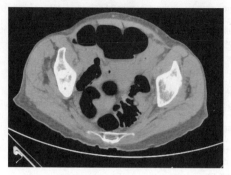

**Fig. 1.5** A soft tissue mass is seen projecting into the lumen of the sigmoid colon. Biopsy confirmed malignancy.

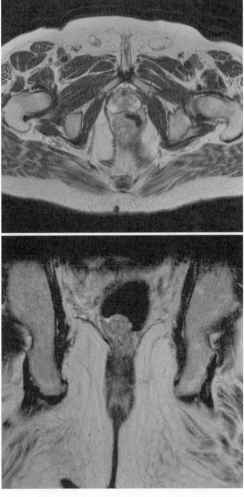

**Fig. 1.6** Axial and sagittal T1W with gadolinium contrast MRI demonstrating a 3.7cm low rectal tumour.

# Carcinoma of the anal region

- Rare. 2% of large bowel malignancies.
- Originate anywhere between anorectal junction and anal verge (Fig. 1.8).
- Patients with biopsy-proven anal cancer need imaging to assess local extent of disease prior to chemoradiation and to identify distant metastases.
- Imaging required to plan radiotherapy.

## CT

- Abdomen and pelvis imaged including groin areas.
- Main role is to detect spread.

## MRI

- Abdominopelvic surface coil T2 sagittal, axial 5mm slices to localize tumour and ascertain size, as well as detect pelvic disease.
- T2W 3mm slice thickness oblique axial and coronal series to delineate spread of tumour in relation to sphincters.

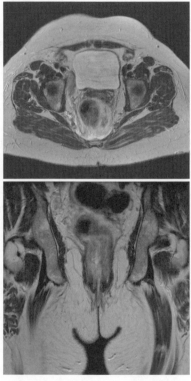

**Fig. 1.7** Sagittal and coronal sections of anorectal carcinoma with lymphadenopathy.

# Renal cancer

### Renal cell carcinoma

- Various types of renal tumour occur with RCC being far more common (80–90% of primary malignancies) than TCC in adults.
- 30% found incidentally on imaging.

### Imaging

#### IVU

- Reduced function due to parenchymal replacement and/or hydronephrosis.
- In case of renal vein occlusion, reduced contrast excretion.
- If tumour necrotic it may fill with contrast – pyelotumoural backflow.

#### Ultrasound

- Hyperechoic mass in 50–61%.
- Iso/hypoechoic usually in larger tumours.
- Can be cystic.
- Inhomogenous appearance in cases of necrosis, haemorrhage, etc.
- Can detect tumour extension into IVC and right atrium.

#### CT

- Investigation of choice for staging and detecting metastases.
- Staging accuracy of 72–90%.
- Unenhanced scans, cortico-medullary phase (30s post-IV contrast) and 65s post-contrast imaging is required. For further lesion characterization, 80–100s post-contrast scans for a true nephrographic phase.
- Tumour usually shows heterogenous enhancement due to areas of necrosis with enhancement >12HU.
- 65s scan allows for detection of renal vein and IVC infiltration (low attenuation filling defect, change in vein calibre, enhancement of malignant thrombus, collateral veins).

#### MRI

- Usually used as problem-solving tool.
- Protocols not agreed, but axial T1W, T2W, T1W with Fat Sat, T1W with Fat Sat and gadolinium contrast 6mm slice thickness images, as well as T1W sagittal/coronal images are advised.
- For renal vein/caval assessment: 3D fat saturated GE sequence with data acquisition post gadolinium contrast at 20, 50, and 80s.

#### [18]FDG-PET-CT

- Not used for primary tumour assessment as [18]FDG is excreted in urine and can mask uptake by tumour.
- Used to detect metastatic diseases and lytic bone metastases.

### Transitional cell carcinoma

- Extrarenal pelvis is more common site of renal TCC compared with infundibulocaliceal region.
- In ureter lower 1/3 (70%) > mid 1/3 (15%) > upper 1/3(15%).

## IVU

*Renal*

- Single or multiple filling defects – papillary or flat, often with irregular stippled appearance.
- Can cause dilated calyx due to calyceal, or infundibular stenosis, or tumour mass growth (oncocalyx).
- Caliceal amputation caused by obstruction of infundibulum (phantom calyx).
- Hydronephrosis with renal enlargement if tumour obstruction of ureteropelvic junction.

*Ureteric*

- Ureteric TCCs may cause hydronephrosis and hydroureter.
- Single/multiple filling defects.
- Irregular strictures with proximal dilatation.
- Non-functioning kidney if tumour advanced.

## Pyelography

- Similar appearances to IVU.
- Additional signs include 'goblet sign', i.e. focal expansion of ureter around mass.

## CT

- Technique as described above with an excretory phase scan at 3–5 min post-IV contrast.
- Filling defect in opacified collecting system.
- Focal areas of wall thickening.
- Infiltrative growth into parenchyma (T3).
- Variable enhancement of tumour.

## MRI

No significant role in the staging of upper urethelial tumours as it's accuracy is no better than CT.

## $^{18}$FDG PET-CT

Not useful for assessment ass radiotracer is excreted within urine physiologically.

# Adrenal malignancy

### Adrenocortical carcinoma
- Majority of adrenocortical tumours are non-functioning and benign.
- Adrenal cortical carcinoma is rare – 0.05–0.20% of all cancers.
- Excess hormone production in >50%.
- Cushing's syndrome is the most common endocrine abnormality.

### Imaging
*CT*
- Able to detect 5mm adrenal masses.
- Oral contrast, unenhanced CT, post-IV contrast, and delayed imaging is undertaken.
- Adrenal cortical carcinomas usually large at presentation – average size 9cm.
- Heterogenous appearance when they enlarge with calcification in 30% (usually central).
- Commonly invade draining vein and extend up IVC.
- Common site of metastases is liver and lungs.
- Liver metastases tend to be hypervascular.

*MRI*
- Used as a complementary tool to CT.
- Body coil can be used, but phased array surface coils are preferred.
- Axial T1W, T2W, post-contrast imaging, and chemical shift imaging using gradient echo in and out of phase T1W sequences are used.
- Heterogeneous signal intensity.
- **T1W:** iso-intense or slightly low signal lesion, but can have high central signal if haemorrhage.
- **T2W:** increased signal intensity and heterogenous.
- **Chemical shift MR:** no uniform loss of signal on out of phase T1WI due to lack of intracystoplasmic lipid.
- Post-contrast imaging shows peripheral enhancement.

### Radionuclide imaging
- Complementary to biochemical test and CT/MR imaging.
- 131 I-6-beta-iodomethyl-19-norcholesterol (NP59) or 75SE-6-selenomethyl-19-norcholesterol concentrate in steroid hormone producing tissue – reduced uptake suggests ACC or phaeochromocytoma (sensitivity – 100%, specificity 71%).
- Further biochemical testing, MIBG scanning, and biopsy is then required to distinguish between the two.

### [18]FDG PET-CT
- Malignant adrenal lesions show increased uptake.
- Extra-adrenal tumour sites can be identified allowing for accurate staging of malignant tumours.
- 100% reported sensitivity of [18]FDG PET in distinguishing benign from malignant disease, 80–100% reported specificity.

*Ultrasound*
- Useful in children or slim adults.
- Smaller lesions are of low echogenicity and larger lesions are more heterogenous with areas of central necrosis or haemorrhage appearing echo free.

## Phaeochromocytomas
- Arise from chromafin cells. May be adrenal or extra-adrenal.
- 90% of adrenal and 50% of extra adrenal phaeochromocytomas are hormonally active.
- Diagnosis made by measurement of urinary free catecholamines.

### *Imaging*
*CT*
- Similar technique to that used for ACC is employed.
- Sensitivity of 93–100% for detection of phaeochromocytomas.
- Precontrast scanned tumours are of soft tissue density. May show central low attenuation due to cystic change.
- Calcification in 12%.
- Marked enhancement following IV contrast medium.
- If non-ionic low osmolar contrast agents are used no premedication is required as it is does not cause an increase in catecholamines.
- Extradrenal paragangliomas (10–15% of chromaffin tumours) usually closely related to aorta and IVC following aorto-sympathetic chain.
- Usually large and heterogenous on non-contrast CT with marked enhancement post-contrasts. Smaller lesions are more homogenous.

*MRI*
- Same scanning technique used as with ACC.
- *T1W:* similar signal or slightly lower intensity to liver.
- *T2W:* hyperintense – 'light bulb' appearance, although the majority are heterogenous (helps distinguish from benign adenoma).
- Enhancement is progressive following IV contrast.
- No loss of signal intensity on out of phase imaging (Fig. 1.9).

*Radionuclide imaging*
- Meta-iodobenzylguanidine concentrates in sympatho adrenal medullary tissue.
- [123]I-MIBG is first choice to image phaemochromocytomas as paragangliomas. (sensitivity 90%), specificity 92–99%).
- [111]In-pentetrotide can also be used – sensitivity 97%, but high uptake in kidneys can mask smaller lesions.
- [131]I-MIBG is used therapeutically.

*PET-CT*
- Increased uptake of [18]FDG in majority of phaeochromocytomas – greater uptake in malignant that benign.
- Other agents used include [11]C-hydroxyephedrine, 6-([18]F)-fluoro-dopamine and [18]F-dopa.
- [18]F-dopa has 100% sensitivity and specificity for detecting phaeochromocytomas, and is superior to scinitgraphy.

*Ultrasound*
Cannot distinguish between ACC and phaeochromocytomas.

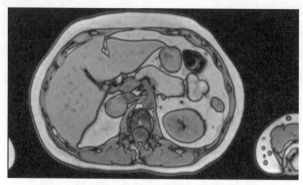

**Fig. 1.8** Right adrenal carcinoma. 36-year-old, incidental finding.

# Bladder cancer

- Commonest tumour of urinary tract.
- 90% are TCC of lateral bladder walls and trigone.
- 1/3 have multifocal disease at presentation.
- Diagnosis established from cystoscopic biopsy.

## Imaging

### Ultrasound

- Transabdominal US not used for staging as results inaccurate.
- Intravesical US is superior to transabdominal US and is accurate for early stage tumours, but rarely used as clinical staging is highly accurate.
- Echogenic focal wall thickening and/or mass protruding into lumen.
- US unable to accurately assess deeply infiltrating tumours and lymph node status.

### CT

- Full bladder desirable.
- Oral and IV contrast.
- Intraluminal mass or focal wall thickening that enhances following IV contrast to a greater degree than normal bladder wall.
- Early tumour spread beyond bladder wall is difficult to identify on CT.
- T1, T2, and T2a tumours difficult to distinguish.
- Oedema after cystoscopic resection, co-existent infection can also cause bladder wall thickening.
- Tumours in diverticula difficult to assess.

### MRI

- Superior to CT for staging.
- Can demonstrate muscle wall invasion and penetration, and allows accurate assessment of adjacent organ tumour involvement.
- Anti-peristaltic agent is helpful.
- T1W axial whole pelvis (6mm slice thickness) with large field of view for nodal and bone assessment, T2W axial/coronal/sagittal 3.5mm slices for primary tumour assessment, T1W gradient echo axial/coronal/sagittal with fat suppression pre- and immediately post-gadolinium contrast to assess tumour depth/invasion/transmural and extravesical spread, T2W axial scans with large field of view for lymph node, hydronephrosis, and ascites.
- TCC is iso-intense on T1WI to bladder wall and hyperintense on T2W.
- Enhancement can be plotted in relation to time – tumour shows greater enhancement than surrounding tissues.

### [18]FDG-PET-CT

Not useful due to radiotracer excretion in urine.

## Follow-up
- CT is primary imaging modality used.
- Reassessment CT at 6 months following treatment and at 1 year is often undertaken.

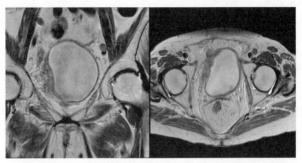

**Fig. 1.9** Carcinoma of the right side of the bladder in a 91 year old. G3pT3 cancer at dome. Irregular wall thickening. Treated with DXT. Seen on T2 coronal and T2 axial.

# Prostate cancer

- Second commonest cause of male cancer death.
- One out of 11 males develop it.
- Clinical management remains controversial.

## Ultrasound

- Transrectal US provides detailed morphology of prostate and seminal vesicles.
- The most important role is guidance for transrectal biopsies.
- Only peripheral zone lesions can be reliably diagnosed.
- Tumour hypoechoic in 61% and not detectable (iso-echoic) in 35% of cases.
- Tumour may present as asymmetric enlargement of gland or deformed contour of prostate.
- Seminal vesicle involvement suggested by asymmetry of size, shape, and echogenicity.

## CT

- Not recommended for T-staging prostate cancer.
- Can be useful in the assessment of nodal status and metastatic bone disease.
- Used for radiotherapy planning.

## MRI

- Imaging technique of choice.
- Anti-peristaltic agent used. 1.5 Tesla (minimum) scanner with surface pelvic-phased array coil. T1W and T2W 3mm axial prostate images, T2W coronal (3mm), T2W-FSE axial abdomen and pelvis (5–6mm slice), and T1W-SE axial pelvis imaging advised.
- Dynamic contrast enhanced T1W may help localize tumour in gland.
- MR spectroscopy with endorectal coil has role in pretreatment assessment for brachytherapy and intensity modulated radiotherapy.
- MR lymphography using super-paramagnetic iron oxide particles (USPIOs) shows promise for nodal evaluation, but not commercially available yet.
- Tumour shows low-signal abnormality with normally high signal glandular tissue on T2W (Fig. 1.11).
- Seminal vesicle involvement suggested by low signal on T2WI.
- Extracapsular extension signs include bulge of contour of gland, thickening and retraction of capsule, and stranding of soft tissue around prostate.

## [18]FDG PET-CT

- No current role.
- Newer isotopes like [11]C-citrate and [11]C-choline are in development and their role is not fully defined.

## Follow-up

- Depends on treatment.
- If rising PSA, MRI is used to assess prostate bed. Contrast may help distinguish scar tissue from active disease.

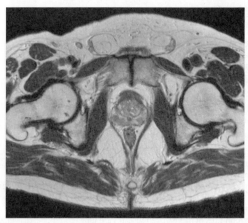

**Fig. 1.10** Carcinoma of the prostate Gleason 7 T2 axial image. Showing reduced T2W signal in the peripheral zone.

# Testicular cancer

- Most common malignancy in males between 15 and 34 years.
- Diagnosis usually established at orchidectomy.
- Imaging has key role in establishing presence of metastatic disease (lymph node, lung, liver).
- Imaging used to assess treatment response.

### Plain chest radiographs

- Can detect lung metastases greater than 1cm.
- Cost effective way for follow-up.

### CT

- Primary imaging modality for staging.
- IV and oral contrast-enhanced CT of thorax, abdomen, and pelvis.
- Primary tumour not assessed by CT (or MRI).
- Seminoma lymph node metastases, usually masses of soft tissue density and non-seminomatous germ cell tumours often contain cystic areas giving them a heterogenous appearance.
- Common sites of haematogenous sites are lung (commonest), liver, brain (usually haemorrhagic metastases that can be asymptomatic), bone.

### MRI

- Similar sensitivity to CT for detecting nodes in retroperitoneum.
- Primary use is in detection of brain metastases and spinal cord disease.
- May also be used to resolve specific problems, e.g. fistulae.

### Ultrasound

- Used in specific situations only.
- Can distinguish between cystic and solid lesion in testis.
- Can assess contralateral testis for synchronous tumours.
- Image guidance for biopsy of metastases if indicated.

### $^{18}$FDG PET-CT

- Not currently used for routine staging.
- Increased uptake in most testicular cancers.
- Sensitive technique for detection of metastases.

### Follow-up

- CT recommended 3-monthly up to 12 months, and 6-monthly up to 2 years for NSGCT.
- Surveillance programmes not usually used for seminoma.
- If tumour markers are rising further imaging with CT of chest, abdomen, and pelvis, and US of remaining testicle is done. If no new disease identified MRI brain is indicated to rule out occult metastatic disease and $^{18}$FDG-PET-CT considered.

# Neuroendocrine tumours

Carcinoid tumours
- Arise from diffuse neuroendocrine system, and can secrete variety of peptides and amines, e.g. serotonin, ACTH, histamine, etc.
- Account for 2% of GI tract malignancy, can occur in bronchus, thymus, and stomach amongst other places.
- Most common primary tumour of small bowel and appendix.

*Imaging*
- Primary diagnosis may be made at endoscopy or bronchoscopy.
- Imaging used for localization and staging of tumour.
- 80% of bronchial carcinoid in central or middle third of lung.

*Plain chest radiograph (bronchial carcinoid)*
- May demonstrate bronchial carcinoid as notched ovoid mass.
- If central in location, signs of airway obstruction, lobar collapse, central smooth lobulated mass.

## CT

*Bronchial carcinoid*
- Most sensitive technique available.
- Mass seen within lumen if central.
- If peripheral appears as solitary lung nodule.
- Round/ovoid mass with lobulated border.
- 30% calcified.
- Collapse/air trapping.
- Marked enhancement post-IV contrast.
- Nodular adrenal hyperplasia if lesion secretes ACTH.

*Thymic*
- Anterior mediastinal mass that may be calcified.
- Bilateral adrenal hyperplasia if ACTH secretion.
- Sclerotic bone metastases, lung, and liver metastases.

*Gastric*
Multiple gastric wall masses.

*Midgut*
- Primary bowel wall tumour rarely demonstrated.
- Secondary features may be seen, e.g. liver metastases, desmoplastic fibrosis with tethering of small bowel mesentery, bone, and lung metastases.

*Hindgut*
Used to stage lymph node and metastatic disease.

## MRI
*Bronchial*
High signal on T2W and STIR images.

*Midgut:*
- Post-gadolinium T1 fat-suppressed image, best sequence for demonstrating primary tumour.
- Moderate/intense enhancement post-gadolinium contrast.

*Hindgut:*
Generally not used for local staging, but used to stage lymph node and metastatic disease.

### Angiography
Superior and inferior mesenteric artery angiography can be used to localize primary midgut tumour, and lymph node and liver metastases

### Barium studies
**Follow through:** distortion of bowel loops in midgut carcinoid if there is fibrotic/desmoplastic reaction within mesentery.

### Scintigraphy
- Radiopeptide or radio-iodinated meta-iodobenzylguanidine scintigraphy ($^{123}$I-MIBG) can be employed to localize carcinoids.
- Radiopeptides used are radiolabelled somatostatin analogues (e.g. $^{111}$In-octreotide) taken up by somatostatin receptors in carcinoid tumours.

### $^{18}$FDG PET-CT
Only taken up by aggressive neuroendocrine tumours.

## Pancreatic neuroendocrine tumours
- Rare.
- 70–85% are functioning.
- Tumours arise from islet cells of Langerhans.
- Various types including gastrinoma, glucagonoma, insulinoma (most common), VIPoma, PPoma, somatostatinoma.

### Imaging
*Ultrasound*
- Transabdominal US is the first line of investigation.
- Endoscopic US is invasive, but provides better image resolution.
- Well defined lesion, homogenously hypoechoic +/− hyperechoic halo and distortion of gland.
- Vascular on Doppler imaging.

*CT*
- Stomach distended with water and anti-peristaltic agent given. Precontrast, arterial phase, and portal venous phase imaging.
- Tumours are isodense on precontrast and due to hypervascularity. In most cases they show greater enhancement than normal pancreas especially in arterial phase.
- Cystic lesions are rare.
- Malignancy suggested by large size, calcification, local invasion, and necrosis.

*MRI*
- T1W fat suppressed axial spin-echo and gradient echo, T2W axial fast spin-echo, axial dynamic contrast-enhanced gradient echo imaging is used.
- Tumours are low signal on T1 and high on T2WI. Marked homogenous enhancement following IV gadolinium.

*Angiography*
Arterial angiography, transhepatic portal venous sampling, arterial stimulation venous sampling are additional techniques for tumour localization, but rarely used.

*Scintigraphy*
- Radiopeptide and [123]I-MIBG scintigraphy can be used to identify neuroendocrine tumours.
- If MIBG uptake is demonstrated, therapy with [131]I-MIBG may be appropriate.

# Soft tissue sarcomas

- Heterogenous group of tumours arising from connective tissues other than bone.
- Malignant fibrous histiocytoma most common type in adults.
- Rhabdomyosarcoma most common tumour in paediatric age group.

## Imaging

- Required to identify local extent of tumour.
- Define spread.
- Identify metastases.
- Plan biopsy.

### Plain radiograph

- Initial investigation.
- Tumoural calcification may suggest histological diagnosis, e.g. synovial sarcoma.
- Identify underlying skeletal deformity.

### MRI

- Imaging modality of choice due to superior soft tissue contrast.
- Poor at soft tissue calcification or gas detection.
- Suggested protocol is T1W and T2W 6mm sagittal/coronal images, 8mm T2W and T1W axial slice images, STIR and T1W with contrast enhancement.

### CT

- Thoracic CT to detect pulmonary metastases.
- In certain tumour types, e.g. rhabdomyosarcoma of lower limb CT of abdomen and pelvis may be indicated for nodal staging.

### Ultrasound

Used for biopsy guidance.

### PET-CT

- Uptake of [18]FDG varies according to histological type and grade.
- Can be useful to define extent of disease prior to surgery in certain instances.

## Follow-up

MRI is used to identify local recurrence.

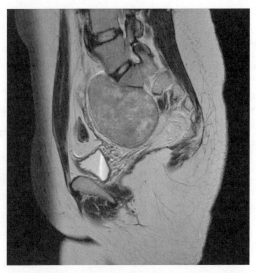

**Fig. 1.11** Pelvic/abdominal retroperitoneal sarcoma. 27 yr old. MRI revealed extensive retroperitoneal mass distinct from large bowel, rectum and pelvic organs.

# Skin cancers

- Collectively, skin cancer is most common human malignancy.
- Various types that are classified according to cellular origin.
- Basal cell carcinoma is commonest skin cancer.
- Separate staging systems are used for the various types.
- Local staging is pathological.

## Imaging

- Indicated in certain circumstances only, e.g. stage I or IIA melanoma needs no imaging investigation (only IIB and above).
- CT (chest, abdomen, and pelvis) and $^{18}$FDG PET-CT are the primary imaging modalities of choice for investigation of metastatic disease.

# 3. Cancer and interventional radiology

## Fine needle aspiration cytology and percutaneous biopsy

- Diagnostic tissue samples can be obtained from most sites in the body under fluoroscopic, US or CT guidance.
- US is preferred imaging modality as it allows real-time guidance and no radiation dose to patient. CT-guided biopsy or EUS used where poor visualization and accessibility.
- Local pathology service should be consulted as to whether FNA or a core biopsy is required.
- FNAC sample only contains few cells. Low risk. Specimen contains only few cells. Cytologist should be consulted regarding specimen preparation.
- Cutting needle biopsy obtains larger specimen. Needle comes in various sizes, e.g. 14–20G with specimen lengths of 1 and 2cm.
- Contraindications:
  - INR > 1.5, platelet count <50,000 (consider FFP +/– platelets);
  - vascular lesions, e.g. renal cell tumour metastases – avoid large vessels and be prepared to embolize if necessary;
  - obstructed system – best to drain system before biopsy as biopsy target may be site of fistula or intra-abdominal leak;
  - uncooperative patient – consider anaesthesia and sedation.
- In cases of coagulopathy transjugular or 'plugged' (where the biopsy tract is occluded with embolic material) biopsies allow tissue samples to be taken with relative safety.

# Radiotherapy planning

X-ray and conventional CT simulators are used to plan the radiation field.
PET/CT usage increasing as well.

# Radionuclide therapy

- Malfunctioning cells are targeted and destroyed using radiation.
- Radioisotope is localized in the required organ through a radioactive element following its usual biological path or by attaching it to a suitable biological compound.

  Common radiopharmaceuticals used in cancer treatment include:
- **Radioactive iodine ($^{131}$I sodium iodide):** remnant ablation is used to destroy residual thyroid tissue after surgical resection of papillary or follicular thyroid cancer.
- $^{32}$**P-chromic phosphate:** treatment of lung, ovarian, uterine, and prostate cancers.
- $^{32}$**P – sodium phosphate:** bone metastases.
- $^{131}$**I-labelled anti-CD20 antibody:** B-cell lymphoma.
- $^{89}$**Sr – strontium chloride:** palliation of bone pain caused by prostate and breast cancer metastases.
- $^{153}$**Sm – samarium lexidronam:** bone metastases from prostate cancer.
- $^{186}$**Rh and $^{188}$Rh – rhenium:** bone metastases.

## Developments

- Considerable medical research is being conducted worldwide into the use of radionuclides attached to highly specific biological chemicals, such as immunoglobulin molecules (monoclonal antibodies).
- The eventual tagging of these cells with a therapeutic dose of radiation may lead to the regression or even cure of some diseases.

# Central venous access for chemotherapy

- *Aim:* placement of catheter tip in central vein, vena cava, or right atrium.
- *Multiple configurations:* silicone or polyurethane, end hole (can be trimmed) or valve tipped (prevent blood reflux into lumen).
- Inserted peripherally or via neck or chest wall, tunnelled or non-tunnelled, and accessed via a subcutaneous port.

## Peripherally inserted central catheters: PICC lines

- Intermediate length of use maximal 3–6 months.
- Inserted via antecubital vein, cephalic, or basilic vein.
- Externally secured.
- Easily replaced, but require intact upper limb venous anatomy.
- Relatively fragile and narrow gauge 2–7F.
- Risk of thrombophlebitis and axillary vein thrombosis.

## External chest wall catheters

### Non-tunnelled
Intermediate use, useful in coagulaopathic and thrombocytopenic patients.

### Tunnelled
- 'Hickman line' most commonly used device.
- Single to triple lumen, silicone or polyurethane, end hole, or valve tipped.
- Tissue in-growth cuff prevents slippage through subcutaneous tunnel. Fully stable in 4–6 weeks.
- Long-term use months to years.
- Clot occlusion and line infection principle problems mandating removal. Peripheral and central cultures taken if in doubt. Tip sent for MC&S if removed.
- Risk of pneumothorax and haemothorax on insertion.

## Subcutaneous ports

- Catheter attached to stainless steel or plastic subcutaneous port.
- Port placed in forearm, upper arm, or chest.
- Metallic ports – CT artefact therefore seldom placed in chest wall.
- Single or dual chambers.
- Access to port via single or dual catheters with non-coring needle through superficial tissues and a silicone septum by trained individuals.
- Access 2000–4000 times possible.
- Long-term use months to years.
- Cost effective if used >6 months.

## Access

- *Internal jugular or subclavian vein.*
- *Blind puncture – SCV:* 3–12% haematomas, 2.5% haemo- or pneumothorax. IJV: success 88%, 3% neck haematomas due to carotid artery puncture.

- *Sonosite:* risk of Pneumothorax, haemothorax, and neck haematoma almost eradicated. Reduced risk of 'pinch off' syndrome – medial placement of SCV catheter leads to compression from subclavius muscle and costoclavicular tendon on arm movement.
- *Anatomy:*
  - **SCV:** axillary vein formed from confluence of the basilic and brachial veins at the lateral margin of teres major; this becomes the SCV at the lateral margin of the first rib. SCA lies posterior to SCV separated by the anterior scalene muscle. SCV lies between the lateral border of the first rib and the clavicle terminating at its junction with the IJV posterior to the sternoclavicular joint.
  - **IJV:** passes from the jugular foramen to its confluence with the SCV at the sternoclavicular joint. Lies within the carotid sheath with the carotid artery and vagus nerve. Relationship to artery: superior neck: posterior. Lower neck: 70% anterolateral, 14% lateral, 14% anterior, 2% medial, or posterior.

## Sonosite approach

Sonosite covered in sterile sheath.
- **IJV:** low anterior approach. IJV identified transversely between heads of sternocleidomastoid. Needle advanced into IJV under direct vision. Posterior approach: transverse visualization. Needle inserted parallel to transducer behind SCM into vein, then angled superiorly to insert guide wire in direction of right atrium.
- **SCV:** longitudinal approach. Compressible SCV is identified anterior to SCA at lateral aspect of clavicle. Needle is advanced parallel to transducer at 45° to pierce SCV. Transverse approach allows continuous visualization of SCA.

## Tunnelled catheter insertion

- 3 stages: venous access, tunnel formation, catheter insertion.
- Venous access as above. A guide wire and transition dilator are passed. Intravascular distance to the right atrium is established by withdrawing the guide wire to the entry point of the dilator if an end-hole catheter is to be placed. The transition dilator is sealed and left *in situ* during tunnel formation.
- Tunnel formation: a parasternal or upper lateral chest wall position is commonly selected according to patient accessibility and comfort
- A skin incision is made and Roberts forceps are used to dissect subcutaneously to the entry point used for venous access to the IJV or SCV.
- A tunnelling device is passed to exit at the insertion site.
- A stiff guide wire is passed through the tunnel and the transition dilator. The transition dilator is replaced by a peel away sheath.
- The definitive catheter is placed over the guide wire, placing the cuff 2cm from the skin incision and exit point. The sheath is removed.
- The skin incision is sutured.

# Vascular embolotherapy

- Used to cause deliberate occlusion of tumour feeding vessels.
- Can be an adjunct to surgery, and for treatment of benign and malignant tumours.
- Choice of embolic agent used, e.g. polyvinyl alcohol, sclerosants, adhesives, coils, etc., depends on the individual case.

### Indications

- Renal cell carcinoma patients with gross haematuria who are not fit for surgical intervention and prior to surgical resection of large paravertebral metastases.
- Transcatheter chemoembolization for unresectable liver tumours: a chemotherapeutic agent is mixed with small sponge particles and injected into the artery that supplies the tumour. This allows use of far lower dosages of the chemotherapeutic agent and the sponge particles cause vascular stasis, which has an ischaemic effect on the tumour as prolonging the time that the chemotherapy agent is in contact with tumour cells. It is especially useful in patients with primary hepatocellular carcinoma and in patients with hypervascular metastases that are confined to the liver.
- Radioactive microspheres for treatment of unresectable HCC. Again relies on the preferential hepatic arterial supply of HCC as opposed to the preferential portal vein supply of normal parenchyma. Yttrium-90 is the active agent in the microspheres.
- Yttrium-90 radioembolization for the treatment of unresectable liver metastases.
- Embolotherapy for the treatment of neuroendocrine hepatic metastases.
- Portal vein embolization: to allow for curative resection of large liver tumours that will require extensive resection. This is achieved by embolization of the intrahepatic portal branches of the future resected liver, thereby causing redistribution of portal blood flow containing hepatotrophic factors exclusively towards the future remnant liver.
- Palliation of pain caused by bone metastases.
- Uterine fibroid embolization.

# Tumour ablation

There are three main categories of percutaneous tumour ablation:
- Freezing (cryotherapy).
- Injection (ethanol, hot saline, acetic acid).
- Heating (radiofrequency, high-intensity focused US electrocautery, interstitial laser therapy, microwave coagulation therapy):
  - reduced morbidity and mortality, lower cost, and the ability to perform procedures on an outpatient basis are all advantages of this method over surgical resection;
  - these techniques induce cell death by coagulative necrosis.

## Radiofrequency ablation

- A relatively new technique used for primary and secondary liver or lung tumours, renal cell carcinomas, and some soft tissue or bone tumours.
- A small (14–18-gauge) needle attached to a radiofrequency device, is inserted into a tumour using US or CT guidance (see image).
- Radiofrequency waves cause resonance of the molecules in the tissue around the tip of the needle.
- This results in localized friction, which heats and causes coagulation necrosis of the surrounding tumour.

### Indications

- Patients with limited, but inoperable colorectal or breast metastases to the liver.
- Primary liver cancer where transplantation is not possible.
- Inoperable lung primaries or metastases.
- Renal cell carcinomas in cases with multiple tumours, previous contralateral nephrectomy, reduced renal function. or patients unable to undergo surgery for other reasons.

### Contraindications

- General:
  - Coagulopathy;
  - active infection.
- For lung ablation: poor respiratory reserve. FEV1 < 1.0.
- For liver ablation: advanced cirrhosis (Child Pugh class C).
  Percutaneous tumour ablation by injection of sclerosing agents (e.g. absolute alcohol) into tumours may be used where RFA is not possible.

## Other methods

- **Percutaneous ethanol injection:** effective in the treatment of hepatocellular carcinoma (HCC) with long-term survival rates of PEI-treated patients similar to those of patients treated surgically. But, RF ablation (see below) is the preferred modality for treatment of HCC as PEI shows similar results, but more sessions are required for small tumours (<2cm) and results are worse for tumours larger than 2cm.
- **Cryoablation:** used for many years during open surgery and is an effective method of tissue destruction. Currently, small size probes for effective percutaneous therapy are not widely available.

- ***Microwave ablation:*** may have theoretical advantages over RFA (if technical difficulties can be overcome) regarding uniformity and shape of thermal lesion. The thermal lesion heats up more uniformly, and is less dependent upon thermal conduction and surrounding blood flow than RFA.

# Percutaneous drainage procedures

- *Pleural effusion/empyema:* symptomatic pleural effusions are easily drained under US or CT guidance. Following drainage chemical pleurodesis to be performed as a palliative measure in cases of malignant effusions.
- *Abscesses:* post-operative complications may result in abscess formation, which can be punctured and aspirated under radiological guidance. Examples include pelvic collections, drained PR or through the anterior abdominal wall. A drainage catheter may be left *in situ* post-aspiration.

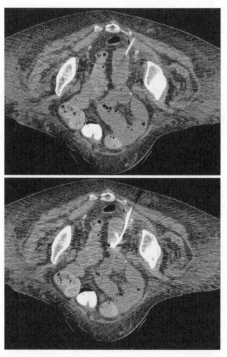

**Fig. 1.12** CT-guided drainage of a collection post-Hartmann's procedure for perforated sigmoid Ca.

## Renal tract

Percutaneous nephrostomy placement under radiological guidance is used in the management of malignant obstruction of the urinary tract and haemorrhagic cystitis secondary to chemotherapy, where it is desirable to divert the urine to 'rest' the bladder, and in patients with recto-vesicle or recto-vaginal fistulae caused by pelvic malignancy. Diversion of urinary flow may assist in healing of the fistulas and ease nursing problems.

### Procedure

- LA lidocaine 5mL 1%.
- Adequate guidance: fluoroscopic or USS 3- or 5MHz curvilinear transducer.
- Posterior calyx for puncture identified for access to the appropriate segment of the kidney and the safe creation of a tract.
- Collecting system of the kidney punctured by a needle introduced below the 11th rib posterior calyx punctured by a 20–30° posterior oblique approach to avoid renal vessels.
- The nephrostomy can be placed through any posterior calyx within the kidney.
- Lower-pole calyx usually infracostal reduces risk of pneumothorax/hydrothorax. A supracostal puncture of the middle or upper kidney may be needed for tumour removal.
- After entering the collecting system the obturator of the needle is removed and 3–5mL of contrast injected to check placement.
- Guidewire (0.035inch) introduced into the collecting system and needle removed.
- Lumbodorsal fascia incised and tract dilated with a dilating catheter passed over the guidewire.
- A nephrostomy catheter (8–14F)placed over the guidewire and secured. catheter. A larger catheter is used for tumours (14–22F).
- Guidewire removed after fluoroscopic check.
- Use a pigtail with a lock; most nephrostomy catheters have a locking mechanism to prevent displacement.
- Bleeding during nephrostomy placement may respond to clamping the tube for 30–40 min and IV furosemide.

## Biliary tree

Malignant biliary tract obstruction that cannot be relieved by ERCP internal drainage can be relieved by percutaneous drainage by 2 approaches.

### External drainage

- Percutaneous drain placed above obstructing lesion.
- Sterile procedure. INR should be <1.5. Antibiotic prophylaxis.
- Local anaesthetic + midazolam sedation.
- 15cm 22G Chiba needle inserted 1 ICS above the costophrenic angle in the mid-axillary line pointing between the xiphisternum and lateral border of T10. A duct is entered by injection or aspiration under fluoroscopic guidance. An initial PTC performed.
- Duct selected – peripheral duct with horizontal course preferable (lower risk of bleeding and ease of cannulation) 18G Longdwell needle inserted.

Inner needle removed and replaced with a guidewire. Outer sheath removed and Kumpe catheter inserted over guidewire
- Attempt is made to traverse the malignant stricture. An external drain is placed when this is not possible.
- Internal drainage preferable. External drains prone to being dislodged, and implicit fluid and electrolyte loss if bile drained externally.

### External/Internal drainage
- Percutaneous drain inserted to traverse the obstructing lesion with the tip placed in the duodenum.
- Procedure is the same as external drainage, but the stricture is negotiated and a long 8F external/internal catheter is placed
- This can be followed by placement of a metallic stent across the site of obstruction. (see Fig. 1.14) A hybrid endoscopic rendezvous is a method involving guide wire insertion percutaneously under fluoroscopic guidance to traverse a malignant stricture. The guide wire enables stent placement by ERCP.

### Biliary drains
- Straight or pigtail tip.
- External/internal catheters are designed with side holes to be positioned either side of a stricture to bypass bile.

### Biliary stents
- Polythene or metallic, balloon expandable and self-expanding, external/internal or entirely internal.
- Useful in palliation.
- Self-expanding metal stents provide effective palliation of malignant biliary strictures: alternative to open surgery.
- Metallic are more expensive and permanent. Longer patency. A single session of metal stenting often sufficient.
- Hepatic duct bifurcation tumours (Klatskin tumour): stents placed in both right and left intrahepatic ducts to provide decompression.
- Open mesh metal stents occlude by tumour in-growth. Covered self-expanding metal stent reduces this.
- Placement executed in stages liver tract is dilated gradually to pass the optimal size stent.
- Percutaneous therapy associated with a 5–10% rate of major complications.

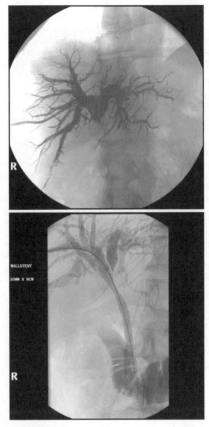

**Fig. 1.13** A 10mm × 9cm Wallstent was placed percutaneously in this patient with gastric cancer related extrinsic compression of the CBD.

# Pain control

- *Regional analgesia with neurolytic blocks:* e.g. brachial plexus blocks, sympathetic chain blocks. Pain can be caused by local spread of a tumour, such as invasion of the coeliac plexus or splanchnic nerves in upper gastrointestinal or pancreatic cancer. Ablation with a sclerosing agent, e.g. ethanol or phenol can be performed under CT guidance. (see Fig.1.15)
- *Percutaneous alcoholization of bone metastases:* used in cases of very painful osteolytic metastases where chemotherapy, radiotherapy, and conventional analgesia has failed. The procedure is performed under general anaesthesia in most cases with CT guidance.
- *Thermal radiofrequency ablation of bone metastases* (see 'Vascular embolotherapy').
- *Percutaneous cementoplasty of bony metastases:* Acrylic cement is injected into metastases under fluoroscopic or CT guidance to consolidate bone and treat pain.
- *Vertebroplasty/kyphoplasty:* Involves the percutaneous injection of polymethylmethacrylate into a vertebral body (see Fig. 1.16) to relieve pain and strengthen bone in cases of vertebral fracture due to osteoporosis or malignant infiltration. It can be performed under fluoroscopic or CT guidance. Up to 80% of patients with pain unresponsive to conventional treatment experience significant pain relief.

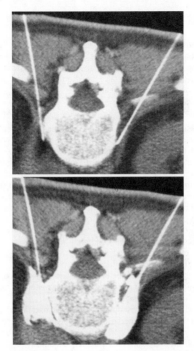

**Fig. 1.14** Splanchnic nerve block performed under CT guidance via a posterior approach.

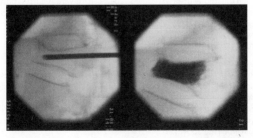

**Fig. 1.15** Vertebroplasty of T12 wedge compression fracture under fluoroscopic guidance.

# Feeding techniques

*Percutaneous gastrostomy:* enteric feeding is preferable to parenteral feeding in patients who cannot eat normally. Percutaneous gastrostomy feeding tubes can be safely placed under fluoroscopic guidance. Gastrojejunostomy tubes can also be used in cases of gastric outlet obstruction or gastro-oesophageal reflux.

*Procedure*
- Push, (Sacks-Vine) or pull, or Ponsky–Gauderer technique.
- *Push technique:* feeding tube pushed though abdominal wall over a guidewire into the stomach under fluoroscopic guidance. Loop catheters or balloon catheters placed. Peel-away sheath frequently used.
- *Pull technique:* feeding tube advanced from mouth into the stomach and retrieved by pulling through the abdominal wall using a snare introduced by direct gastric puncture under fluoroscopic guidance. Mushroom or bumper, catheters placed.
- Particularly useful in placement of large-bore gastrostomy or gastrojejunostomy catheters in children.
- Local anaesthesia or sedation if required.
- NG tube gas insufflation aids fluoroscopic puncture.
- USS used to delineate left lobe liver edge and transverse colon.
- *Oesophageal strictures:* gastric distension via needle introduced into the stomach under guidance.
- Oblique and lateral fluoroscopy guides needle insertion. A guidewire is introduced through this needle and gastropexy anchors may be placed. Abdominal wall and gastric wall dilatation can be achieved by using either serial Teflon dilators or angioplasty balloons.
- A hybrid CT/fluoroscopic pull technique has been described. This involves insertion of a guide wire through a sheathed needle directly into the stomach percutaneously under CT guidance. The stomach is then inflated with air via an NG tube. A snare wire is passed down the NG tube into the stomach where the snare is used to retrieve the percutaneous guidewire under fluoroscopic guidance. This wire is brought out orally. A conventional PEG tube is attached and drawn out through the stomach and dilated abdominal wall tract

*Venous access*
Patients with terminal disease may require central venous access for chemotherapy, total parenteral nutrition (TPN) and delivery of analgesia. Various long-term venous access systems, such as tunnelled central venous catheters, Hickman lines, peripherally inserted central catheters (PICCs) and venous ports are available, and can be placed under fluoroscopic and US guidance (see above).

# Oesophageal stenting

- Dilatation alone is unlikely to be effective in malignant strictures and is usually followed by some form of stenting.
- Self-expandable metallic endoprostheses are available covered and uncovered, some of which have anti-reflux valves.
- Over 95% of patients with inoperable oesophageal strictures can be palliated successfully with these devices (see Fig. 1.17).
- Principally used to palliate dysphagia due to primary tumour or anastomotic recurrence. May be used for extrinsic mediastinal compression.
- Retrievable oesophageal stents available if stenting is required as a bridge to future surgery or when complications occur as a result of surgery.
- Self-expanding metallic stents are inserted using small calibre delivery systems and often do not require pre-dilatation.
- **Tracheo-oesophageal fistulae and oesophageal perforation.**
  - Covered stents used with success rates of 80–100%.
  - Stent insertion may not preclude further treatment with either chemoradiotherapy or more definitive surgery.
  - Large bore stents (20–25mm) often necessary to adequately cover fistulae or perforation in patients following attempted recanalization of malignant strictures. To ensure adequate anchorage of the stent a temporary plastic balloon-expandable oesophageal stent (Wilson–Cook) placed endoscopically may be preferable to a metallic stent.
- *Early complications:* chest pain 90% (prolonged in 13%), bleeding, perforation, aspiration, fever, and fistulae occur in 10–20% of patients, 30-day mortality is reported to be as high as 26%, incidence of stent migration for uncovered stents is low (0–3%), rising to 6% at cardia, but 30% covered stents particularly at cardia.
- *Late complications:* restenosis and tumour overgrowth 60%, haemorrhage (3–10%), oesophageal ulceration (7%), perforation or fistulae (5%), stent torsion (5%), stent migration (5%), and stent fracture (2%).
- This may be a temporary measure allowing stabilization of the patient prior to definitive surgery or, alternatively, in patients who are not surgical candidates, the stent may provide adequate palliation.

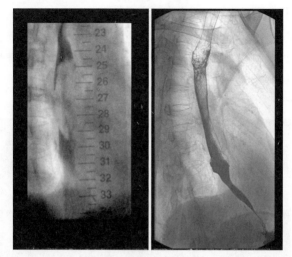

**Fig. 1.16** A 26mm × 12cm self-expanding nitinol stent has been placed over a mid/distal oesophageal malignant stricture.

# Tracheobronchial stenting

- Self-expanding metallic stents provide good palliation in cases of unresectable tracheobronchial malignancy.
- Covered stents are also very effective in managing tracheo-oesophageal fistulas unsuitable for treatment with covered oesophageal stents.
- Stents are inserted under general anaesthesia or sedation with local anaesthetic using combined fluoroscopic and bronchoscopic guidance.

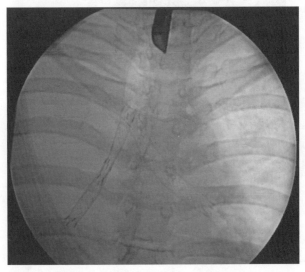

**Fig. 1.17** Bronchial stents (Niti-S): two 12mm × 40mm right bronchial stents and a 14mm × 50mm left bronchial stent.

# Malignant central venous obstruction

- Superior vena cava syndrome due to mediastinal neoplasia can be very distressing.
- It is caused by SVC compression or invasion by the tumour, and is often complicated by venous thrombosis.
- Metallic stent placement can restore flow and provides rapid relief from symptoms. Malignant inferior vena cava obstruction can be similarly treated.

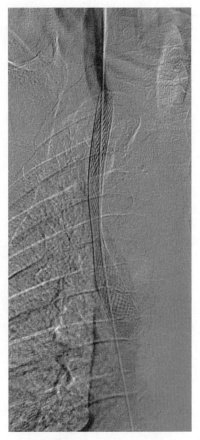

**Fig. 1.18** Wallstent (22mm × 7cm) inserted for SVC obstruction.

# Breast intervention

- Galactography is used in cases of persistent nipple discharge in absence of obvious lesion. This may demonstrate intraductal carcinomas, papillary carcinomas, papillomatosis, papillomas. Duct can be marked with permanent dye to facilitate surgical excision.
- US and mammography guidance can be used for fine needle and large core biopsy under LA. FNAB is usually sufficient.
- Stereotactic mammography provides excellent accuracy for localization of lesions. Equipment accommodates aspiration needles and automated biopsy guns.
- US and stereotactic mammography are used for needle localization and hookwire deployment in breast lesions prior to surgery to reduce amount of tissue excised.

# Breast cancer

# Breast cancer epidemiology, aetiology, and risk factors

## Epidemiology

Breast cancers are among the top 2 cancer killers in the western world with a worldwide incidence 1 million new cases per year (10% of all new cancers). Lowest incidence is in the African and Asian population.

The incidence has been steadily rising and is the commonest cancer in the UK (16%) with an annual incidence of 44,000 (US 240,000; commonest non-skin female cancer, EU 430,000). The annual breast cancer related mortality in the UK is over 12,000 (US 40,000).

80% occur above the age of 50, with a peak incidence at 50–70 years. The lifetime risk in women is 10%. 1% of breast cancers occur in men.

An increasing proportion of cancers are diagnosed by screening now (30–40%; in the UK in 2005–2006 15,944 cancers were diagnosed) and the rate of DCIS has increased from 4% (of symptomatic cancers) to 20% (screening cancers).

Mortality in the UK has fallen by 30% over the last 20 years. Currently, there is an overall 5-year survival rate of 80–85% and a 20-year survival of 50–65%.

## Breast cancer aetiology and risk factors

### Age

Risk increases with age (doubling every 10 years up to menopause) with the curve flattening after menopause. 80% of breast cancers occur above the age of 50, with a peak incidence at 50–70 years (50%). Under 30 years this drops to <2%.

### Diet and exercise

Alcohol is commonly implicated and may potentiate other risk factors. Data on saturated fats and red meat is, at best, weak. Physical activity decreases risk of breast cancer, as well as the risk of dying from cancer.

### Social

Higher incidence in higher social classes, later stage in lower social classes.

### Endogenous hormones

*Early menarche* and *late menopause* increases risk (RR increases by 3% per year of menopause delayed). *Multi-parity* protects, as well as earlier age of first childbirth (RR increases by 3% per year of delay in first childbirth). *Breast-feeding* and the length of feeding protect. (As a general rule, breast cancer risk is increased by longer the duration of uninterrupted menstrual cycles, i.e. oestrogen exposure).

*Oophorectomy* in pre-menopausal women reduces risk of Ca (especially oophorectomy at <35 years). Prophylactic oophorectomy in high risk BRCA mutation women may reduce breast Ca risk by 50%.

### Exogenous hormones

*HRT* increases risk of breast cancer and decreases sensitivity of mammography. HRT presents no increased risk for women under 50 (the same risk as having normal menstruation). In post-menopausal women the overall RR is 1.66 (66% higher than never users). Combination (oestrogen and progesterone) worse than oestrogen alone (RR – 2.0 vs. 1.3). Relative risk for each year of use is 1.023. In current users of more than 10 years the RR is 2.31. Risk returns to normal 5 years after stopping HRT (RR - 1.01). HRT best advise – probably best not to use more than 5 years (>5 years use = breast cancer risk over shadows potential benefit of reduction of hip fractures and colorectal cancer)

*OCP* has conflicting data. Some studies show no increased risk, while a meta-analysis (54 studies in the *Lancet*) showed RR increases to 1.24, but returns to normal risk 10 years after stopping. Specifically higher risk in patients with positive family history and age above 35 years. OCP in BRCA1 patients increase breast cancer risk, but protects against ovarian cancer.

### Body habitus

• *Obesity:* moderate increase of post-menopausal breast cancer incidence.
• *Mammographic breast density:* increased risk of breast cancer (4–6×) independently and decreased sensitivity of imaging. (density increases with HRT usage).

### Family history and genetic predisposition

5–10% of all breast cancers are hereditary. (see 'Familial breast cancer and genetics', p. 84–85 ).

Predisposing family history includes first degree relatives with young age of onset, bilateral breast Ca, ovarian Ca, male breast Ca, multiple cancers, other cancers (sarcoma, adrenocortical Ca, glioma in younger age group), and Ashkenazi Jewish (commonly eastern European) ancestry (2.5% population have a 5–10× greater risk of BRCA mutations).

#### Genetic prediliction

Commonly mutations of BRCA1, BRCA2, and TP53. Klinefelter's syndrome presents an increased risk of male breast cancer.

### Previous breast pathology

• *Benign disease:* fibroadenoma – no increased risk. Proliferative disease without atypia – 2-fold increased risk. Atypical epithelial (ductal/lobular) hyperplasia – 3–5-fold increased risk.
• *Breast cancer:* LCIS increases risk in either breast (see 'Non-invasive breast cancer: DCIS and LCIS). DCIS may progress to invasive cancer.
• *Previous invasive cancer:* 2–6-fold increased risk of a new cancer (the younger the age of previous cancer, the higher the risk). Previous ovarian/endometrial cancer carries 2× risk.

### Radiation exposure

- Mantle radiation for Hodgkin's and nuclear fall-out exposure is considered to double the risk, with a strong relation to age at exposure.
- Other: thymic radiation in infants, multiple diagnostic X-rays (e.g. skeletal/spinal disease). Diagnostic X rays may contribute to an extra 29 cases of breast cancer per year (UK).

### Risk prediction models

- *Gail model (1989) risk prediction:* provides a rough estimate of risk (next 5 years and lifetime) by taking into account current age, age at menarche, age at first parturition, number of previous breast biopsies, number of biopsies showing atypical hyperplasia, and family history of breast cancer in first-degree relatives. (Not validated in non-Caucasian population).
- *Other systems* include Claus (1994), BRCAPRO (1997), Cyrillic and Tyrer-Cuzick, Amir (2003), Antoniou models among others. NCI-NSABP risk calculator (http://nci.nih.gov/bcrisktool/)

### Further reading

Amir E, Evans DG, Shenton A, Lalloo F, Moran A, Boggis C, *et al.* Evaluation of breast cancer risk assessment packages in the family history evaluation and screening programme. *J Med Genet* 2003; **40(11)**:807–14.

Berry DA, Iversen ES, Jr., Gudbjartsson DF, Hiller EH, Garber JE, Peshkin BN, *et al.* BRCAPRO validation, sensitivity of genetic testing of BRCA1/BRCA2, and prevalence of other breast cancer susceptibility genes. *J Clin Oncol* 2002; **20(11)**:2701–12.

Claus EB, Risch N, Thompson WD. Autosomal dominant inheritance of early-onset breast cancer. Implications for risk prediction. *Cancer* 1994; **73(3)**:643–51.

Gail MH, Brinton LA, Byar DP, Corle DK, Green SB, Schairer C, *et al.* Projecting individualized probabilities of developing breast cancer for white females who are being examined annually. *J Natl Cancer Inst* 1989; **81(24)**:1879–86.

# Familial breast cancer and genetics

- Only 5–10% of breast cancers considered hereditary/genetic (up to 25% of young age onset cancers).
- Factors in family history considered to increase risk: young first degree relatives with breast cancer, higher number of relatives with breast cancer in the same side of the family, bilateral breast cancer, breast and ovarian cancer, male breast cancer, Ashkenazi Jewish heritage.
- Presence of affected relatives on either parental side of family will not be additive but paternal side history is important as 50% of inherited Ca will be from the paternal line.
- 85% of individuals with a close relative with breast cancer never develop the disease.
- Mutation carriers have 1–4% annual breast cancer risk.

## Common gene mutations

- BRCA1: (17q21) (1994) – tumour suppressor oncogene. Seen in up to 40% of hereditary breast cancers. Also increases risk of ovarian, colon and prostate cancer. Autosomal dominant. 50% penetrance, 65–85% lifetime risk, 20–50% ovarian cancer risk. When cancer develops, it tends to be high grade, steroid receptor and Her-2 –ve, and occur earlier (average age 45 years) with a higher incidence of bilaterality. Men with BRCA1 have a higher risk of developing breast cancer.
- BRCA2: (13q) (1994) – in 30% inherited breast cancers. Also male breast cancer, ovarian, prostatic, pancreatic cancers. 50% penetrance, 40–85% lifetime risk of breast cancer and 20–50% ovarian cancer. Autosomal dominant inheritance.
- TP53: tumour suppressor gene – Li-Fraumeni syndrome. Autosomal dominant. Lifetime risk ~100%

## Other mutations

PTEN, STKII/LKB, ATM, CHK2, MSH2/MLH1, CDH1 (see Table 2.1).

## Gene testing

High risk individuals are identified on the basis of family history and offered tertiary referral to a genetics clinic. Detailed analysis of risk is then made (e.g. Manchester scoring system) and genetic testing will be discussed if appropriate (>20% chance of finding mutation).

Detailed counselling should precede and follow gene testing. Psychosocial and management ramifications of the process of testing, as well as results of testing (negative, positive, ambiguous) on the individual and family should be discussed. Informed consent is needed.

In the USA, the law protects against insurance discrimination based on genetic testing.

*Molecular genetic testing* is by targeted mutation analysis or comprehensive analysis. Requires identification of the relevant mutation in the affected relative (>500 mutations known in each BRCA).

If positive, screening protocol and risk reduction measures should be discussed (see Management of breast cancer risk, p. 164).

**Table 2.1** Breast cancer risk mutations

| Gene | Syndrome | Inheritance | Main cancer risk |
|------|----------|-------------|------------------|
| BRCA1 | Breast/ovarian | AD | Breast, ovarian |
| BRCA2 | Breast and multiple cancer | AD | Breast, uterine, ovarian, prostate, gastric pancreatic, melanoma |
| TP53 | Li-Fraumeni syndrome | AD | Early onset breast Ca, childhood cancers. Brain, soft tissue sarcomas, lung, eukemia, adrenocortical Ca (no ovarian) |
| PTEN | Cowden disease | AD | Breast (very early), ovary, endometrial, follicular thyroid, colon, renal |
| STKII/LKB1 | Peutz–Jegher syndrome | AD | GI, breast Ca |
| CDH-1 | Hereditary diffuse gastric cancer | AD | Gastric, colon, breast |
| ATM | Ataxia-telangiect-asia | AR | Breast, NHL |
| CHK2 | Site-specific | AD | Breast. Activates actions of BRCA1 and P53 (subset of Li-Fraumeni syndrome results from CHK2 mutation) |
| MSH2/MLH1 | Muir–Torre syndrome | AD | Colorectal, breast, BCC |

# Pathology and biology of invasive breast cancer

The majority of symptomatic breast cancers are invasive ductal adenocarcinomas. The incidence of DCIS has increased with the advent of screening (DCIS – 20% in screen detected and 4% symptomatic cancers).

**Breast cancer: pathological groups**

## Morphological varieties

### Epithelial invasive cancer
- Invasive ductal carcinoma (80%). Morphological varieties.
- No Special Type (NST/NOS).
- Tubular 2–3%.
- Mucinous/colloid 5%.
- Medullary 3%.
- Invasive cribriform and papillary 1–2%.
- Invasive lobular carcinoma (5–15%; 1–4% in male breast cancer).
- Mixed ductal and lobular.
- Inflammatory carcinoma.
- Adenoid cystic carcinoma.
- Metaplastic carcinoma (<1%).
- Paget's (with invasive carcinoma, 1–5%).

### Epithelial non-invasive
- DCIS (4%; 20% of screen detected cancers).
- Papillary, micropapillary, cribriform, comedo, solid.
- LCIS.
- Paget's (with intraductal carcinoma, 1–5%).

### Non-epithelial tumours
- Phylloides.
- Sarcoma.
- Lymphoma.
- Squamous cell carcinoma.
- Secondary carcinoma.

- *Invasive (infiltrating) ductal carcinoma*: most common, found in all ages, hard in consistency, solid core, DCIS may co-exist. Lymph node and metastatic spread common.
- *Ductal carcinoma in situ (DCIS)*: in situ cancer arising from the ductal epithelium. Found by itself or co-existing with invasive cancer. Four morphological varieties. Contained within ductal basement membrane – no stromal invasion. Central necrosis can occur and may later undergo dystrophic calcification – microcalcifications on mammography. DCIS can transform into invasive cancer often maintaining the same morphology (e.g. a low grade papillary DCIS transforms into low grade ductal-papillary invasive cancer). Grades – low, intermediate, and high grade.

- *Invasive lobular carcinoma:* invades stroma in a single file pattern (indian file). Ill-defined lesions. Stage for stage, has the same prognosis as ductal cancers, but there is a propensity for multicentricity and bilateral cancers.
- *Lobular carcinoma* in situ *(LCIS):* does not behave like a cancer and is considered only a marker for high risk. Neoplastic cells distend the acini preserving the general architecture of the lobule. ER +ve. More frequent in premenopausal women (see 'Non-invasive breast cancer: DCIS and LCIS', p. 154).
- *Tubular carcinoma:* well differentiated – tumour propagates in a tubular fashion, histology shows predominantly (>75%) multiple single cell layered tubules. Tend to be low grade, with a better prognosis, ER/PR +ve.
- *Mucinous carcinoma:* tumour cells float as clumps in a sea of mucin. Better prognosis.
- *Medullary carcinoma* : large undifferentiated cells with pleomorphic nuclei and lymphocytic infiltration. Tend to be low grade with better prognosis. Usually steroid receptor –ve.
- *Inflammatory breast carcinoma:* characterized by skin oedema and redness due to involvement of dermal lymphatics. Poor prognosis (see 'Breast cancer: special conditions', p. 156).
- *Paget's:* breast carcinoma in which cancer cells invade the epidermis of the nipple producing ezcematoid changes and eventually destruction. Underlying cancer is invasive 90% (if palpable) or DCIS (see 'Other breast cancers and pathology, p. 162).
- *Adenoid cystic carcinoma:* (see Other breast cancers and pathology, p. 162).
- *Metaplastic:* rare (0.2–1%) breast cancer with epithelial and mesenchymal elements. Often presents at later stages, and tends to be higher grade and hormone receptor –ve. Nevertheless, stage for stage prognosis and behaviour is similar to breast adenocarcinomas and treatment is identical.

## Tumour biology/natural history

Arise from a single cell undergoing malignant transformation. Generally impalpable below 1cm size. Size doubling time depends on cell proliferation vs. destruction. Average doubling time 120 days (1 month–3 years). To reach 1cm$^3$ volume requires about 30 doublings, i.e. 5–8 years.

### Mode of spread
- **Contiguous:** direct infiltration.
- **Lymphatic:** primarily to axillary LN (I–III). Smaller proportion to the internal mammary nodes. Secondary sites supraclavicular. Generally contiguous spread, but non-contiguous LN spread can occur. LN state and number, and sites involved have significant bearing on prognosis and is reflected in staging systems.
- **Haematogenous spread:** e.g. skeletal, lung, liver.

## Tumour size

**Size at diagnosis:** prognostic factor; predicts for regional spread and metastasis.

## Tumour grade

Based on mitotic rate, tubule formation (% of tumour occupied by tubular structures) and nuclear pleomorphism impacts on prognosis.

Table 2.2 Modified (Elston–Ellis) Scarff, Bloom, and Richardson grading

| Score | Mitotic rate | Tubule formation | Nuclear pleomorphism |
|-------|--------------|------------------|----------------------|
| 1 | $\leq 7$ | > 75% | Small, uniform cells |
| 2 | 8–14 | 10–75% | Moderate variation |
| 3 | > 15 | <10% | Marked variation |

*Grade 1:* well-differentiated (Score 3–5, 10-year survival 85%).
*Grade 2:* moderately differentiated (Score 6–7).
*Grade 3:* poorly differentiated (score 8–9, 10-year survival 40%).

## Steroid (oestrogen and progesterone) receptor

The actions of oestrogen (which regulate the growth and differentiation of normal and breast cancer cells), are mediated through the oestrogen receptor (ER), a nuclear transcription factor. Two isoforms – ER-$\alpha$ and ER-$\beta$. PR receptor (PR-A and PR-B isoforms) is a similar nuclear transcription factor.

Around 70% of breast cancers are ER +ve, half of which are also PR+. 5% are ER and PR –ve. Steroid receptor positive cancers tend to have a better prognosis.

*ER and PR scores:* H score or Allred score (0–8) sum of percentage of cells stained (0–5) and intensity (0–3). Score ≥3 considered positive.

## HER-2 (HER-2-neu, c-erb-B2) receptor

• One of 4 trans-membrane epidermal growth factor receptors (1–4).
• Activation results in tyrosine kinase-mediated downstream signalling, controlling cell proliferation, invasiveness, and angiogenesis.
• Over-expression of HER-2 is associated with more aggressive disease.
• Test positive immunohistochemistry (IHC) 3+ or fluorescent *in situ* hybridization (FISH) positive. When IHC 2+, proceed to FISH test. If FISH borderline – retest, count additional cells, or IHC testing.

## Lymphovascular invasion

Presence of tumour emboli in microvascular or lymphatic channels. Predicts lymph node status and is an independent prognostic factor.

# Breast screening

- A key strategy for reducing breast cancer mortality is early detection.
- Major land mark trials have shown the benefits of breast screening
  – e.g. **Swedish two counties trial** (RCT) – 77,080 in screening arm
  and 55,985 non-screening arm. Data from 20 years before and after
  screening was introduced (1977), showed a 27% mortality reduction
  in the screening invited population. **New York Health Insurance
  Plan (HIP) project** (RCT) – 60,000 participants (1963), 30% mortality
  reduction.
- Mammography fulfils the criteria for a good screening test: high
  sensitivity and specificity, ability to recognize early lesions, effective
  treatment for early disease, relatively minimal adverse effects, significant
  improvement in mortality and morbidity on early detection, good
  compliance/participation rate and acceptable cost benefit ratio.
- Per exposure 2mGy. Breast cancer risk – 1 per 100,000 mammograms.
- Screening saves an estimated average 1400 lives annually in the UK.
  (2003 stats) with the average cost per life year saved being £3000 (UK).
- **UK:-** following Forrest report 1986 (Professor Sir Patrick Forrest),
  the NHS Breast Screening Programme (NHSBSP) was established in
  1987/1988, completing national rollout by 1992/93.
- Women are invited for the first screening between their 50th and 53rd
  birthdays, and then every 3 years until the 70th birthday. Above this age
  screening is available on self-referral.
- In the new cancer reform strategy the screening invitations age group
  will be extended to 47–73 years. (UK).
- **US:** ACS guidelines, from 40 years annual mammogram and clinical
  exam. No upper age limit. Uptake ~60% (20–40 years – 3-yearly clinical
  exams). In high risk cases, start at 25 years or 5–10 years earlier than
  youngest family history case.
- Screen detected cancer now account for a third of cancers detected.
- 95% of women are reported as normal after the first mammogram.
  5-7% will be recalled for further evaluation/investigation. (Of those
  recalled - around one in eight will be found to have cancer.
- Mammographic features of cancer: irregular mass, spiculation,
  architectural distortion, microcalcifications (DCIS is associated
  with microcalcifications in 90% of cases) 60–80% of lesions will be
  impalpable.
- DCIS accounts for 21% of screen detected cancers.
- Single view mammography is 90% sensitive and 95–99% specific.

**NHSBSP screening standards (UK, Quality Assurance Framework)**

- Few examples.
- ≥ 70% uptake in the screening population.
- All films are double read. <10% recall rate (first invitation).
- ≥80% of Ca should be diagnosed by non-surgical biopsy (FNA, Core).
- Rate of benign biopsy should be <3.6/1000 (prevalent) and <2/1000 (incident screen).
- Mean dosage limit of radiation ≤2.5mGy.

*Negative aspects of screening*

Anxiety and morbidity from unnecessary biopsies in benign cases. Some low grade DCIS may never progress to cancer, and resection may represent over-diagnosis and treatment.

# Evaluation of breast cancer

## Modes of presentation
- *Screen detected:* e.g. mammography.
- *Symptomatic.*
- *Incidental:* found during examination/investigation/imaging for another condition. At presentation breast cancer may be *early* (mostly stage I and II) or *advanced* (mostly III and IV)

## Presenting symptoms
Lump, nipple discharge (especially unilateral, single duct, and older age), nipple inversion, distortion, breast pain, breast/areola contour change, skin changes (peau'd orange, dimpling, discolouration, prominent veins, direct skin involvement, ulceration, nodules), inflammatory changes, cysts (bloody aspirate, persistent mass after aspiration, recurrent refilling of cysts), breast abscess, post-trauma discovery of lump (may be initially dismissed as bruise/fat necrosis), axillary involvement (palpable nodes, skin changes, upper limb oedema), symptoms from metastasis (e.g. bone pain, fractures, vertebral collapse, liver, lung, brain, skin nodules, non-axillary lymph nodes, contralateral breast/axilla). Only 10% of attendees in a breast symptomatic clinic will turn out to have cancer.

## Breast mass differential diagnosis
Benign breast tumours/abnormalities of normal ductal involution 'ANDI' – fibroadenoma, fibroadenosis, cysts, hamartoma, abscess, sclerosing lesions (radial scar, complex sclerosing lesion, fat necrosis).

## Evaluation of breast lesion
- *Physical exam.*
- *Imaging:* mammography and/or USS.
- *Pathology.*
Combining the above 3 modes of evaluation (triple assessment) results in ~99% accuracy and is now considered the standard of care. Accuracy rates are lower in the younger patient. Suspected cases should be urgently referred and evaluated in a 'one stop clinic' (Fig. 2.1). (The primary investigations of a triple assessment should be completed with a majority of patients reaching a diagnosis during the same visit and benign cases reassured.)

## History
*Presenting symptoms:* onset, duration, other details.
*Past history:* breast and general medical-related (including biopsies, previous breast cancer). Radiation exposure.
*Reproductive history:* menarche, number of pregnancies, age of first pregnancy, breast feeding, menstrual cycles, menopause, OCP, HRT use.
*Family history:* number and age of relatives with breast cancer. Other cancers – ovarian, colonic. Ashkenazi Jewish ancestry (for other risks, see 'Breast cancer epidemiology, aetiology, and risk factors, p. 80).

## Physical examination

Examine both breasts, including nipple and areola, axillae, further lymph nodular regions and perform a general examination. The characteristics of the lump should be recorded, including size, location consistency, fixity, skin changes, nipple-areolar changes. Nipple discharge may be uni- or bilateral single or multi-duct, and may be serous, milky, discoloured, or bloody. Recording should be standard and consistent location may be quadrant-based (combination of upper, lower, inner, outer, and central) or clock face-based. Size and distance from nipple should be recorded. A palpation score (P1–P5) should be accorded:

### Palpation scoring
- **P1:** normal breast.
- **P2:** benign lump.
- **P3:** borderline.
- **P4:** suspicious.
- **P5:** malignant.

## Imaging

Mammography and ultrasound are the primary modalities. (see 'Investigations: imaging, p. 100, for further details). A radiology score is given (R1–R5) or U1–U5 (USS) and M1–M5 (mammography).

## Pathology

A FNAC or tissue (core/mammotome) biopsy is taken. Freehand or image-guided. A cytology (C) score or biopsy (B) score is given. Note that a score of C1 does not indicate normality (see 'Investigation: cytology and histology', p. 96).

## Other tests

- **Blood tests:** blood counts, liver function tests, bone profile.
- **Staging investigations:** as appropriate (see 'Investigations: imaging, p. 100).

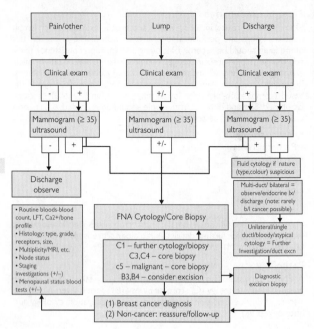

**Fig. 2.1** Breast cancer referral evaluation.

# Investigations: cytology and histology

Techniques for obtaining tissue for diagnosis are: fine needle aspiration cytology, core biopsy, mammotome biopsy and open/excisional biopsy. Biopsy may be free hand in palpable lesions or USS-guided or stereotactic (under X-ray guidance) in non-palpable lesions.

Fine needle aspiration cytology

- Use a 21–23 gauge needle. Make several passes through the lesion maintaining negative pressure (see Fig. 2.2). Specificity >95%. Sensitivity 70–90%.
- Accuracy >90% when concordant with triple assessment.
- A simple procedure, with quick same-visit reporting. Diagnosis and steroid receptor status are possible, but exact tumour type and other characteristics will require more tissue. The tumour can be graded (e.g. Robinson's, Mouriquand's grading systems), but some amount of discordance with final histology occurs.

Cytology scoring

- *C1:* inadequate cells/artefacts (will require further cytology/biopsy).
- *C2:* benign.
- *C3:* atypical, borderline, indeterminate.
- *C4:* atypical cells suspicious of malignancy.
- *C5:* malignant.

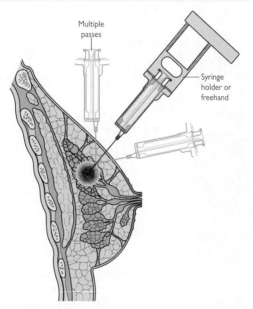

**Fig. 2.2** Fine needle aspiration.

**Nipple discharge/nipple scraping cytology/duct lavage**

- *Suspicious discharge:* unilateral, single duct, unexpressed discharge, older age, sero-sanguinous, black, brownish colour (occasionally clear).
- >85% accuracy, but using cytology for all unselected cases of discharge may result in high proportion of confounding results and unnecessary invasive procedures.
- *Duct lavage:* trial setting mainly, not in widespread routine use.

**Core biopsy**

- Freehand or under ultrasound/mammographic (stereotactic) guidance.
- 14G (22mm) needle used. Usually automated instrument. Local anaesthesia, 2–3mm skin incision. (see Fig. 2.3).
- Core of tissue available – better diagnosis, histological grade and type assessment as well as steroid receptor and Her-2 status – also useful in assessing response to neo-adjuvant therapy.
- 90–95% sensitivity. Specificity ~100%. Scored from B1 to B5.

**Histology scoring**

- *B1:* normal tissue.
- *B2:* benign.
- *B3:* borderline.
- *B4:* suspicious.
- *B5:* B5a, *in situ* disease; B5b, invasive disease.
- Usually at least 4 cores are taken to reduce sampling error.

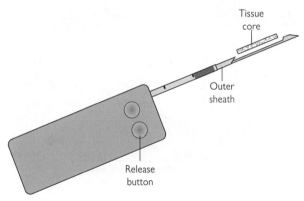

**Fig. 2.3** Automated core biopsy needle.

**Vacuum-assisted mammotome biopsy**
- 14, 11, and 8 G sizes (see Fig. 2.4). A larger volume of tissue decreases sampling error.
- Usually performed under USS guidance and provides confirmation to prevent sampling error. Diagnostic specificity ~100%. Close to 98% sensitive.
- Complete excision of benign lesions possible (usually up to 3cm).

**Open biopsy**
- Considered when needle/core biopsy fails or histology is equivocal.
- Specimen should not weigh more than 20/30g for a diagnostic biopsy (UK guidelines: 80% of diagnostic biopsies should weigh <20g) and incision oncologically and cosmetically placed (incision should not prejudice future therapeutic excision or reconstructive surgery).
- In impalpable or difficult to palpate lesions, ultrasound marking, or insertion of one or more guidewires, or radiolabelled dye is pre-operatively done. Intraoperative ultrasound may further aid localization.
- Specimen radiography is essential to confirm removal of small or impalpable lesions.

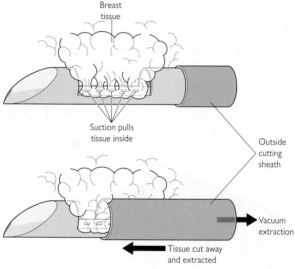

**Fig. 2.4** Mammotome excision.

## Histological analysis

- Report should be standardized and contain information on histological type, grade/differentiation, size, multifocality (multiple lesions
  – same quadrant/>5cm apart), multicentricity (multiple lesions
  – usually different quadrants/<5cm apart), status of margins, steroid receptor status, HER-2 status, determination of micrometastases by immunohistochemistry (cytokeratins CK19 and CAM 5.2), PCR, and RT-PCR, etc.
- Mixed invasive (ductal + lobular) and metaplastic cancers should be graded according to the ductal component. (the non-ductal component does not alter prognosis/treatment).
- RT-PCR assay (gene) may be used to predict recurrence and direct adjuvant chemo and endocrine therapy in equivocal cases.
- In neo-adjuvant chemotherapy, pretreatment histology including receptor status is considered more reliable (pre-operative chemotherapy may have altered histological features in the excision specimen) and is used for planning post-operative adjuvant treatments.

## Tumour genetic profiling

Gene expression profiling of the cancer by various techniques can provide prognostic and predictive information, and is likely to have increased use in the future (e.g. chemotherapy decision-making). Results from randomized trials are awaited.

Techniques include DNA micro-array technique, RT-PCR (reverse transcriptase – polymerase chain reaction). Scored as low, intermediate, or high risk..

## Five major subtypes based on gene profiling

Five major tumour sub-types have been identified currently. These are likely to undergo further/revised characterization in the future as trials data accumulate).

- *Luminal A:* ER+, HER-2 –ve with good prognosis (survival >5 years).
- *Luminal B:* ER+, HER-2 –ve with poor prognosis (survival <5 years).
- *Basal subtype:* ER –ve, PR –ve, HER-2 –ve.
- *HER-2 + subtype:* ER –ve, HER-2 +ve.
- *Normal:* ER –ve, HER-2 –ve.

# Investigations: imaging

Mammography
- *Overall sensitivity:* 75–95% and specificity 50–95%.
- Sensitivity is directly related to breast density and age (sensitivity drops from ~95% in >60 years age to ~50% in <40s (hence, not used in those under 35 years).
- Units are gradually moving from analog to digital mammography.
- Up to 10% of cancers may not be visible on mammography. Use other modalities if mammogram is negative, but clinical suspicion persists.
- *Screening:* 2 views – cranial-caudal (CC) and medio-lateral-oblique (MLO) views. Diagnostic mammography: 2 views + additional views if indicated (e.g. medio-lateral, magnification, and spot compression views).
- Mammographic features of cancer: calcifications (often fine <0.5mm), densities, ill-defined margins, spiculation, focal asymmetry, and associated features – architectural distortion, skin thickening, and retraction. Change/enlargement over time.
- *Scoring:* BI-RADS system (American College of Radiology).

Category 6: known biopsy proven malignancy Breast Imaging Reporting and Data System (BI-RADS) scoring

Adapted for mammography, USS, and MRI.
- *Category 1:* negative, normal appearance.
- *Category 2:* benign.
- *Category 3:* probably benign (<2%malignant). Follow-up mammogram at 6 months.
- *Category 4:* suspicious abnormality, needs bx (subdivided A, B, C).
- *Category 5:* highly suggestive (>95%) of cancer – for bx/treatment.
- *Category 0:* incomplete, needs further evaluation.

Ultrasound
- *Malignant lesions:* 70–98% sensitive and 50–75% specific. Sensitivity drops in very dense breasts (~40%).Overall, 80–90% of breast lesions are visible on USS.
- High frequency USS probes are used (>7.5 MHz). ~5cm penetration.
- Calcifications are poorly delineated on USS. Highly sensitive for cysts.
- *USS:* particularly useful when mammography relatively contraindicated or of poor yield – young age, presence of implants, less accessible sites e.g. axillary tail/axilla, male breast, avoiding multiple X-ray exposure.
- *Diagnostic information:* diagnosis, number, extent, and position of breast lesions and axillary nodes, and correlation and delineation of mammographic findings.
- *Interventional procedures:* FNAC (breast lump, axillary node), core biopsy, mammotome excision, pre-operative localization(guidewire/skin marking), USS guided radionuclide injection prior to SNB, marker placement (radio-opaque or sono visible markers) prior to neo-adjuvant therapy, intraoperative localization, cyst/abscess drainage.

- **USS features of cancer:** solid mass, hypoechogenicity, irregular shape and margins, acoustic shadowing, anterior echogenic rim, shape – taller than wider orientation (may be reversed in advanced stages).
- Doppler US demonstrate increased vascularity. Locate vascular pedicle.
- Currently not recommended as a primary population screening tool (ongoing trial results awaited), but may form adjunct to mammography.

## MRI

- Using dedicated breast coils. Sensitivity – 90–100% (invasive cancers), 80–90% for DCIS. Specificity lower. Not useful for micro-calcifications. Also MRI-guided needle sampling and wire localization.
- Uses paramagnetic contrast administration (e.g. gadolinium).
- **Advantages:** specifically useful in sizing lesions, detecting multi-focality/centricity. Breast with implants. Lobular carcinoma detection (USS and mammo negative in ~20%). Also provide information on axillary disease, internal mammary nodes and distant metastasis (especially spinal disease) and response to neo-adjuvant therapy. Surgical clips OK.
- **Disadvantages:** cost, availability, patient size limitations, long scan time, unnecessary extra examinations and biopsies due to lower specificity.
- **MRI features of cancer:** solid mass, irregular margins, rim enhancement, contrast enhancement, and washout pattern/curve.
- Useful in younger women and has been recommended for screening in high-risk patients (NICE recommendations, 2006; ACS guidelines, 2007) For example, BRCA1 and 2 mutation carriers between 30 and 49 years, and TP53 carriers >20 years (see 'Management of breast cancer risk', p. 164)

## CT imaging

Generally no role in primary breast evaluation, but may incidentally pick up breast lesions when performed for other conditions. Useful in staging for chest and abdominal metastasis.

## Ductography (and ductoscopy, ductal lavage)

Useful in evaluation of nipple discharge, but use is not widespread. Newer 0.9mm scopes have improved efficiency.

## Specimen radiography

- **Wide excision specimen:** for per-operative assessment of margins.
- **Core bx:** to ensure bx is representative of lesion (microcalcification).

## Staging investigations

- **Loco-regional staging:** tumour characteristics
  - *Size:* USS gives accurate pre-op size measurement or MRI; final size is from histology;
  - *Regional nodes:* axillary clearance; sentinel node assessment;
  - *Imaging/biopsy* (FNAC/open) of non-axillary nodes in appropriate situations.
- **Staging investigations for metastatic disease:**
  - *Lung:* chest X-ray/CT/PET.
  - *Liver:* USS/CT.

- *Skeletal:* isotope bone scan, skeletal survey/X-ray; CT/PET/other as appropriate for other viscera according to symptoms.
- No universal consensus on when to initiate metastatic staging investigations. The usual indications are:
  - presence of significant nodal disease;
  - large/aggressive tumour, locally advanced;
  - symptoms/signs of possible metastatic disease;
  - when contemplating major extirpative/reconstructive procedures, e.g. mastectomy, flap reconstruction;
  - biologically poorer prognosis tumours, e.g. steroid receptor negative, young patients, inflammatory cancer;
  - onset of recurrent disease.

# Staging of breast cancer

Staging/scoring systems provide prognostic and treatment planning information. Include: AJCC/UICC system, NPI, and VNPI.

## Van Nuys Prognostic Index for DCIS (1996) (2003 – 'age' added)

Score of 1–3 (good to poor) for each of four predictor variables
- **Tumour extent/width** (≤15, 16–40, ≥41mm).
- **Excision margin** (≥10, 1–9, < 1mm).
- **Nuclear grade** (Van Nuys Group 1, non-high nuclear grade without necrosis; Group 2, non-high nuclear grade with necrosis; Group 3, high nuclear grade with or without necrosis).
- **Age** (39 or less, 40–60, 61 and above).

### Scores
- **4–6:** good prognosis, managed by excision alone.
- **7–9:** reduction in recurrence rates if local radiotherapy (RT) added to excision.
- **10-12:** high incidence of local recurrence even if RT added – consider mastectomy.

## Nottingham Pr0ognostic index

NPI = 0.2 × tumour diameter (cm) + grade (1–3) + LN stage (1–3)
(Lymph node: no nodes = 1, 1–3 nodes = 2, 4, or more nodes = 3.)

### Prognostic groups
- **Excellent**: 2.0–2.4 (91–95% 10-year survival with treatment).
- **Good**: 2.41–3.4 (82–87%).
- **Moderate1**: 3.41–4.4 (75–80%).
- **Moderate2**: 4.41–5.4 (55–75%).
- **Poor:** 5.41–6.4 (25–50%).
- **Very poor**: >6.41 (<20%).

## AJCC/UICC System (TNM)

UICC/AJCC (TNM system) – was first introduced in 1958 (UICC) and 1977 (AJCC). The current version is the 6th edition (combined UICC/AJCC) incorporating new developments such as SLNB (sn), IHC, RT-PCR (mol +/–)and distinguishing between micrometastasis (pN1mi, size 0.2–0.02mm) and isolated tumour cells [pN0(i+), size <0.2mm].

Stage-related 5-year approximate survival rates following treatment are as follows:
- Stage **0 -** 100%
- Stage **I -** 98%.
- Stage **IIA -** 92%.
- Stage **IIB -** 81%.
- Stage **IIIA -** 67%.
- Stage **IIIB -** 54%.
- Stage **IV -** 16%.

**Table 2.3** AJCC/UICC stage groupings

| Stage | Tumour (T) | Node (N) | Metastasis (M) |
|---|---|---|---|
| Stage 0 | Tis | N0 | M0 |
| Stage 1 | T1 | N0 | M0 |
| Stage IIA | T0 | N1 | M0 |
| | T1 | N1 | M0 |
| | T2 | N0 | M0 |
| Stage IIB | T2 | N1 | M0 |
| | T3 | N0 | M0 |
| Stage IIIA | T0 | N2 | M0 |
| | T1 | N2 | M0 |
| | T2 | N2 | M0 |
| | T3 | N1, N2 | M0 |
| Stage IIIB | T4 | Any N | M0 |
| | Any T | N3 | M0 |
| Stage IV | Any T | Any N | M1 |

## AJCC/UICC TNM nomenclature (clinical TNM)

### T: tumour size
- **TX:** primary tumour cannot be assessed.
- **T0:** no evidence of primary tumour.
- **Tis:** *in situ* cancer – DCIS, LCIS, Paget's disease of the nipple (with no associated invasion, or palpable mass).
- **T1:** 2 cm or less in diameter:
  - T1mic: ≤0.1cm;
  - T1a: >0.1–≤0.5cm;
  - T1b: >0.5–≤1cm;
  - T1c: >1–≤2cm.
- **T2:** >2–5 cm in diameter.
- **T3:** more than 5 cm in diameter.
- **T4:** any size with chest wall or skin involvement:
  - T4a: extension to the chest wall (ribs, intercostal, serratus anterior, but not pectoralis muscle);
  - T4b: skin involvement – oedema/peau d'orange, ulceration, ipsilateral satellite skin nodules (skin dimpling, nipple retraction not included);
  - T4c: both T4a and T4b;
  - T4d: inflammatory carcinoma.

### N: lymph nodes (regional)
- **Nx:** regional lymph nodes cannot be assessed (e.g. previous excision and no details).
- **N0:** no lymph node metastases.
- **N1:** mobile metastatic ipsilateral axillary lymph nodes.
- **N2:** fixed or matted ipsilateral axillary lymph nodes or ipsilateral internal mammary nodes* (without axillary involvement):
  - N2a: axillary lymph nodes (fixed or matted);
  - N2b: internal mammary nodes (no axillary involvement).
- **N3:** ipsilateral Infraclavicular or supraclavicular nodes (with or without involved axillary lymph nodes), or ipsilateral internal mammary lymph nodes* with involved ipsilateral axillary lymph nodes:
  - N3a: infraclavicular lymph nodes;
  - N3b: internal mammary with axillary lymph nodes;
  - N3c: supraclavicular lymph nodes.

*By clinical examination or imaging other than scintigraphy

### M: metastasis
- MX: metastasis cannot be assessed.
- M0: no distant metastasis.

### TNM versions
- **cTNM:** clinical (preoperative).
- **pTNM:** pathology.
- **rTNM:** for recurrent tumour.
- **aTNM:** post-autopsy detected cancers.

*pN : lymph node – pathological status*
- *pNx:* axillary nodes cannot be assessed (not available for examination).
- *pN0:* no metastases.
  - (i-): histologically negative and negative IHC;
  - (ii): histologically negative, positive IHC, but IHC cluster >0.2mm.
- *pN0 (mol–):* histologically negative and negative molecular tests – RT-PCR.
- *pN0 (mol+):* histologically negative, positive RT-PCR.
- *pN1:* 1–3 axillary lymph nodes have metastases or internal mammary lymph nodes with microscopic disease detected by sentinel node method, but not clinically apparent.
  - pN1mi: micrometastasis >0.2mm, but <2.0mm;
  - pN1a: metastases in 1–3 axillary lymph nodes;
  - pN1b: internal mammary lymph nodes with microscopic disease detected by sentinel lymph node (SLN) dissection but not clinically apparent;
  - pN1c: metastases in 1–3 axillary lymph nodes and in internal mammary lymph nodes with microscopic disease detected by sentinel node dissection, but not clinically.
- pN2: 4–9 axillary LN or mets in internal mammary LN (clinically evident and axilla clear):
  - pN2a: mets in 4–9 axillary LN;
  - pN2b: internal mammary (clinically evident) LN mets (and no axillary mets).
- pN3: ten or more axillary LN mets (at least 1 mets >2mm) or infraclavicular LN or ipsilateral internal mammary LN (clinically evident) with 1 or more axillary node mets or > 3 axillary LN with clinically negative microscopic metastases in internal mammary lymph nodes, or ipsilateral supraclavicular lymph nodes.
  - pN3a: 10 or more positive axillary LN or positive infraclavicular lymph nodes;
  - pN3b: mets in internal mammary lymph nodes (clinically evident), plus 1 or more positive axillary lymph nodes or internal mammary mets (clinically not evident, but detected by lymphoscintigraphy), plus more than 3 axillary lymph nodes;
  - pN3c: mets in ipsilateral supraclavicular LN. By clinical examination or imaging other than scintigraphy.

When axillary status is based only on sentinel node surgery (not followed by ANC), a further postfix (sn) is added (e.g. pN0 (i+) (sn))

# Prognostic factors

- *Prognostic factors* help provide information on survival and likelihood of recurrence, as well as identify patients requiring adjuvant treatment.
- *Predictive factors* predict likelihood of response to treatment.
- Many of these factors are incorporated in the various staging systems.

## Lymph node metastasis

*Lymph node metastasis:* 10-year survival reduces from an overall 60–75% in node free to 25–30% when metastatic nodes are present. Probably the most significant single prognostic factor.

## Tumour size

*Tumour size:* the rate of lymph nodular and distant metastasis is proportional to size of the primary tumour. (LN positive ~20% at <1cm to ~50% at 3cm).

## Tumour grade/differentiation

*Tumour differentiation:* 10-year survival falls from 85% in well differentiated to 45% in poorly differentiated cancer.

## Steroid receptor status

- ER expression correlates with response to endocrine therapy. ER status has direct relation to survival in the first 5 years.
- ER and PgR receptors are steroid receptors located in the cell nucleus. [Detected by radiolabelled ligand binding or currently by immunohistochemistry (IHC)]. Tumours with moderate/high ER levels and positive PgR expression have an 80% response rate to endocrine therapy and correlates with survival rates in different cancers (section3 p. 88)

## Growth factor receptors

- *HER-2 (erbB2neu):* 15–30% expression in invasive breast cancer and 80% of DCIS, associated with poor prognosis in invasive breast cancer.
- Best detected by FISH.
- When positive, targeted therapy using Trastusumab now available.

## Distant metastasis

Stage IV disease (see section 8).

## Histological type

Tumour type and subtype. (see section 8).

## Lymphovascular invasion

Lymphovascular invasion correlates with lymph nodular involvement and prognosis. However, inter-observer variation exists in its reporting.

## Other serum/molecular markers

- Not in routine use, awaiting more trial data/approval.
- Insulin-like growth factor peptide, S-phase fraction, DNA ploidy, p53mutations (poor prognosis), p27, urokinase plasminogen activator, and inhibitor. Gene expression profiling (see 'Investigations: cytology and histology', p. 96).

# Management of early breast cancer

After confirmation, the diagnosis of breast cancer should be given to the patient sensitively and in an appropriate setting. A named breast specialist nurse or other supportive staff should be available. Treatment planning and decision making may involve multiple clinic visits. All major management decisions should be made in multidisciplinary meeting settings.

Pre-treatment variables that can influence treatment include:
- Age.
- Previous cancers and adjuvant treatments.
- Co-morbidities or other conditions, such as pregnancy, location, and size of tumour.
- Breast size and relative tumour size.
- Axillary status.
- Distant disease.
- Type and grade of tumour.
- Receptor status.
- Possibility of post-operative radiotherapy.

*Key questions for decision making:*
- Is neo-adjuvant treatment (e.g. chemotherapy, endocrine treatment) indicated?
- Primary surgery or primary endocrine treatment?
- Which surgical procedure:
  - breast: BCS or mastectomy;
  - axilla: no surgery, sentinel node or clearance?
- Is reconstruction to accompany primary surgery?
- Post-surgery: what adjuvant treatment? (chemotherapy, trastusumab, endocrine treatments, radiotherapy).

The various management modalities and aspects are outlined below. For further details refer to the appropriate sections that follow and see the general management algorithm for breast cancer (Fig. 2.5).

## Neo adjuvant chemo/endocrine therapy

*Benefits*
- To down-size tumours allowing breast conserving surgery (BCS).
- To render inoperable locally advanced tumours operable.
- Response to a particular modality/drugs can be assessed (which is not normally possible after resection) and can direct post-operative use.

## Primary endocrine therapy

When surgery is contraindicated, hormone receptor positive tumours can often be kept in abeyance for long periods with endocrine therapy.

## Breast conserving surgery

Primary or following neo-adjuvant treatment to downsize. Larger tumours or masses in difficult locations can still undergo BCS by judicious use of volume displacement or replacement oncoplastic techniques (see 'Reconstruction in breast conserving surgery', p. 132). All BCS for invasive cancer must be followed by RT.

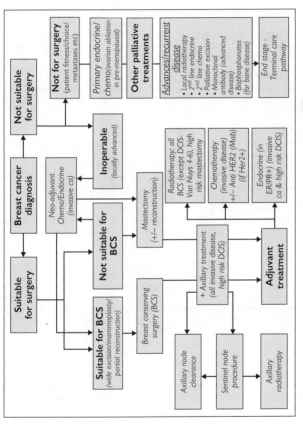

**Fig. 2.5** Principles of breast management.

### Mastectomy

Removal of the whole breast (see 'Mastectomy', p. 126). Expertise for reconstruction should be available and discussed in all cases.

### Post-mastectomy reconstruction

- *Using myocutaneous flaps:* e.g.: latissimus dorsi (LD), free or pedicled transverse rectus abdominis myocutaneous (TRAM), free deep inferior epigastric perforator (DIEP), free superficial inferior epigastric artery (SIEA) flaps. Less common are rubens, gluteal, thigh and omental flaps.
- Implant based reconstruction or flap + implant

### Axillary clearance (ANC)

All invasive cancers must have their axilla staged. Routine axillary node clearance has many side effects and may be over treatment in 50–70% cases.

### Sentinel node biopsy (SNB)

Avoids some of the complications of ANC. Removal of one or more representative LN using blue dye and radiolabelled tracer will accurately predict the status of the axilla. If positive, treat further by ANC or axillary radiotherapy. SNB and sampling are generally not indicated in DCIS except probably in high risk cases (e.g. high grade, large tumours).

### Axillary sampling

Removal of a four node sample from the axilla can also accurately predict axillary status. Blue dye or radiotracer can be used to direct this sampling. Further treatment as in SNB.

### Adjuvant radiotherapy

- *All BCS for invasive cancers, DCIS (Van Nuys 7-9):* breast radiotherapy (RT) and tumour bed boost. Supra-clavicular RT when ≥4+ nodes
- *Post-mastectomy radiotherapy:* (chest wall and supraclavicular) Indications – >5cm tumour size, ≥4 node positivity, and margin involvement (usually deep). (Other factors – tumour grade 3, lymphovascular invasion positive and younger age.)

### Adjuvant chemotherapy

Post-surgical poly-chemotherapy reduces relapse by 5–15% (absolute risk reduction). Probable indications – node positive, receptor negative, young age, lymphovascular invasion, large tumour size, higher grade (2,3).

### Adjuvant endocrine therapy

Tamoxifen or AI (post-menopausal) when steroid receptor positive.

### Newer drugs – monoclonal antibody therapy

Trastuzumab is used with in HER-2 positive tumours in conjunction with chemotherapy. Cardiotoxic.

## Patient support

Breast care nurse services, information sources, psychological support, and support from patient groups should be available throughout the patients' journey through cancer treatment.

## Follow-up

Generally, follow-up is continued for 5–10 years with clinical examination and yearly mammography. Look for local recurrence, contralateral disease, metastasis, and treatment-related complications (see 'Post-treatment follow-up and surveillance', p. 150)

### Menopause definition for AI use (based on NCCN, 2008)

- Profound and permanent decrease in ovarian oestrogen synthesis.
- Prior bilateral oophorectomy.
- Age ≥60 years.
- Age <60 years + amenorrhoea ≥12months (in the absence of chemotherapy/anti-oestrogen/ovarian suppression).
- Age <60 years + anti-oestrogen/ovarian suppression (FSH) and oestradiol in post-menopausal range. Post-chemotherapy – serial estimation (FSH + oestradiol). Not reliable on LH–RH agonist/antagonist therapy.

## Further reading

NCCN (2009) (breast):
http://www.nccn.org/professionals/physician_gls/PDF/breast.pdf

# Surgical anatomy: breast and axilla

**Breast**

- A modified apocrine sweat gland. Breast volume varies from person to person, but base area remains reasonably constant – almost circular with a vertical extent – 2nd to 6th rib in the mid-clavicular line and transverse extent – overlies the pectoralis major from just lateral to the midline across the muscle and extends on to overlie part of the serratus anterior and external oblique inferiorly. An axillary tail (of Spence) extends from the upper outer aspect of the gland entering the axillary space. There may be asymmetry between either side.
- Male breast and female pre-pubertal breast are similar. The areola is fully formed and glandular breast tissue does not normally extend beyond the areolar margins. Nipple is small.
- *Structural anatomy – ductoglandular tissue:* 15 major ducts radiating out from the nipple and branching several times before ending in individual lobules. The breast gland is cushioned within subcutaneous fat of the anterior chest wall. A layer of fat of variable thickness is found between the breast and the skin. There is an inconsistent filamentous whitish areolar layer (more evident in the upper hemisphere), which may serve to define the plane of dissection for the mastectomy flap. There is no subcutaneous fat beneath the nipple and areola. On the deep aspect, a condensation of fascia (continuation of Scarpa's fascia) defines the posterior capsule of the breast. Deep to this is the pectoralis fascia (deep fascia overlying pectoralis major). The space between these two fasciae is relatively bloodless, and serves as the deep dissection plane and pocket for sub-mammary prostheses. Coopers ligaments– fibrous tissue strands running from the sub-mammary deep fascia through the breast inserting into the skin, provides natural support and shape to the breast. Contraction of these fibres results in the skin puckering associated with some breast cancers. Laxity in later life results in breast ptosis (Fig. 2.6).
- **Blood supply**:
  - lateral thoracic artery (branch of 2nd part of axillary a) – travels along the inferior border of the pectoralis minor and travels anteriorly around the lateral edge of pectoralis major branching to supply the breast;
  - thoraco-acromial artery (branch of 2nd part of axillary a) – pierces the clavipectoral fascia to divide into 4 branches – pectoral branch supplies the upper breast;
  - internal mammary artery (branch of 1st part of subclavian artery) – branches pass through inter-costal spaces (2 and 3 are the largest) to supply the medial breast;
  - smaller contributions from branches of the intercostal arteries and underlying muscular arteries; veins follow the arteries.
- **Innervation:** anterior and lateral cutaneous branches of the corresponding intercostal nerves (2–6). Nipple T4 spinal dermatome.
- **Lymphatic drainage:** majority (75–97%) of drainage from the breast parenchyma occurs primarily into the axilla flowing mainly flowing via the subareolar, subdermal, subcutaneous, submammary or parenchymal

lymphatic channels. A portion of the drainage occurs into the internal mammary nodes also. Less common pathways include passage into the supra- and infraclavicular nodes, cervical nodes, opposite breast, and peritoneal cavity via the rectus sheath. Experimental studies have shown that drainage first occurs into an identifiable single node in the axilla and is the basis of sentinel node sampling surgery. Additionally, in an individual, the same lymph node acts as the sentinel node, irrespective of the site/quadrant within the breast in >90% of cases.

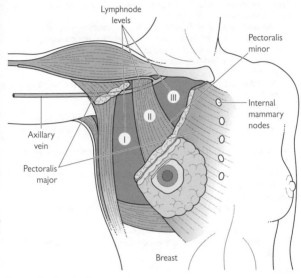

**Fig. 2.6** Breast and axilla: anatomy.

## Axilla

- Forms an oblique pyramidal space. The base is formed by the axillary fascia – deep fascial continuation of the clavipectoral fascia. The anterior wall comprises the pectoralis muscles and clavipectoral fascia, while the posterior wall comprises the teres major and subscapularis, and part of the tendon of latissimus dorsi. The medial wall is the lateral chest wall and overlying serratus anterior muscle up to the 4th rib. The anterior and lateral walls form an edge at the medial border of the humerus. The apex opens into the posterior triangle of the neck.
- **Contents:** loose areolar fat, lymphatics, lymph nodes (variable number, 10–50), neurovascular structures.
- **Lymph node groups:** in modern oncological breast surgery, and with the advent of lymphatic mapping and sentinel node surgery, this separation is less relevant. Anatomically the groups are:
  - apical – at the highest point of the axilla closely related to the axillary vein;
  - central or medial – nodes on the chest wall side of the axilla;
  - pectoral or anterior – along the lateral border of the pectoralis minor.(draining the breast mainly);
  - subscapular or posterior – posterior wall of the axilla along the border of the subscapularis in the posterior axillary fold (draining the posterior shoulder);
  - humeral or lateral – lateral wall around and behind the axillary vein (drains the arm);
  - inter pectoral or Rotter's nodes – between the pectoralis major and minor muscles.
- **Lymph node levels:**
  - I – all axillary nodes lateral to the lateral border of the pectoralis minor;
  - II – nodes posterior to the pectoralis minor;
  - III – apical nodes medial to the medial border of the pectoralis (Fig. 4.7).

## Nerves

- **Long thoracic nerve (nerve of Bell):** medial wall of the axilla along the lateral thoracic wall overlying and innervating the serratus anterior muscle; division results in winging of the scapula.
- **Thoracodorsal nerve (nerve to latissimus dorsi):** enters the axilla posterior to the axillary vein crossing the axilla laterally to travel along the medial border of the latissimus dorsi muscle along with the thoracodorsal vessels. Division leads to loss of latissimus dorsi function- the 'climbing' muscle.
- **Medial pectoral nerve:** curving around the lateral border of pectoralis minor muscle along with the vascular bundle (innervates the pectoralis major). [Note that the medial pectoral nerve is 'laterally' located.]
- The above 3 nerves should be preserved during axillary dissection. Intercosto-brachial nerves- sensory nerves passing out from the intercostal space, traversing the axilla to innervate the skin of the medial upper arm and adjacent chest wall. Division may be inevitable in axillary dissection resulting in cutaneous anaesthesia/chronic pain. Sentinel node procedure reduces this complication.

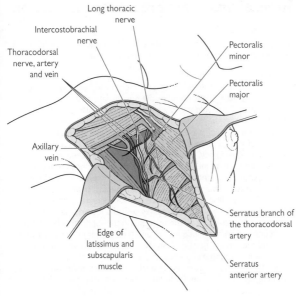

**Fig. 2.7** Axillary dissection anatomy.

# Surgical anatomy: breast reconstruction

## Myocutaneous flap

A flap consisting of vascularised muscle with a paddle of overlying skin kept viable by perforating musculocutaneous vessels.

## Latissimus dorsi muscle

- Largest muscle in the body with a wide origin and narrow insertion. Size around 20 × 40cm. Overlies the posterolateral thorax. Powerful adductor of the shoulder and a climbing muscle. Also extends and medially rotates the humerus.
- The latissimus dorsi is a very versatile muscle, and can be used as muscle or myocutaneous or osteo-myocutaneous flap for breast, as well as head and neck, and axial reconstructive procedures.
- *Extent and origin:* medially originates from the spinous process and supraspinous ligaments of the lower thoracic (from the 7th), lumbar and sacral vertebrae, and inferiorly from the posterior third of the outer lip of the iliac crest. The inferomedial corner is aponeurotic. Superior border is horizontal, passes over the lower pole of the scapula, and is overlaid by the trapezius in the superomedial corner. The lateral border is oblique first, and then travels up vertically winding around the teres major becoming tendinous and gaining insertion into the intertubercular groove of the humerus. At the level of the 10/11th rib there is a firm thick attachment to the underlying serratus muscle that needs to be divided to prevent detachment of the serratus anterior along with latissimus dorsi elevation. Muscular fibres also attach to the lower four ribs.
- *Innervation:* thoracodorsal nerve (branch of the posterior cord of brachial plexus). It enters and traverses the axilla to lie on the inside (medial) aspect of the anterior border of the distal part of the latissimus dorsi and entering it.
- *Vascular supply:* thoracodorsal artery (branch of the subscapular artery in turn a branch of the 3rd part of the axillary artery) measures 1.5–3mm in diameter traverses the axilla and continues alongside the nerve giving off a serratus branch anteriorly before entering the inner/medial aspect of the muscle (about 10cm below the axillary artery), then dividing into lateral and transverse branches. Perforating branches from the posterior intercostal and lumbar arteries compliment the blood supply. The serratus branch is able to support the muscle by flow reversal in cases where the main trunk is interrupted (Fig. 2.15 Thoracodorsal pedicle ).

## Transverse rectus abdominis myocutaneous (TRAM) flap

- The superiorly based pedicled TRAM flap is a myocutaneous transposition flap based on the rectus abdominis muscle with a transverse skin paddle overlying it. (see Fig. 2.8 and Fig. 17.03 ).
- Vascularity is based on the superior epigastric artery. The normal blood supply to this skin and fat paddle in the lower abdomen comes from the deep inferior epigastric artery (main), as well as the superior epigastric artery and the intercostal arteries.

- Loss of abdominal wall strength is inevitable and has led to the development of an inferiorly-based muscle sparing free TRAM/DIEP/DIEA flap with a similar skin and fat paddle. Based on the proximity of the tissues to the muscle or vascular pedicle, the flap can be divided into 4 zones in decreasing levels of predicted survival allowing the safe use of the appropriate tissue areas in the reconstruction
- For the free flap technique the recipient vessel for microvascular anastomosis is either the thoracodorsal artery and vein (above the serratus branch) or the internal mammary vessels (usually exposed deep to the 3rd costal cartilage; see Fig. 2.8).

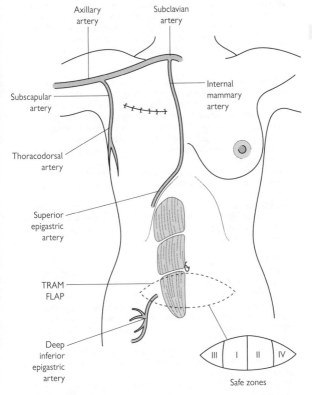

**Fig. 2.8** TRAM/DIEP flap: basic anatomy.

# Breast conserving surgery

Radical mastectomy was popularized by Halsted in the 1890s and its modifications remained the procedure of choice for all breast cancers into the latter part of the last century, until the advent of breast conserving procedures. Over 40–60% of breast cancers are now being treated with breast conservation and mastectomy rates are falling worldwide.

Several randomized controlled trials [e.g. NSABP B-06 (1976), Milan trial (1973), Danish Trial DBCCG (1983), EORTC 10801 (1980), NCI (1979)] have shown that **survival** is identical after breast conservation and mastectomy (>25 years survival data) in early invasive breast cancer. However, breast conserving procedures are associated with higher ipsilateral local recurrence rates, which may have an overall survival implication. To counter this, the conserved breast should receive **post-operative radiotherapy** (45–50Gy) breast +/– local tumour bed boost (reduces local recurrence by 40–75%) along with the usual **adjuvant systemic treatment**.

## Types of procedures

- **Wide local excision** is the primary procedure combining tumour excision with adequate margins maintaining the cosmetic integrity of the breast. Variations/synonyms (see Fig: 2.9) include partial mastectomy, segmentectomy (excision using a wedge/segment of breast parenchyma in a radial fashion from the centre of the breast ), quadrantectomy (similar to segmentectomy but including the overlying skin).
- **Therapeutic mammoplasty** (see 'Reconstruction in breast conserving surgery' p. 132).
- Wide excision combined with **volume replacement** (partial flap reconstruction) or **local volume displacement** techniques (see chapter #).
- **Impalpable tumours:** localization of the tumour may be aided by preoperative placement of guidewires, or ultrasound skin marking or intralesional radioisotope injection (ROLL – radioisotope guided occult lesion localization).

## Indications

- Usually, for single tumours up to 3–4cm in size when conservation surgery will not result in unacceptable cosmetic morbidity. Size relative to natural breast volume (usually up to 5–15%) and location within the breast are, however, more important than absolute tumour diameter.
- Some would consider a centrally located tumour a contraindication, although a central wide local excision is feasible with or without a mammoplasty technique for reconstruction.
- When relative size is large and precludes conservation, neo-adjuvant treatment (chemotherapy/endocrine) can be used to downstage and downsize the tumour to enable conservation.
- All decisions must be made in a multi disciplinary setting, taking into consideration the patients views after counselling regarding cosmesis and oncological implications.

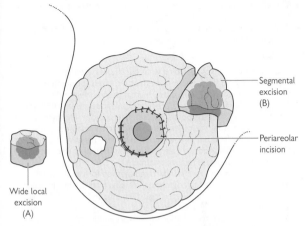

**Fig. 2.9** Breast local excision: (A) wide local excision and (B) segmental excision.

## Contraindications

- *General contra-indications to breast conservation surgery:* large relative size of tumour and predicted poor cosmetic outcome, multifocal disease (unless tumours are very close to each other and adequate clearance can be obtained), extensive *in situ* component/microcalcification. Locally advanced/infiltrative disease and distant metastasis.
- *Contraindication to local radiotherapy* (heart and lung disease, connective tissue disease): previous radiotherapy (moderate–high dose). Initial trimesters of pregnancy (due to potential delay of radiotherapy).
- *Patient preference for mastectomy:* patients with high-risk family history or genetics may prefer mastectomy for risk reduction.

### Pre-operative

Counselling, MDT discussion, consent, side/incision marking. Pre-operative guidewire insertion, US marking.

## INCISION

Avoid upper hemispheric (especially medial) skin incisions for obvious cosmetic reasons. A circum-areolar incision should allow access to all regions of the breast. Other acceptable incision sites are infra mammary crease, lateral vertical, axillary incisions (Fig. 2.10). In unavoidable circumstances, when the above incisions are not possible, place the incision along skin tension lines.

### Excision

- Skin flaps are first raised and excision with adequate margin is aided by palpating the tumour through the breast parenchyma avoiding direct contact with the tumour at all times. In non-palpable tumours, the guidewire or ultrasound will direct localization.

- The excision should be orientated and labelled (radio-opaque markers for specimen X-ray +/− suture tags for pathologist.
- Post-excision specimen X-rays prior to wound closure will reveal necessity for further excision/shave.

**Margins**

- There is no consensus regarding what constitutes adequate margins. A positive margin (i.e. tumour present at the inked specimen margin) warrants further excision. A 'close' margin (tumour within 1 or 2 mm of the inked surface) may be a predictor of residual disease with varying estimates (0-30%) of the possibility of finding tumour if further excision were carried out. At the other end of the spectrum some would advocate using 5-10mm or even more to achieve negative margins. For DCIS the Van Nuys scoring (see section 8, p. 104) takes into account margin width to dictate further treatment.
- Pathologists must follow a standardized method for reporting on margins. Margin width at geographical margins (radial, superior, inferior, medial, lateral, nipple-end, superficial, deep etc) and type of disease at/close to margin should be reported.
- A balance has to be struck between cosmesis and oncologic safety in establishing the criteria for adequate margin width and advocating further excision, mastectomy or controlling disease with local radiotherapy.
- Factors which may predict residual disease or local recurrence are younger age, features of aggressive disease, extensive in situ component, lobular carcinoma, proximity to excised margins and area of tumour exposed or close to the resection margins.
- Normally the width of the deep and superficial margins are of no concern, providing the excision is carried out to the anterior and posterior capsule of the breast and no gross disease was seen infiltrating superficially into the skin or deeply into muscle or chest wall.

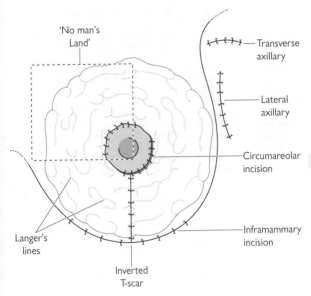

**Fig. 2.10** Breast: common cosmetic incisions.

### Closure
- Meticulous haemostasis is mandatory as breast tissues do not tamponade well. Avoid drains if possible.
- Best cosmetic results are obtained if breast parenchymal flaps (pillars) can be safely mobilized and approximated to close the excision defect beneath the skin. Failure to close the defect may lead to significant distortion especially in lower polar tumours.

### Complications
Bleeding, infection, positive margins (requiring further excision/mastectomy), scarring, deformity, recurrence.

### Post-operative
- To ensure that a mammographically detected DCIS is completely excised after BCS – a post-procedure ipsilateral mammography can ensure completeness in the absence of any mammographic lesions. Alternatively specimen X-rays along with histology can provide evidence of complete excision.
- If margins are inadequate or disease is extensive a further wide excision or mastectomy may be needed. Positive margins or residual disease after complex volume displacement techniques can be salvaged only by mastectomy in most cases. Patients should be pre-operatively counselled regarding this possibility.

- Adjuvant radiotherapy to breast: Following BCS in invasive disease and high risk DCIS (Van Nuys score 7–9)
- **Endocrine treatment:** post-operative tamoxifen or AI in steroid receptor-positive cancers reduces recurrence by 40–60%. Strong evidence for tamoxifen after BCS and RT in DCIS.
- **Following neo-adjuvant chemotherapy:** no role for post-operative chemotherapy unless the full course of chemotherapy was not completed pre-operatively.
- Delayed cosmetic deformity especially in post-radiation cases may necessitate corrective surgery later.
- **Follow-up:** clinical and mammographic surveillance to detect recurrences is generally continued for 5 years or more (DCIS – clinical examination 6–12-monthly × 5 years, then annually, mammogram annually – NCCN 2008) Longer follow-up in higher risk cases. Following BCS +RT ~1% recurrence rate per year.

# Mastectomy

Types of mastectomy

- *Mastectomy:* complete excision of the breast, including the nipple and areola along with a variable amount of surrounding skin to leave a flat mastectomy bed and scar, allowing comfortable placement of an external prosthesis.
- *Skin sparing mastectomy:* mastectomy with preservation of the whole skin envelope except the nipple and areola. *Types:* circum-areolar, circum-areolar with lateral extension (when areolar diameter is small) and reduction pattern (for large ptotic breasts; see Fig 2.11).
- Nipple areola preserving mastectomy.
- More radical procedures are historical in early breast cancer:
  - radical mastectomy – mastectomy with excision of the pectoralis major and minor with axillary clearance;
  - modified radical mastectomy – preserving the pectoralis major- and its variations;
  - Patey's mastectomy (level 3 axillary clearance resecting the pectoralis minor);
  - Scanlon's procedure (dividing the pectoralis minor insertion preserving the muscle and the medial pectoral nerve);
  - Auchincloss method (ANC with retraction of the pectoralis minor, preserving it completely) continues to be used today.

Indications

- *Early breast cancer:* large relative size of tumour and predicted poor cosmetic outcome for BCS, multifocal disease, extensive *in situ* disease/micro-calcifications, contraindications for local radiotherapy (heart and lung disease, connective tissue disease) precluding BCS, high risk DCIS (Van Nuy's score 9–12), positive margins after 2 or more wide excisions, or following complex flap displacement reconstruction after BCS. Patient preference for mastectomy at the outset.
- *Advanced disease:* locally advanced/infiltrative disease. Local recurrence.
- Patients with **high-risk,** e.g. family history or gene mutations (risk reducing mastectomy; see 'Management of breast cancer risk', p. 164).

Medical contraindications to surgery

- Elderly frail patients' where a hormone responsive tumour can be kept in abeyance by endocrine therapy.
- Widespread disease in near-terminal patients.
- When expected survival is shorter than expected loss of local control.

Pre-operative

- Counselling, MDT discussion, consent, side/incision marking.
- All patients undergoing mastectomy must be offered a choice of reconstruction (NICE – UK guidelines).

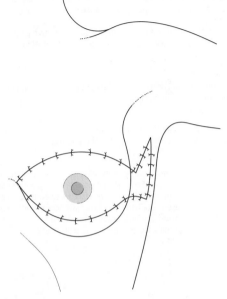

**Fig. 2.11** Simple mastectomy with lateral 'fish tail' extension (to remove redundant lateral skin flap).

## Procedure

- Supine position/arm in extension (GA).
- **Incision:** transverse elliptical incision (Fig. 2.11) including nipple and areola as well as previous excision/biopsy sites. Lateral extensions (see Fig. 14.2) – 'fish tail', 'hockey stick', may be added to minimize a fatty lateral fold and dog ear.
- Skin flaps are raised passing through the dissection plane (see Surgical anatomy: breast and axilla', p. 114) to reach the pectoralis fascia above the superior limit of the breast and inferiorly to the infra-mammary crease. The breast is now lifted off the pectoralis and chest wall muscles by dissecting through the sub mammary plane. Medially avoid reaching the midline when raising the flap. The 2nd and 3rd internal mammary perforators are large vessels and must be controlled carefully to avoid post-operative haemorrhage. If there is extension into pectoralis muscle a portion of the muscle may be shaved/excised along with the breast.
- Additional axillary procedures as indicated.
- Meticulous haemostasis is necessary.
- Suctions drains are usually placed in the breast bed and axilla to allow apposition of the flap to the breast bed and control seroma formation.
- **Closure:** in 2–3 layers with absorbable sutures. The wound may be sealed with glue, adhesive strips, or clear occlusive dressings to allow inspection.

- Adequate skin excision will result in a moderately tight flap and will produce an even bed for the successful use of an external mammary prosthesis.
- Local anaesthetic infiltration to mitigate post-operative pain (this is sometimes unnecessary as the extensive flap mobilization often results in sensory loss).

### Complications

Bleeding, seroma, infection, wound disruption, anaesthesia, chronic pain, decreased shoulder mobility, poor cosmesis, keloid/hypertrophic scar, recurrence.

### Immediate post-operative period

Drain and wound surveillance, shoulder physiotherapy.

### Post-mastectomy management

- *Post-mastectomy radiotherapy* (high risk cases – loco-regional risk >20%): main indications - >5cm tumour size, ≥4 node positivity and margin involvement (usually deep). Other factors to consider are tumour grade (grade 3) presence of lymphovascular invasion and younger age.
- Adjuvant hormone and chemotherapy as indicated.
- Mammographic surveillance of the contralateral breast.

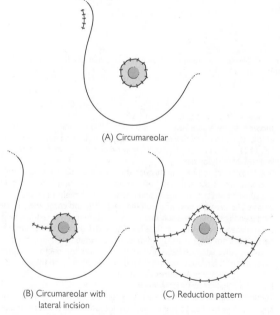

(A) Circumareolar

(B) Circumareolar with lateral incision

(C) Reduction pattern

**Fig. 2.12** Skin sparing mastectomy (types/incisions).

**Axillary surgery**

- Axillary nodal clearance (ANC) has been the gold standard for the primary management of the axilla in all cases of invasive breast cancer up to the late nineties. Axillary surgery allows loco-regional control and provides powerful prognostic data directing adjuvant therapy.
- However, a full axillary clearance results in considerable morbidity, including chronic lymph oedema (5–25%), nerve injuries, shoulder dysmobility (5–15%) among others. Moreover, the axilla may not contain positive nodes in 50–70% (~50% symptomatic and 80% screening) of cases making routine axillary clearance an over treatment.
- Sentinel node biopsy (SNB/SLNB; removing a representative LN from the axilla localized by injection of radiotracer and/or blue dye) and/or axillary sampling (removing a 4-node sample from the lower axilla with or without dye injection) avoids the morbidity of routine ANC and helps predict the status of the axilla. If the sentinel/sample node is positive the axilla is treated by clearance or radiotherapy. SNB technique has been validated by several studies and is over 90–95% accurate in predicting the status of the axilla.
- SLNB and axillary sampling may be undertaken as a stand alone procedure or combined with BCS or mastectomy.

**Sentinel lymph node biopsy (SLNB/SNB)**

- Indications: All invasive breast cancers (including micro-invasive). Relative indication- high risk DCIS (large/extensive tumour e.g.>5cm, high grade disease, palpable DCIS). As a stand alone procedure prior to commencement of neo-adjuvant chemotherapy. (as neo-adjuvant treatment may decrease the accuracy of later SNB)
- **Contraindication:** dye allergy, pregnancy, locally advanced cancer. Relative contraindication: previous axillary surgery, post-neo-adjuvant chemotherapy. Axilla already proved positive (e.g. by USS and FNA). Routine axillary USS +/− FNA will reduce number of unnecessary SNB.
- **Preparation:** counselling, MDT-based decision, consent, same day or previous day admission for radiotracer injection
- Radiolabelled dye: can be performed in accredited institutions (protocol for radioisotope handling should be in place). The radio tracer (e.g. 2mL of $^{99m}$Tc colloid albumin is injected peritumorally the day prior (40MBq) or the same day (20MBq), and imaged (2–3h later) with a gamma camera. The sentinel node location is marked on the skin.
- **Blue dye injection:** immediately before the start of the procedure 1.5–2mL of blue dye (Patent V blue, methylthioninium chloride (methylene blue), or isosulfan blue) is injected either peritumorally or peri-areolarly in the subcutaneous or subdermal plane followed by 5–10min of massage.
- **Procedure:** the scintigraphy pictures are displayed. A small transverse or vertical or skin crease incision is made as directed by the skin marking and gamma probe signal is made and deepened to pass through the axillary fascia. Using the hand held gamma probe the dissection is continued to the sentinel node. Blue-stained lymphatics may be traced to the sentinel node and the blue-stained node itself may be visible through the axillary fat. (~1–4 nodes are removed).
- The nodes are sent for routine histology (standardized protocol) including IHC (full significance of IHC only positive axilla not known).

Frozen section/imprint cytology may be used to determine axillary status per-operatively, proceeding to ANC accordingly.

- **Internal mammary nodes SNB:** no clear recommendation or evidence of benefit. Some centres routinely biopsy IMN if scintigraphy reveals drainage. (IMNs show up only when tracer injection is peri-tumoural)
- **Complications:** all the complications of ANC can occur, although considerably reduced. Lymphoedema – up to 6%. Blue dye reaction can occur in 0.5–1%. False negative rate – 2–15% (all techniques).

## Axillary sampling

- Small axillary incision is made to remove 4 lymph nodes in the lower axilla. This may be aided by blue dye and or radioisotope injection.

## Axillary node clearance (ANC)

### Indications

- Positive axilla proved by USS/FNAC or SNB assessment.
- SNB contraindicated (e.g. pregnancy) or when no sentinel node was identified at SNB procedure.
- Post-chemotherapy when SNB was not undertaken prior to neo-adjuvant chemotherapy.

### Relative contraindications

- Elderly patients (or severe co-morbidities) with good prognosis tumours where axillary status will not influence adjuvant treatment/prognosis. Local factors – previous axillary RT/complicated surgery, which may result in poor yield/unacceptably high complications.
- Transverse or vertical axillary incision. Deepen to reach the axillary fascia first identifying the lateral border of the pectoralis major which is the anterior limit of the excision. (Posteriorly the anterior border of latissimus dorsi serves as the posterior border of the ANC.)
- Dissection is continued posteriorly to the level of the pectoralis minor preserving the medial pectoral nerve and lateral thoracic vessels. The muscle is retracted and dissection continued posteriorly over the serratus fascia preserving the long thoracic nerve to reach the subscapularis muscle.
- Dissect carefully superiorly to identify the axillary vein. Keep to the inferior aspect of the vein sweeping the axillary contents down. Control the vessels taking care to identify, and preserve the thoracodorsal vessels and nerve.
- At the posterior aspect sweep the axillary tissue laterally preserving the thoracodorsal pedicle to reach the anterior border of the latissimus.
- Superiorly proceed toward the apex keeping below the axillary vein to complete a level II or III dissection. (See 'Surgical anatomy: breast and axilla', p. 114.) A full level 3 dissection is avoided unless there is gross disease extending into level 2. The apex of the specimen may be marked with a stitch.
- **Closure:** meticulous haemostasis, suction drain.
- **Complications:** seroma, lymphoedema (5–25%), nerve damage (sensory – intercostobrachial nerve, motor – long thoracic (climbing/

adduction), long thoracic nerve to serratus anterior (scapular winging), brachial plexus, shoulder stiffness. Angiosarcoma may develop within chronic lymphoedema.
- Axillary radiotherapy should be avoided after ANC due to the unacceptably high incidence of chronic lymphoedema (~40%).

# Reconstruction in breast conserving surgery

## Principles of reconstruction in BCS

- Smaller tumours (5–15% of breast volume) can be excised with minimal cosmetic deformity. Larger tumours can still be amenable to BCS by either using neo-adjuvant therapy to reduce tumour volume or using volume replacement techniques. Upper medial quadrant and lower pole locations – result in higher rate of cosmetic defects.
- The resultant defect can be compensated by volume displacement (mobilizing local breast tissue/flap) or by volume replacement techniques.
- A further alternative in a large breasted woman would be to excise the tumour by breast reduction techniques, combined with symmetrization surgery contralaterally.
- It is also important to consider the possible effects of the inevitable radiotherapy treatment on the proposed oncoplastic procedure following breast conservation. Additionally, the patient must be warned of the possibility of mastectomy if the primary excision is inadequate, especially if a complex volume displacement has been undertaken.

## Volume displacement techniques

The simplest procedure is mobilizing tissue on either side of the defect and closing the dead space. This will often require wide skin (subcutaneous plane) and breast flap (sub mammary plane) mobilization, whilst not compromising flap viability.

## Mammoplasty

Inferior pedicle type procedure to tackle upper breast tumours and superior pedicle based for lower tumours (see Figs 2.13 and 2.14). For example, Wise pattern, vertical technique/Lejour, Grisotti advancement/B-technique and modifications (for central tumours), Benelli round block technique While mobilizing flaps, for aesthetic reasons the nipple areola complex should remain inferolateral to the upper medial quadrant (16cm below the sternal notch and 7cm lateral to the midline) - 'No mans land'.

## Volume replacement techniques

Partial flap-based procedure - latissimus dorsi, rectus abdominis, and omentum. A sub-pectoral implant can be used to augment the volume loss, but will be subject to the side effects of the radiotherapy following breast conservation.

## Correctional surgery

Following BCS around 10–20% of patients may end up with cosmetic deformities (Type 1 – some skin and breast parenchymal defect, Type 2 – severe skin and parenchymal defect, and some associated nipple areolar distortion, Type 3 – significant skin, parenchymal and nipple areolar defects).

Minor defects – corrected by local techniques. Major defects – will require autologous flap based reconstruction.

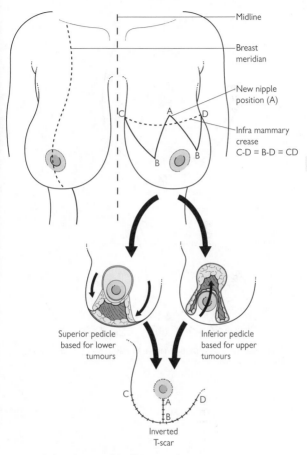

**Fig. 2.13** Reduction mammoplasty (Wise pattern).

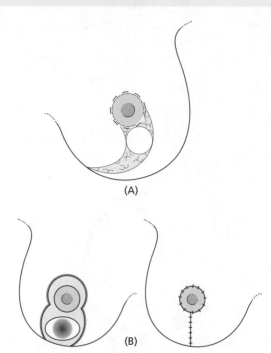

**Fig. 2.14** Other techniques: (A) B-technique for central breast excisions/defects.
(B) Vertical scar mammoplasty.

# Post-mastectomy reconstruction

**Principles of total breast reconstruction**

- **3 types:** (1) implant only; (2) myocutaneous/fasciocutaneous (skin + fat)/muscular-facial flap based on a vascular pedicle; (3) flap + implant.
- **Immediate or delayed reconstruction:** in immediate reconstruction – native skin is preserved – better cosmesis. Also psychological benefits, reduced number of operations and hospital stay. However, possibility of post-mastectomy radiation and its effects on the flap must be considered. Another alternative is to use an implant as a spacer initially, preserving the skin followed by delayed reconstruction after radiotherapy. A further factor is axillary surgery – treatment must be complete before flap reconstruction – as later return to axilla may not be possible/may affect flap. Delayed reconstruction, generally 3–6 months or later after completion of adjuvant chemotherapy/radiotherapy.
- **Flap based:** myocutaneous (e.g. latissimus dorsi, rectus abdominis) pedicled or free flap. Flaps provide additional skin. Generally, flaps may lose up to 20% of volume over time. Volume loss and distortion may be accelerated by radiotherapy.
- **Autologous flap or implant augmented flap:** autologous flaps (no implant) achieve and maintain natural ptosis (also mirror changes in body weight and ageing) and texture, and generally tolerate radiotherapy better. An autologous flap may not be possible in every case as quantity of donor site tissue is variable. Abdominal wall flaps generally yield higher donor site volumes.
- **Perforator flaps:** based on perforator vessels, conserving muscle.
- **Relative contraindications:** smoking, presence of vasculopathy/collagen disease, radiotherapy increase risk of flap complications/loss. Previous abdominal surgery may preclude the use of abdominal flaps.
- **Complications/adverse effects:** decreased shoulder strength, mobility. Abdominal wall hernias, flap/skin loss, donor site morbidity (seroma, wound breakdown, infection).

**Latissimus dorsi myocutaneous flap reconstruction (LD flap)**

- Main workhorse for breast reconstruction, very robust.
- Latissimus dorsi muscle, and overlying fat and skin paddle is dissected out (see 'Surgical anatomy: breast reconstruction', p. 118) and rotated anteriorly around the chest wall after undermining the skin to overlie the mastectomy bed.
- To improve flap mobility the tendon insertion may be divided.
- The flap may be used alone (autologous/extended LD reconstruction) or supplemented with an implant. An autologous flap will tolerate post-operative radiotherapy better. Marking and technique (see Fig. 2.15).

## Pedicled and free **TRAM flap** (see Fig 2.16)

- Abdominal wall is weakened by loss of rectus muscle.
- Previous abdominal surgery precludes the use of this flap
- TRAM flap yields higher volume of tissue. Further advantage – patient will benefit from an abdominoplasty.

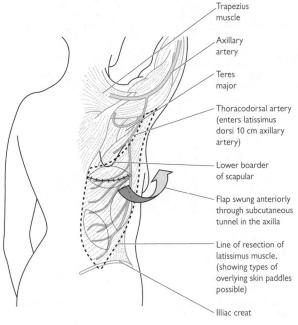

Trapezius muscle

Axillary artery

Teres major

Thoracodorsal artery (enters latissimus dorsi 10 cm axillary artery)

Lower boarder of scapular

Flap swung anteriorly through subcutaneous tunnel in the axilla

Line of resection of latissimus muscle, (showing types of overlying skin paddles possible)

Illiac creat

**Fig. 2.15** Latissimus dorsi flap.

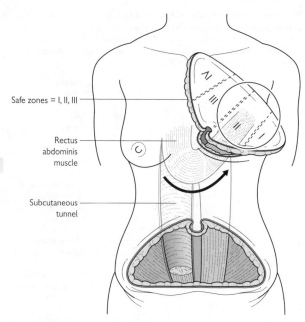

Safe zones = I, II, III

Rectus abdominis muscle

Subcutaneous tunnel

**Fig. 2.16** TRAM flap.

**Free deep inferior epigastric perforator (DIEP) flap (without rectus)**

- Micro-vascular anastomosis to the internal mammary artery and vein, or thoracodorsal vessels.
- Avoids the donor site morbidity of a weakened abdominal wall.

**Other flaps**

Free superficial inferior epigastric artery (SIEA) flap, gluteal (see Fig. 2.17) [superior and inferior gluteal artery perforator (GAP)], thoracodorsal artery perforator (TAP), thigh, rubens, TUG and omental flaps.

**Implant reconstruction**

- *Types:* round or anatomic shaped, smooth or textured, single or dual chambered (gel/saline, Becker, e.g. 35:65, 50:50, or 25:75), and saline, silicone gel, or combination filled. Implant only or flap with implant procedures. The silicone implant consists of a shell (silicone elastomer rubber-like silicone) and silicone gel content [silicone oil + cross-linked cohesive silicone (20% in standard and 60% in cohesive implants)].
- Concerns over silicone implants in the early nineties led to its dramatic fall in use (being replaced by saline) in the USA for pure cosmetic use, although it continued to be used in most of Europe.

However, more recent reviews and discussions have allayed many of the fears with its use. Silicone gel filled implants are approved for use in the reconstruction setting in the USA and is considered by many to be cosmetically superior to other fills.

- **Advantages:** avoids major surgery (flap procedure) complications, easier to perform. Ideal in small/medium-sized breasts without ptosis and when no radiation needed. **Disadvantages:** complications, no natural ptosis and warmth, may require future replacement in young patients.
- **Technical aspects:** implant only reconstruction – placed subpectorally . (see Fig. 2.18) – pectoralis detached laterally, inferiorly, and partially medially. Serratus elevated laterally and sutured to lateral edge of pectoralis to complete pocket. May be combined with a myocutaneous/ de-epithelialized flap. Adjustable/expander implants are filled in stages to over inflation (will improve shape and dispel skin folds) before reducing to appropriate volume followed by injection port removal in 3–6 months. The expander may be replaced with a permanent implant.
- **Complications/adverse effects:** infection, bleeding, change in skin and nipple sensation (increased/decreased), seroma, skin scarring, pain, wrinkling/rippling, implant/port displacement, extrusion, capsule formation and contracture(~20%; textured implants are considered to reduce capsule formation), implant rupture (with leak of oil/gel), deflation (saline implant, 10% in 10 years) and cosmetic dissatisfaction. A further procedure will be required in 10–40% of patients. (For implant augmentation – patients should be warned about impact of the implant on future mammography). **Risk of cancer** (silicone implants) – several studies have now failed to demonstrate any increased risk of cancer or autoimmune disease.

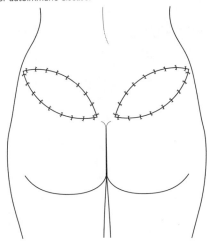

**Fig. 2.17** Gluteal flap.

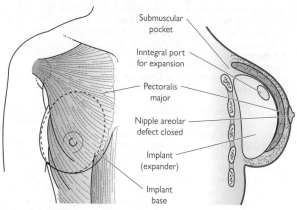

**Fig. 2.18** Implant reconstruction post-skin sparing mastectomy.

Nipple areola reconstruction
- *Local skin flap-based reconstruction:* CV flap, Bell flap, double opposing flap, star flap, Skate flap (fig: 2.19).
- *Nipple sharing graft.*
- *Nipple areolar tattooing:* 3–6 months after reconstruction.

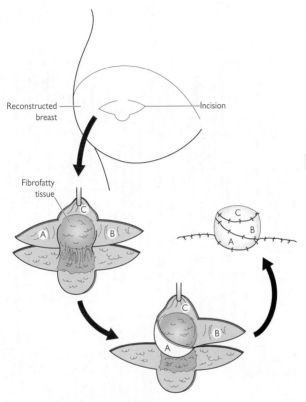

**Fig. 2.19** Nipple reconstruction C–V flap.

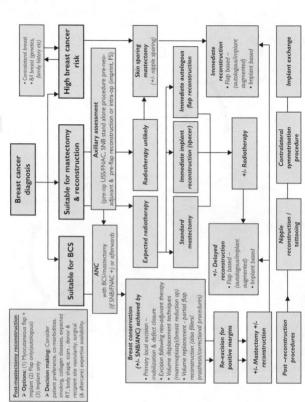

**Fig. 2.38** General algorithm for breast treatment options

**Post-mastectomy reconstruction**
➤ **Options:** (1) Myocutaneous flap + implant (2) Flap only(autologous) (3) Implant only
➤ **Decision making:** Consider patient preference, co-morbidities, smoking, collagen diseases, expected RT, body shape, scars, donor & recipient site vascularity, surgical (& aftercare) expertise availability.

**Breast cancer diagnosis**
- Suitable for BCS
- Suitable for mastectomy & reconstruction
- High breast cancer risk
  - Contralateral breast
  - B/l breast (genetics, family history etc)

**Axillary assessment**
(pre-op USS/FNAC, SNB stand alone procedure pre-neo-adjuvant & pre-flap reconstruction or intra-op (imprint, FS))

**ANC**
with BCS/mastectomy (if SNB/FNAC +) or afterwards

- Expected radiotherapy
- Radiotherapy unlikely
- Skin sparing mastectomy (+/- nipple sparing)

- Standard mastectomy
- Immediate implant reconstruction (spacer)
- Immediate autologous flap reconstruction

+/- Radiotherapy

**Immediate reconstruction**
- Flap based – (autologous/implant augmented)
- Implant based

**Breast conservation** (+/- SNB/ANC) achieved by
- Primary local excision – mobilization & defect closure
- Excision following neo-adjuvant therapy
- Volume displacement techniques (mammoplasty/breast reduction op)
- Volume replacement – partial flap reconstruction (also fillers/prosthesis/correctional procedures)

Re-excision for positive margins

+/- Mastectomy +/- reconstruction

+/- Delayed reconstruction
- Flap based – (autologous/implant augmented)
- Implant based

Post–reconstruction procedures

Nipple reconstruction / tattooing

Contralateral symmetrisation procedure

Implant exchange

# Systemic endocrine treatment

- 60–80% of breast cancers are steroid receptor positive. When both ER and PR are positive, 70–80% of cancers are responsive to hormone therapy, falling to 50–60% when ER+ only and 30–40% when PR alone positive. <10% response when ER/PR –ve.
- Standard first line endocrine treatment in hormone receptor positive invasive cancers is 5 years of tamoxifen (20mg/day) in pre-menopausal women. In post-menopausal women 5 years of upfront tamoxifen or aromatase inhibitors (AI) or switching (2–3 years tamoxifen then switching to AI for 3–2 years – will combine the benefits and cancel out the some side effects of either agent). Extended treatment (>5 years) AI may be considered in higher risk cases, but is now increasingly taken up.
- **DCIS:** risk reduction for ipsilateral recurrence and contralateral d/s, but no survival advantage. Therefore, individualize decision making.
- Generally endocrine therapy is not given concurrently with chemotherapy (endocrine to follow chemotherapy), but is acceptable concurrently with radiotherapy (NCCN).
- Adjuvant tamoxifen may be avoided in extremely good prognosis invasive disease (e.g. small <1cm or micro-invasive, grade1, node negative disease). DCIS unless increased risk (e.g. Van Nuys >6).

## Tamoxifen

- Oestrogen promotes breast cell proliferation and tumourogenesis.
- Tamoxifen is an anti-oestrogen with partial agonistic activity [antagonist activity – breast cancer tissue. agonist activity – endometrium (vaginal bleeding, cancer), bone, lipid metabolism.]
- Tamoxifen (5 years) reduces the risk of recurrence by 40% and mortality by 30%. Overall recurrence rates after 5 years of tamoxifen – 2% per year in node negative and 4% in node positive. Benefit continues for a further 5 years afterwards. Treatment beyond 5 years – no evidence of benefit shown yet. Benefits both pre- and post-menopausal women.
- Tamoxifen also reduces incidence of contralateral new cancers.
- **Other benefits:** reduces bone resorption and decrease fracture rates. (Hip fracture rate reduced by 30%.) Also has lipid lowering effect.
- **Side effects:** hot flushes, night sweats, weight gain, oligomenorrhoea, atrophic vaginitis, vaginal discharge, bleeding, and endometrial cancer (NCCN 2008 – annual gynaecological assessment if uterus intact). Increases risk of thromboembolic events.
- **Newer agents:** raloxifene, toremifene.

## Aromatase inhibitors

- In post-menopausal women ovaries cease oestrogen synthesis, but smaller amounts are produced by peripheral (subcutaneous fat, skin, bone, muscle, liver, breast tissue) aromatization of adrenal and ovarian androgens. AIs block this oestrogen production by >95%.
- The AIs in current use are 3rd generation consisting of the non-steroidal anastrozole (1mg/day) and letrozole (2.5mg/day), and steroidal exemestane (25mg/day). AI may also be used in women proven (biochemically) to be post-menopausal following chemotherapy

(in women who become post-menopausal following tamoxifen
– FSH and oestradiol levels should be continually monitored, as a
subset of patients relapse to pre-menopausal state – AI will need to
be discontinued). Exemestane binds irreversibly to aromatase, while
anastrozole and letrozole bind reversibly.

- **Other benefits:** reduces endometrial cancer risk, thromboembolic and
  ischaemic cerebrovascular events, vaginal bleeds/discharge, hot flushes.
- **Side effects:** increased bone mineral loss, hypercholesterolemia, slight
  increase in cardiovascular events (may not be a direct effect, but rather
  loss of agonistic action of tamoxifen in comparative trials).
- There is significant increase of fracture incidence when pretreatment
  bone density is low. Therefore, all patients should undergo pretreatment bone densitometry (DEXA scan+/– skeletal survey X-rays).
  A reduction of BMD (bone mineral density) by 10% corresponds to
  a t-score change of –1 equating to a doubling of hip fracture risk. At
  risk patients should receive nutritional supplement (calcium, Vit D),
  lifestyle advice (regular weight-bearing exercise, bone safety, smoking
  and alcohol cessation). May further require bisphosphonate, regular
  monitoring (DEXA scan) and specialist referral. Note: same concerns/
  management in patients with early treatment-induced ovarian failure.

### Neo-adjuvant and primary endocrine Rx

**Neo-adjuvant hormone therapy** may be used with a view to down stage
disease prior to definitive management in appropriate. It is less toxic
compared with chemotherapy and can be continued peri-operatively, but
is slower acting and is only applicable to receptor positive cancers. No
difference in DFS and DDFS between chemotherapy and endocrine
therapy. Additionally, hormone responsiveness can be determined pre-
operatively and can help direct post-surgical adjuvant therapy. However,
more long-term data is awaited.

In elderly patients and where surgery is contraindicated **primary endocrine treatment** can keep the disease in abeyance for several years in
receptor positive patients.

### Second/third line endocrine therapy

- Used on failure of primary therapy, or as adjuncts in aggressive,
  recurrent or advanced disease.
- Progesterones (medroxy progesterone, megestrol acetate), ovarian
  ablation (surgical – oophorectomy; radiotherapy; medical - Goserelin
  GnRH analogues – gonadotrophin-releasing hormone), Fulvestrant
  (pure anti-oestrogen – no agonistic activity – acts by receptor
  blockade and down-regulation. Licensed for advanced breast cancer
  in post-menopausal receptor positive women – 4-weekly injections).
  Aminogluthemide (non-selective first generation AI – adrenal blockade-
  medical adrenalectomy), B/L adrenalectomy, hypophysectomy.
- Ovarian ablation (surgery or radiotherapy – same results and effects)
  in <50 years significantly improves survival in both LN + or – patients
  [better results in pts who did not have chemotherapy] with early breast
  cancer (EBCTG – Cochrane review). However, ABC-OAS trial did not
  show a benefit, although longer-term follow-up data is awaited.

# Chemotherapy and other systemic therapy

- Chemotherapy reduces the relapse rate in breast cancer by ~10–15% (node negative – node positive) in the <50-year group and by ~5% in the 50–70-year group (EBCTCG overview 1998) translating into a similar 10 year survival advantage . Higher response in ER/PR –ves.
- In general chemotherapy is instituted in node positive (not micro-metastasis (≤2mm) especially if <T1c, gr1, receptor positive) or high risk cases. Online tools such as 'adjuvantonline' (based on SEER database – approx 10% of cancers in the US and overviews/trial data) can help make informed decisions on chemotherapy (chemo useful when >3–5% estimated survival benefit, >10% relapse risk at 10 years). Gene expression profiling can also help predict benefit of chemotherapy.
- In the elderly (e.g. >70 years) risks may outweigh benefits, and treatment has to be individualized according to co-morbidities and general fitness.
- Chemotherapy and endocrine treatment are not given concurrently, but sequentially for better results (effects on cell cycle phase).
- The CMF regimen that was the mainstay in breast chemotherapy has largely been supplanted by anthracycline-based regimens in the nineties and has been followed by the introduction of taxanes in the late nineties. CMF – 2/3 rd become amenorrhoeic.
- In general, chemotherapy is started within 4–6 weeks of surgical treatment and lasts for 3–8 cycles (months) followed by RT if indicated.

## Anthracyclines

- Doxorubicin/adriamycin, mitomycin-C, mitoxantrone, daunorubicin.
- Anthracycline-based regimens have improved (or, at worst, similar) DFS and overall survival compared with CMF.
- Act as intercalating agents inhibiting DNA/RNA replication in rapidly growing cancer cells. Also release free oxygen radicals damaging cell membranes and DNA.
- *Side effects:* general chemotherapy side effects + cardiotoxicity (arrhythmias, cardiomyopathy, failure) + bone marrow effects.
- Polyethylene glycol (PEG) liposome encapsulated doxorubicin: improved cell penetration and reduced tumour cytotoxicity with reduced systemic toxicity.

## Taxanes

Docetaxel, paclitaxel. Acts by binding and stabilizing microtubules causing cell cycle arrest and death. Used in higher risk patients.

## Alkylating agents

Cyclophosphamide, cisplatin, carboplatin.

## Antimetabolites

Methotrexate, 5-flurouracil, gemcitabine, capecitabine (a prodrug – gets enzymatically converted to 5-FU within the tumour).

## Vinca alkaloids

Vinblastine, vinorelbine (mitotic inhibitor – microtubule disruption). Second line agents.

## Some common polychemotherapy regimens

- *CMF:* cyclophosphamide, methotrexate, 5-FU.
- *EC:* epirubicin, cyclophosphamide.
- *AC:* adriamycin (doxorubicin), cyclophosphamide.
- *FEC:* 5-FU, epirubicin, cyclophosphamide.
- *AC→T:* adriamycin, cyclophosphamide→taxane +/− trastuzumab.
- *CAF:* cyclophosphamide, adriamycin, 5-FU.
- *GT:* gemcitabine, paclitaxel.

## Neoadjuvant chemotherapy

- *Aka:* preoperative or induction or upfront chemotherapy. Also primary chemotherapy (generally when surgery is not contemplated).
- Chemotherapy prior to surgery to facilitate breast conservation or operability by down-sizing and down staging.
- No survival disadvantage. Higher rate of breast conservation (68% vs. 60% – NSABP-B18-doxorubicin + cyclophosphamide). Trials of taxane containing regimens appear to show equal or better response rates. Consider trastuzumab with HER-2 +ves. Highest response in ER/PR −ves. Invasive ductal cancers respond better than lobular.
- Provides information on chemosensitivity of tumour. Survival rates (overall and DFS) are higher in pathological complete responders (pCR).
- In general, excision is still required after complete response as assessment for residual disease may not be completely accurate.
- Sentinel node sampling/axillary surgery must be undertaken prior to chemotherapy as post-treatment accuracy of SLNB may be diminished.
- Non responders- use further/other agent chemotherapy +/− RT.
- *Disadvantages:* after a complete response there may be difficulty in locating the tumour for resection (advisable to prior mark site of tumour with radio opaque markers, skin tattooing). In partial responders it may not be possible to determine if tumour has shrunk concentrically (as opposed to a patchy response). Post-treatment sentinel node sampling may be inaccurate. Also significance of post-treatment excision margins and histological features (e.g. grading) not fully known.

## Trastuzumab

- Monoclonal antibody (against the extracellular domain of HER-2; humanized mouse antibody; see 'Pathology and biology of breast cancer', p. 86).
- HER-2 is over-expressed in 14–30% of breast cancers indicating poorer prognosis. Improved survival when given with taxane-based chemotherapy in adjuvant setting. Usual duration of therapy – 1 year.
- Action additive with chemotherapy. DFS and DDFS significantly improved. Approved in early breast cancer along with chemotherapy in HER-2 +ves. Survival improved in metastatic cancer. Monotherapy licensed if chemotherapy given previously for metastatic disease.
- Main side effect cardiotoxicity, an additive when administered with anthracyclines. Contraindicated when ejection fraction <55% (NICE, 2006).
- *Indications:* currently licensed in the metastatic and adjuvant setting (in HER 2 positive cancer receiving chemotherapy). Primary/neoadjuvant setting – response improved by addition of trastuzumab in trials.

## Further reading

NICE (2006) (Trastuzumab):
http://www.nice.org.uk/niceMedia/pdf/2006-038LaunchOfHerceptinGuidance.pdf

# Adjuvant radiotherapy

## Standard external beam radiotherapy

### Indications

- **Following BCS:** (whole breast RT +/– local tumour bed boost- for high risk Ca) recurrence risk is reduced to a 3rd/5th when adjuvant RT is given (e.g. NSABP-06 for node positive cancer – lumpectomy with and without RT; recurrence rate – 8 vs. 44%). All BCS should be followed by RT except in low risk DCIS (e.g. Van Nuys score 4–6).
- Following mastectomy : (chest wall +/- supraclavicular RT) in high risk cases reduces recurrence risk by 60%. Indications for RT: >5cm tumour size, ≥ 4 +axillary LN (now being extended to 1-3LN+- NCCN 2008), positive margins. Relative indications: grade 3, lymphovascular invasion, and young age. (RT reduces recurrence risk from 50% to 10%).
- RT may be avoided in elderly (e.g. >70) with good prognosis disease.

### Technical

- Photon field or electron beam (using multiple tangential beams). CT based field planning recommended with shielding (lung and cardiac, etc.).
- A common regimen is 45–50Gy over 5–7 weeks (2Gy fractions) for the entire breast with local tumour bed boost (e.g. 10Gy in fractions).
- **Internal mammary RT:** controversial (NCCN, 2008 – give if clinically/pathologically +).
- Axillary irradiation in SLNB or sampling positive cases when ANC not undertaken. Supraclavicular fossa RT when ≥4 axillary node positive.
- To reduce toxicity chemotherapy and radiotherapy are not given concomitantly, but sequentially in either order. Generally, radiotherapy can be safely delayed until completion (full or part) of chemotherapy.

### Complications

- **Local skin changes:** erythema, dryness, excoriation, pigmentation, microcapillary changes/telangiectasia.
- **Arm lymphodema** following axillary RT (~3-5%)(25-40% if post-ANC).
- **Brachialplexus:** neuropathy.
- **Bone:** rib fracture risk.
- **Shoulder:** skeletal/osteoporotic, nerve-related morbidity.
- **Increased fibrotic changes in breast with cosmetic morbidity and volume loss:** increased capsule formation with implant reconstruction.
- **Second malignancy:** angiosarcoma, leukaemia, melanoma.
- Vascular anastomotic stenosis and compromise in free-flaps.
- Pneumonitis, pulmonary fibrosis, myocardial and vascular fibrosis and ischemia, oesophagitis.

**Partial breast radiotherapy**
- Confining RT to only the high risk area within the breast. The potential advantages- dose reduction and shortened treatment duration.
- *Techniques:* ongoing trials and specialist centre use:
  - 3-D conformational external beam radiotherapy;
  - IORT – intraoperative radiotherapy, single fraction;
  - brachytherapy – multicatheter implant (placed in 2–3 planes), balloon catheter device.

# Post-treatment follow-up and surveillance

- Although advances in treatment have reduced recurrence and mortality a significant proportion of breast cancer patients develop post-treatment recurrence or metastases. It is vital that these events are picked up early and treatment instituted.
- Over 12,000 breast cancer-related deaths occur in the UK annually representing an overall 5-year mortality rate of around 20% and 20-year rate of 35%. Following BCS the recurrence rate is approximately 0.5–2% per year remaining steady for over 10 years (5–20% at 10 years).
- In general, peak incidence of recurrence is in the first 2–3 years (especially post-mastectomy) with the risk falling after 5–10 years, but carrying on through to 20 years. Further long-term recurrences are not unknown. Lifetime risk may approach 30–50%.
- NSABP-B-04 (1971) 25-year results: 25% distant recurrences occur after 5 years, 50% of contralateral cancers detected after 5 years. Only few recurrences after 10 years. Node +ve patients who are disease free at 5 years have same probability of remaining disease free as node –ve pts.
- Local recurrence is an independent risk factor for the presence/development of metastatic disease (~10% after BCS and 25% after mastectomy – metastasis will be present at onset of local recurrence).
- Local recurrence can be focal (better prognosis – salvage resection/excision possible + RT if possible and chemotherapy) or diffuse/widespread (poor prognosis).
- The longer the interval between primary tumour and recurrence the better the prognosis. Also histology of recurrence (invasive vs. DCIS), positive regional LN.
- Factors that determine risk of recurrence and metastatic disease can help categorize low and high risk cases, and frequency and duration of follow-up modified accordingly.

## Low risk disease

Small tumours(<2cm), low grade, absence of lymph node involvement and lymphovascular invasion, absence of extensive intraductal disease or multifocality, steroid receptor positive and HER-2 negative, good resection margins, no residual calcifications, received adjuvant treatment and age >35 years.

## Post-treatment follow-up

- No consensus as to the optimum duration or frequency of follow-up.
- *Usual duration:* 5 years + further 5 years if higher risk.
- Extended further in cases of recurrence and metastatic disease.
- Additionally, patients should have access to breast care nurses and breast outpatient clinics in the interval between follow-ups.
- *Mammography:* annual 2-view bilateral mammography in BCS and contralateral mammography in mastectomy. First post-treatment mammogram to the conserved breast at 6 months. MRI surveillance may be indicated in high risk individuals (BRCA mutation) (NCCN).
- *Clinical follow-up:* 6–12 monthly for 5 years, annually thereafter.

- *Clinical examination and Ix:*
  - for local recurrence – breast and scar clinical examination and mammography;
  - regional lymph node – clinical examination (axilla/SCLN);
  - contralateral breast and axilla – clinical examination and mammography;
  - examination for arm lymphoedema;
  - examination and investigation for metastatic disease as directed by symptoms/findings;
  - examination and investigations for side effects of treatment, e.g. DEXA scan for osteoporosis from AI (US – NCCN – yearly gynaecological exams while on tamoxifen);
  - counselling and psychological support as necessary.

## Loco-regional recurrence

- Confirm by tissue diagnosis followed by staging investigations.
- Hormone receptor status may change in the recurrence.
- Convert to mastectomy when previous BCS. Local resection in other cases (BCS in a previously non-irradiated breast) or post-mastectomy recurrence (resect if focal/isolated recurrence). A reconstructed breast may need to be deconstructed. LN recurrence after sentinel node/axillary sampling – proceed to axillary clearance.
- Radiotherapy if tissue dose limit will not be exceeded. Second line endocrine, chemotherapy.
- Other – interferon, local hyperthermia, miltefosine local application.

## Distant metastasis

- *Bony metastasis (most common site for relapse):* bisphosphonates, palliative local RT (pain control, bone healing variable). Prophylactic orthopaedic fixation to prevent fractures in appropriate cases (e.g. hip).
- Liver metastasis may be amenable to resectional surgery if appropriate.
- Lung (50% isolated lesions from primary lung Ca, rather than breast).
- Chemotherapy, trastuzumab (HER-2 +), second line endocrine.

## Pregnancy after breast cancer treatment/chemotherapy

- 50–90%: ovarian failure after chemotherapy: reversible in 20%.
- Prior chemotherapy does not significantly increase risk of foetal mal development.
- The general advice is to avoid pregnancy for the first 2–3 years post-initial treatment of breast cancer. This will help select out those with aggressive disease as well as allow 2 years of tamoxifen therapy when the benefit is maximum. Tamoxifen can lead to foetal loss and is discontinued ideally from 3 months before conception.
- No contra-indication to breast feeding from the unaffected breast after completion of treatment.
- *Fertility:* embryo, ovum, or ovarian tissue cryopreservation may only have limited success, but may be considered in appropriate circumstances prior to cancer treatment. Exogenous ovarian stimulation during infertility treatment may have an unquantified deleterious effect on a steroid receptor positive breast cancer.

# Management of advanced breast cancer

Advanced breast cancer includes *locally advanced* (5–10%; generally T3, T4) and *metastatic* disease (stage IV). 2–7% of cancers are metastatic at presentation.

## Primary management
- Establish diagnosis, staging, and receptor status – steroid and HER-2.
- Requires multidisciplinary input and discussion.

## Locally advanced cancer
Modalities of management include
- *Neo-adjuvant chemo- or endocrine therapy* to improve operability/ conservation (e.g. inflammatory breast cancer) followed by resectional surgery. This may be followed by chemo (for completion) and RT. Response to pre-operative chemotherapy is an indicator of relapse and survival (NSABP-B18). Common chemotherapy – anthracycline based +/– taxane.
- *Palliative resection*/toilet procedures.
- *Palliative radiotherapy:* for local control. Does not improve survival.
- *Primary endocrine or chemotherapy* in inoperable disease.

## Metastatic disease
- Metastatic disease may be present in ~5% of breast cancers at initial presentation. Additionally up to 40% of early cancers may go on to develop metastatic disease with a median survival of 18 months. Common sites – bone, liver, lung, CNS.
- *Endocrine treatment:* AI considered first line therapy in post-menopausal women. In premenopausal – tamoxifen, ovarian ablation (see 'Systemic endocrine treatment', p. 144). First, second, and third line agents, and endocrine sequencing maybe used.
- *Chemotherapy:* carefully chosen, balancing the risks of toxicity vs. survival and symptom relief benefits, and estimated sensitivity and response. If first line agents have failed judicious use of other agents is indicated. Besides anthracyclines and taxanes, antimetabolites, such as Capecitabine (effective orally) and gemcitabine are effective.
- *Trastuzumab:* monotherapy or in combination with chemotherapy (continued until disease progression). Capcitabine + Lapatinib in recurrent/metastatic disease. Bevacizumab (Mab to vascular EGF, in trials).
- *Symptomatic bone metastasis:* eventually up to 25% of breast cancer patients develop skeletal metastasis.
- *Treatment:*
  - local radiotherapy (e.g. single dose 8–12Gy);
  - bisphosphonates – controls bone pain and hypocalcaemia and reduces incidence of fracture, spinal compression (oral/IV clodronate, IV zoledronic acid, IV disodium pamidronate and ibandronate) and are also used to treat AI induced osteoporosis as well as prevent bone metastasis. (+Vit.D and $Ca^{2+}$);
  - preventive bone fixation.

## Palliative care

Psychological care, pain management, home- or hospice-based care. Use specialized care plans for terminal care (e.g. Liverpool care pathway).

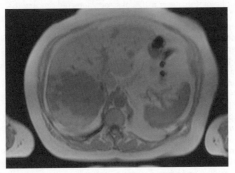

**Fig. 2.21** Liver mets from Ca breast. 56-year-old woman. Largest mass low signal on T2W fat sat images. 10 × 7 cm in segment V.

# Non-invasive cancer: DCIS and LCIS

Ductal carcinoma *in situ* (DCIS)
- 2–4% of symptomatic and 20% of screen detected cancers.
- AKA intraduct cancer/pre-invasive cancer (basement membrane intact)
- **Presentation:** mostly asymptomatic (90%) and screen detected.
  **Symptoms:** nipple discharge, lump, Paget's. May co-exist with invasive cancer.
- **Histological:** *Grades* – low, intermediate, high grade. *Varieties:* papillary, cribriform, solid, and comedo (pure DCIS = Stage 0 disease).
- **Natural history:** spreads along duct. Tumour may be multicentric (20–30% – usually low grade). Over time may progress to invasive cancer (30–40%). 5% risk of invasive disease in contralateral breast.
- **Receptors:** ER +ve 60%, HER-2 positive 60%.
- **Mammographic features:** microcalcifications (dystrophic calcification of necrosis, seen in 90%) alone or with a mass lesion (10–30%).
- **Diagnosis:** mammography, core biopsy, sometimes guided excision biopsy. MRI (100% sensitivity) sometimes used to determine extent. (as lesion may extend beyond mammographically visible calcification).
- **Treatment:** BCS to achieve clear margins (see 'Breast conserving surgery', p. 120)
- **Mastectomy – indicators:** multicentric disease, large tumour (~>4cm), persistent positive margins, recurrence (after BCS and RT), Van Nuys Score 10–12 (see p. 104), and when radiotherapy contraindicated.
- Axillary surgery: not indicated as <1–4% LN metastasis. Relative indications for SLN biopsy/sampling – high grade, large size, multifocal tumour. (*Other:* along with mastectomy, local excision at tail of breast).
- **Adjuvant radiotherapy:** indicated after BCS in high risk cases, e.g. Van Nuys Score 7–9 (close/positive margins, high grade, size, young age; see 'Staging of breast cancer', p. 104). Reduces invasive recurrence by 40%. Survival rate same.
- **Adjuvant endocrine therapy:** tamoxifen (5 years) reduces recurrence by ~30% in ER +ve tumours. It may, however, be an over-treatment in low risk cases (e.g. after mastectomy). More trial data awaited.
- **HER-2:** Trastuzumab – no evidence. Lapatinib–under investigation
- **Follow-up:** overall 10% recurrence at 5 years (50% invasive). Overall survival rate, high nineties (follow-up protocol, see 'Post-treatment follow-up and surveillance', p. 150)

Lobular carcinoma *in situ* (LCIS)
- Seen in 1% of screening and 0.5% of symptomatic biopsies incidentally. Mostly (60–70%) pre-menopausal. Often bilateral, multicentric.
- Not cancer or precancerous directly, but a marker for high risk. (RR-7).
- Future cancers predominantly ductal. 40% *in situ* cancers. 50% contralateral breast. (approximately 1% risk per year; ~20% over 15 years).
- **Management:** if found on core, need to exclude co-existing cancer by excision biopsy/further imaging. If incidentally found in excision specimen, no further action needed, but management needs to be individualized. Occasionally, some patients may choose b/l mastectomy

in the presence of other risk factors (e.g. BRCA or strong family history).
- Tamoxifen can reduce risk of cancer by 50% (NSABP P-1, IBIS trials) (US tamoxifen/raloxifene in post-menopausal; NCCN, 2008 )
- **Follow-up:** clinical exam (6–12-monthly) and mammography (yearly). Risk of finding invasive cancer 1–1.5% yearly (ductal/lobular Ca).

### Further reading

NCCN (2009) (breast):
http://www.nccn.org/professionals/physician_gls/PDF/breast.pdf

# Breast cancer: special conditions

Pregnancy and breast cancer

- 1 in 3000–10,000 pregnancies (~ 1–3% of all breast cancers).
- Challenging management. Multidisciplinary approach is vital – surgeons, oncologists, obstetricians.
- **Pathology:** tend to be ER –ve (50–80%) and PR –ve, and are often HER-2 +ve (30-60%). >80% are ductal invasive. Inflammatory cancers occur in 1.5–4% of cases. Higher rate of node positivity (>60%).
- **Prognosis:** stage for stage, survival is nearly the same as age-matched controls, but the disease tends to be diagnosed at later stages – increased size and node positive (up to two-thirds).
- **Diagnosis:** accuracy of clinical examination decreases during pregnancy. Ultrasound is probably the first choice, although digital mammography with abdominal shielding is safe during pregnancy.
- FNAC has a higher false positive rate owing to the epithelial proliferative changes associated with pregnancy. Core biopsy is the modality of choice. Occasionally, excision biopsy may be required.
- **Staging:** decide on appropriate investigation on individualized basis – multidisciplinary team decision. Chest X-ray (0.008 rad) with abdominal shielding is safe. USS to stage liver, MRI is probably safe (no comprehensive human safety data available – contrast material known to cross placental barrier and cause anomalies in animal tests). Safety of isotope scanning (bone scan – 0.1 rad delivers less radiation than a full skeletal X-ray series) not fully known.
- **Management:** surgery is generally the first line of treatment and safe during all trimesters of surgery. Anaesthetic and surgical consideration regarding the physiological changes in pregnancy. Includes dilutional anaemia, hyper-coagulability, regurgitation and aspiration risk, decreased lung capacity, supine positional hypotension due to the pressure effects of the gravid uterus on venous return (tilt to the left to improve venous return), increased breast vascularity. Obstetrician/neonatologist on standby if surgery in 3rd trimester. If lactating – stopping breast feeding may reduce engorgement and vascularity prior to surgery.
- Generally mastectomy advised as breast conserving surgery will require subsequent radiotherapy, which may need to be delayed until parturition. (Adjuvant RT and endocrine treatment may be delayed till post-partum – NCCN v.2. 2008, e.g. after BCS).
- Neo-adjuvant chemotherapy followed by BCS may be appropriate in certain situations (usual guidelines) in the later trimesters of pregnancy. In this case, timing would be appropriate for radiotherapy to commence after delivery. (avoid chemo >35 weeks/3 weeks prior to delivery– due to haematological complications at delivery).
- **Axillary surgery:** axillary dissection is preferable to SLNB due to safety issues in relation to the administration of radiotracer (especially <30 weeks) and blue dye.
- **Chemotherapy:** safe during 2nd and 3rd trimesters of pregnancy. If the cancer is aggressive/presentation is advanced, and chemotherapy is indicated in the first trimester, termination may be discussed. In general, treatment should not be delayed due to pregnancy. Methotrexate

should be avoided, but anthracycline based chemotherapy (e.g. FAC) can be safely administered. Taxanes have been used in pregnancy, but being newer agents comprehensive safety data is only emerging.

- *Monoclonal antibody:* high rate of HER-2 positivity – Trastuzumab crosses the placental barrier; currently treatment is not recommended as foetal safety not known.
- *Radiotherapy:* generally avoided during pregnancy, although not absolutely contraindicated with appropriately thick lead shielding (keeping a foetal dose <0.1Gy), and after the first and second trimesters. Short delays (e.g. 4–6 weeks) may not significantly affect maternal prognosis and may be acceptable in certain situations.
- *Termination of pregnancy:* although termination will simplify treatment planning there is no evidence that it will affect/improve survival. Non-medical reasons for termination in early pregnancy include patients with very advanced or terminal cancers wishing to terminate for social reasons. A challenging issue is the need for a multidisciplinary approach, including significant input from the patient, as well as close family and relatives.
- *Endocrine treatment:* tamoxifen is contraindicated in pregnancy as it can induce miscarriages and genital tract cancers (animal studies). It is recommended to avoid pregnancy within 2 months of taking tamoxifen.
- In patients wishing to consider future pregnancy after chemotherapy, oocyte preservation may be discussed.

## Inflammatory breast cancer

- Breast cancer accompanied by extensive erythema and oedema (peau'd orange; >1/3rd of breast skin), warmth and breast swelling as a result of dermal lymphatic invasion. May sometimes be mistaken for infection initially. Occurs in 1–4% of breast cancers. Younger patients. Slightly higher incidence in the black population.
- Historically very poor prognosis, but has improved with modern multimodality treatment. Around 50% 5-year and 33% 10-year survival rate.
- Underlying mass may not be evident, and core, punch biopsies, and occasionally incisional biopsies may be needed to diagnose. Investigation work-up may include mammogram, USS, MRI, axillary assessment, and staging investigations.
- Designated T4d, UICC Stage IIIB, and above. Commonly hormone receptor negative, lymph node positive and metastatic at presentation.
- *Management:* neo-adjuvant chemotherapy (60–80% response rate) followed by mastectomy and axillary dissection (rather than SLNB), followed by adjuvant therapy (further chemotherapy, radiotherapy, hormone, and trastuzumab treatment as appropriate).
- Predictors to survival are lymph node status, response to pre-operative chemotherapy, surgical margin involvement, and metastasis.

Male breast cancer

- 1% of breast cancers, <1% of male cancers, average age 5–10 years older than female breast cancer. 1 in 1000 lifetime risk. Peak – 7th decade.
- *Risk factors:* testicular disease and atrophy leading to higher oestrogen: testosterone ratio, obesity, liver disease, breast trauma, radiation exposure, Klinefelter's syndrome (47/XXY, ×50 increased risk), Ashkenazi Jewish ancestry, family history (15–20% have a positive first degree family history) of breast cancer, BRCA2, and p53 mutation. Gynaecomastia does not predispose.
- *Prognosis:* stage for stage, the prognosis is similar to age-matched female counterparts. However, often presentation and diagnosis is delayed (diagnosis at later stages) resulting in lower overall survival rates.
- *Histology:* 85–90% ductal and mostly invasive. DCIS accounts for 10%. Lobular carcinoma is less common 1–3% (minimal lobular tissue), but common in Klinefelter's (hyperoestrogenism). Paget's – 1–4%.
- *Immunohistochemistry:* 80–90% ER +ve, 30% HER-2/neu over-expression.
- *Clinical presentation:* painless mass, nipple distortion, bleeding, nipple discharge, skin infiltration, axillary adenopathy, pain, metastatic disease.
- *Diagnosis:* mammogram, USS, FNAC, core biopsy, occasionally incisional or excisional biopsy.
- *Treatment:* primary modality is surgery – mostly total mastectomy, although rarely a breast conserving excision is possible. Pectoralis fixity is often encountered and may require shaving part of the muscle along with excision to achieve clear margins.
- Neo-adjuvant chemotherapy in locally advanced disease to increase operability followed by surgery.
- Indications for axillary dissection and sentinel LNB (no large scale data) are the same as in women
- Adjuvant treatment (chemotherapy and radiotherapy) guidelines are the same as in female breast cancer, although no large scale data is available. Tamoxifen in ER +ve tumours.
- *Other modalities/second line agents:* orchidectomy/gonadal ablation, LHRH analogues (goserelin and leuprorelin), androgen blockade (flutamide and bicalutamide), progestins. There is insufficient data on the efficacy of AIs, which will not block the production of oestrogen (20%) from the testis. There is no direct trial data available for Trastuzumab in men, but it is likely that it may be of benefit in combination with chemotherapy in HER-2/neu over expressed tumours.
- *Adrenalectomy/hypophysectomy.*

Paget's disease

- 1–5% breast cancers. Breast carcinoma (invasive or DCIS) in which cancer cells invade the epidermis of the nipple-producing eczematoid changes. Tumour cells are considered to have travelled intraductally to reach the nipple. In some instances, no underlying cancer is found, giving rise to the possibility of de novo transformation.
- *Presentation:* median age of presentation 50–60 years. Delay in presentation/diagnosis may occur due to non-specific nature of

symptoms or misleading temporary resolution (e.g. to topical agents). Features include (usually unilateral, although bilateral disease is not unknown) redness, itching, burning, discharge or bleeding and scaling of the nipple progressing to nipple erosion, and distortion, ultimately leading to nipple destruction. A clinically identifiable mass is present in 50–60%.

- When accompanied by a palpable mass, 90% have underlying invasive cancer. No palpable mass – 60–70% DCIS.
- **Differential diagnoses:** nipple eczema, contact/irritant dermatitis (usually bilateral), primary skin cancers.
- **Diagnosis/work-up:** mammography/USS (micro-calcifications, mass lesion), punch biopsy, scrape or discharge cytology, FNAC/core (mass lesion), +/– MRI to determine extent. Examine/investigate carefully for underlying lesion. Characteristic cells are called Paget's cells (large rounded or ovoid cells with clear or eosinophilic abundant cytoplasm with vacuoles and enlarged hyperchromatic nuclei and nucleoli within the epidermis) – CK7. Most often HER-2 positive.
- Classed as Tis(Paget's) or T1–4 if tumour/mass present.
- **Treatment:** mastectomy in many cases. Breast-conserving central wide local excision including the nipple and areola is also possible in some cases when extent is limited. Skin sparing mastectomy and reconstruction can be considered in appropriate cases.
- **Axilla:** ANC or SLNB in invasive disease and SLNB in high grade DCIS, and/or when mastectomy planned.
- **Adjuvant therapy:** similar guidelines as in general breast cancer.
- **Prognosis:** depends on the presence of invasive disease, extent of lesion and presence of underlying mass (no mass – 90% 5-year survival rate, 40% when mass present).

## Axillary metastasis: occult primary

- **Common primary sites:** lymphoma, breast cancer, melanoma, other.
- **Diagnostic work-up:** needle biopsy/excisional biopsy. Histology/ immunohistochemistry to diagnose cancer and categorize possible primary tissue. Steroid receptor status.
- **Breast assessment:** clinical examination, mammography, USS. Further MRI/PET if appropriate.
- Often requires investigations to rule out possible non-breast primary sites. Requires co-ordination with other site-specific oncology specialists relevant inter-multidisciplinary team discussion.
- **Staging investigations:** stage allocation.
- **Treatment:** if suggestive of breast cancer, but no primary seen – mastectomy appropriate after patient counselling (no primary will be found in specimen in a third of cases). Axilla – usual for invasive breast cancer.
- **Adjuvant treatment:** same principles as node positive breast cancer.
- **Prognosis:** similar to usual invasive breast cancer (stage II and above). Limited data.

## Recurrent breast cancer

- Recurrences/relapse may be early or late and be local, regional, or systemic (see 'Other breast cancers and pathology', p. 162).

- Specific management depends on the site and extent of the recurrence: Local excision if feasible, local RT, hyperthermia, bone mets (bisphosphonates), spinal/CNS (e.g. intrathecal chemo), and other site-specific treatments. Second/third line endocrine and chemotherapy. Pain management. Needs multimodality input including psychosocial aspects. If disease progress is unresponsive, avoid further unrealistic aggressive treatment and decide on transition to palliative pathway (e.g. Liverpool care pathway).

# Other breast cancers and pathology

## Phyllodes tumour

- Non-epithelial tumour arising from periductal and interlobular stroma.
- 2.5% of all fibro-epithelial breast tumours (0.5% of all breast tumours).
- **Presentation:** breast swelling, distortion, venous engorgement, and thinning/breakthrough (but no involvement) of overlying skin. Usually, well circumscribed, mobile, and large. Differential diagnosis – fibroadenoma (phyllodes – faster growing and presents – 10–20 years later). Lower age group in Asian population. Higher incidence in Li–Fraumeni.
- **Histology:** mostly benign (grading spectrum – benign 60%, borderline 15%, malignant 25%) – grading is sometimes difficult and is assessed using stromal cellularity, mitotic rate, cellular atypia, stromal/epithelial ratio, boundaries (pushing or infiltrating), necrosis, and Ki67, p53.
- **Recurrence:** local recurrence 15–30% (from benign to malignant).
- **Distant metastasis:** 0–25% (benign to malignant) – lung, liver, bone.
- **Diagnosis:** clinical appearance, rapid enlargement, USS, mammogram, FNAC, core (moderate accuracy), excision biopsy.
- **Treatment:** excision with adequate margin (~1cm) in view of the high local recurrence rate. Larger lesions may require mastectomy.
- Axillary metastases are rare (1%) and axillary surgery is not indicated unless clinically evident adenopathy is present.
- **Metastatic disease:** chemotherapy useful (e.g. doxorubicin, ifosfamide), Radiotherapy of symptomatic deposits. Recurrence: re-excision/mastectomy (+/– rarely RT if multiple recurrences).
- 40–80% ER/PR +ve, but no clear data on hormone therapy benefit.

## Angiosarcoma breast

- Primary (0.04% of breast cancers) or more commonly radiation induced – usually more than 5–10 years post-radiation. Frequency may be radiation dose-related (40–50Gy). May also arise in the post-surgical chronic lymphoedema. Primary breast angiosarcomas arise in the younger premenopausal age group (20–40 years).
- **Presentation:** breast or upper extremity. Primary or secondary (post-surgery or radiation) breast mass (primary tumours), or multiple or single skin nodules (radiation induced), which may be discoloured and often violaceous. May also appear as non-healing ulcers. Nodal dissemination is rare. Haematogenous spread to lungs, bone.
- **Differential diagnosis:** benign radiation changes, skin cancers – amelanotic melanoma, SCC, BCC
- **Diagnosis:** mammography, MRI, core and FNAC (bleeding risk), excisional biopsy of skin lesions. FNAC has a high rate of false negativity (up to 40%). Histological diagnosis may sometimes be difficult, especially in low grade tumours. Immunohistochemistry is useful in these cases – staining for vimentin, factor VIII-related antigen, CD34, and BNH9.
- **Treatment:** primarily surgery followed by adjuvant chemotherapy (in poorly differentiated tumours) and radiotherapy if feasible.

- Mastectomy is preferred in larger tumours, in a central location, and when multifocal or multicentric. Microscopic extent is often beyond the macroscopic edges, limiting the use of breast conserving surgery. Even negative histological margins may not guarantee complete excision.
- Axillary spread is uncommon and axillary surgery is not indicated.
- Neo-adjuvant treatment: neo-adjuvant anthracycline-based chemotherapy may improve operability in extensive high grade tumours and may be combined with radiotherapy.
- Primary chemo- and RT in inoperable tumours.
- *Prognosis:* poor-aggressive tumours. 15–50% 5-year survival rate. Prognosis depends on grade, extent, multifocality. Few long-term survivors.

## Lymphoma

- *Rare:* 0.1–0.5% of breast cancers. 0.5–1% of all lymphomas (NHL extra-nodal, commonly B-cell). May be primary-50%, or secondary-50%.
- *Diagnosis:* mass, mammography (homogenous faint shadow – no microcalcification/speculation), core, or excision biopsy.
- *Investigations:* search for primary. Establish stage as for NHL.
- *Treatment:* commonly excisional surgery precedes diagnosis. Followed by chemotherapy (e.g. CHOP) and RT. Primary localized lymphoma is treated by RT and chemotherapy alone.

## Melanoma

- Metastatic melanoma in breast parenchyma or primary cutaneous.
- *Diagnosis:* excisional or incisional biopsy as appropriate. Core in deep seated lesions.
- *Treatment:* primary cutaneous melanoma – wide excision treatment of choice, staging by thickness and lymph node status (sentinel lymph node biopsy). Axillary clearance if node positive.
- *Adjuvant treatment:* as standard for melanoma.

## Intracystic papillary carcinoma

- *Papillary Ca:* rare (1%). Cystic mass with papillary lesion projecting into lumen. Excellent prognosis.
- *Treatment:* local excision. Nodal surgery in invasive disease.

## Intraduct papilloma and multiple papillomatosis

- Single duct papilloma (central ducts) and multiple papillomatosis (peripheral breast) have 2–10% risk of associated invasive cancer.
- Ductoscopy may help. Treatment: duct excision for single duct papiloma. For papillomatosis, local excision or surveillance is indicated.

## Adenoid cystic carcinoma

- Rare cancer (0.1%) – adenocarcinoma variant resembles adenoid cystic Ca, elsewhere histologically, but better prognosis.
- Commonly tender mass. LN and distant mets rare. ER, PR –ve.
- *Treatment:* mastectomy or wide local excision + RT.

## Secondary breast cancer

From primary–contralateral breast cancer (commonest), lymphoma, melanoma, lung carcinoma, renal cell carcinoma, rhabdomyosarcoma, carcinoid, AML, mesothelioma.

# Management of breast cancer risk

A multifaceted and multidisciplinary strategy is required for the assessment and management of individuals suspected with increased risk of breast cancer.

## Risk assessment

Following preliminary risk assessment, reassurance, and/or referral to specialist units, various risk stratification models (see 'Breast cancer epidemiology, aetiology, and risk factors', p. 80) may be used for formal evaluation.

For assessment of familial breast cancer risk, affected individuals must be blood relatives of the patient and each other, and on the same side of family (maternal and paternal relatives, not additive). Bilateral cancer counts as 2 first degree relatives.

## Familial risk categories

### Population risk (lifetime risk < 17% or 10-year risk <3% in 40–49 years)

*Examples:*

One 1st degree relative (FDR) or 2nd degree relative (SDR) with breast cancer diagnosed at >40 years of age only.

### Moderate risk (lifetime risk 17–30% or10-year risk 3–8% in 40–49 years)

*Examples for at least moderate risk*

- One FDR female with breast cancer diagnosed at <40 years age **or** one FDR male relative with breast cancer – any age, **or** one FDR with bilateral breast cancer, first primary diagnosed <50 years of age.
- Two FDR **or** one FDR **and** one SDR relative with breast cancer at any age.
- One FDR or SDR with breast cancer at any age **and** one FDR or SDR degree relative with ovarian cancer at any age. (at least one should be FDR).
- Three FDR or SDR diagnosed with breast cancer at any age from the same side of the family)

### High risk: (lifetime risk >30% or10-year risk >8% in 40–49 years or >20% risk of BRCA1, BRCA2, or TP53 mutation in family)

*Examples*

- *Female breast cancer:* two FDR or SDR of average age <50 years, **or** three FDR or SDR of average age of <60 years, **or** four relatives of any age
- *Ovarian cancer:* one relative with ovarian cancer at any age **and** one of three
  - one FDR (including the relative with ovarian cancer) or SDR with breast cancer <50 years; **or**
  - two FDR or SDR breast of average age <60 years; **or**
  - another relative with ovarian cancer at any age.
- *Bilateral breast cancer:* one FDR with bilateral breast cancer, average age <50 years, **or** one FDR or SDR with bilateral breast cancer **and** one FDR or SDR with breast cancer of average age <60 years.
- *Male breast cancer:* one male breast cancer **and** one of 2 in the same side of family:
  - one FDR or SDR <50 years; **or**
  - two FDR or SDR average age of <60 years.

## Surveillance

- Mainstay of surveillance is mammography, but has no role in patients aged below 30 years. 30–39 years exceptional cases with high risk/ mutations. Moderate and high risk – annual mammography 40–49 years. Thereafter, 3-yearly mammograms or more frequently in high risk on an individual basis.
- NCCN 2008 guidelines, NICE 2004, 2006 guidelines.
- MRI – role in younger individuals with very high risk.

## MRI: indications for yearly MRI screening (UK, NICE, 2006)

- TP53 gene mutation carriers ≥20 years of age.
- BRCA1 or BRCA2 gene mutation carriers – 30–49 years.
- 30–39 years with >1 in 12 risk (8%) of developing breast cancer in the next 10 years.
- 40–49 years with >1 in 5 risk (20%) of developing breast cancer in the next 10 years [or >1 in 8 risk (12%) in the next 10 years and previous mammograms showing dense breast/unreliable pattern].

## ACS Guidelines (2007)

### Recommend annual MRI Screening (evidence based)
- BRCA mutation.
- First-degree relative of BRCA carrier, but untested.
- Lifetime risk ~20–25% or greater, as defined by BRCAPRO or other models that are largely dependent on family history.

### Recommend annual MRI screening (based on expert consensus )
- Radiation to chest between age 10 and 30 years.
- Li–Fraumeni syndrome and first-degree relatives.
- Cowden and Bannayan-Riley-Ruvalcaba syndromes and FDR

### Recommend against MRI screening (based on expert consensus)
Women at <15% lifetime risk.

### Advice and intervention
- Women should be 'breast aware' and seek advice on any suspicious changes.
- **Exogenous hormones:** in high risk individuals or gene carriers use OCP and HRT with caution. Enhanced surveillance may be indicated.
- Minimize radiation exposure (especially chest), use shields for uninvolved areas, and use low dose equipment.
- Parity especially before age 30 years can reduce risk by 2–3-fold. Breast-feeding protects.
- **Lifestyle and diet:** regular exercise, limiting alcohol and fat intake, and reduction of excess weight reduces risk.
- **Tamoxifen:** although debate continues, tamoxifen may reduce risk in LCIS (NSABP-P1 study by ~55%). Atypical hyperplasia (NSABP-P1 ~85% risk reduction), mutation carriers, and other high-risk individuals. Tamoxifen prevents risk of a second breast cancer by 40%. However, its use must be weighed against the significant side effects of increased DVT, PE, and endometrial cancer incidence. Raloxifene (SERM selective oestrogen receptor blocker) approved for post-menopausal osteoporotic fracture risk reduction. No endometrial cancer risk. DVT risk same as oestrogen. Showed significant reduction in breast cancer incidence (MORE study – secondary endpoint). (Further follow-up of MORE - CORE study, other trials – NSABP-P2).

- *Prophylactic risk reducing mastectomy (and reconstruction):* this is a major irreversible step and individualized multidisciplinary case assessment including psychological counselling is mandatory. Common indications are mutation carriers, high risk (>1in 4 lifetime risk, through family and personal history) and previous unreliable examination, imaging, and biopsy results due to nature and structure of the breasts. Risk reduction is not total, but 90–95% due to inevitable residual breast tissue. Removal of the nipple areola complex improves risk reduction. Reconstruction with expander/implants, or various free or pedicled myocutaneous flaps as a single or two-stage procedure should be available (see 'Post-mastectomy reconstruction', p. 136)
- *Prophylactic bilateral risk reducing oophorectomy:* in BRCA 1 and 2 carriers – along with ovarian cancer, risk of breast cancer is reduced. Recommended as soon as child-bearing is completed. Reduces risk by half.

## Management: familial risk categories

### Population risk
Manage in primary care – offer support mechanisms.

### Moderate risk
Refer to secondary care – mammographic surveillance annually, 40–49 years, and then 3-yearly (NHSBSP). Risk counselling, risk management advice, psychological support.

### High risk
Cared for in tertiary or secondary care with tertiary specialist input. Genetics referral if >20% chance of mutation in the family. Personal risk estimation. Counselling and support. Discuss risk reducing surgery. Mammographic surveillance, 40–49 years, annual mammography (30–39 years in exceptional cases, e.g. mutations). >50 years – 3-yearly (or more frequent, e.g. 18-monthly, tailored individually in high risk). MRI surveillance. (see 'MRI: indications for yearly MRI screening', p. 166).

## Further reading

Saslow D, Boetes C, Burke W, Harms S, Leach MO, Lehman CD, *et al.* American Cancer Society guidelines for breast screening with MRI as an adjunct to mammography. *CA Cancer J Clin* 2007; **57(2)**:75–89.

NCCN guidelines (2008): http://www.nccn.org/professionals/default.asp

NICE (2004). Management breast cancer risk surveillance: http://www.nice.org.uk/nicemedia/pdf/**CG14**fullguidance.pdf

NICE (2006): http://www.nice.org.uk/nicemedia/pdf/**CG41**quickrefguide1.pdf

# Breast cancer: key trials and evidence base

The following are a selection of some of the key trials that have helped change practice in breast cancer management.

Breast cancer risk

- *Million women study (observational study):* $n$ = 1 million women who accepted mammography invitation. Breast cancer relative risk of 2.0 (1.3 for oestrogen only) in current users of combined HRT preparations after 2.5 years.
- *HERS-2 study, WHI study* (randomized placebo-controlled HRT studies): WHI showed increased rate of MI, Strokes, PE, and breast cancer. Hip fractures and colorectal cancers reduced (study terminated early due to risks).

Screening studies

- Swedish two-counties study ($n$ = 133,000), HIP study (60,000; see 'Breast screening, p. 90); UK – Edinburgh trial (237,000); Canada –CNBCS (89,835); Stockholm Mammographic Screening Trial (59,107).
- FH01 (effectiveness of mammographic surveillance in those <50 years with family history): *ACRIN6666* (ultrasound screening), *ACRIN6667* (MRI) **MARIBS** (MRI screening in high risk cases, $n$ = 839).

Breast cancer prevention

- *IBIS-1* ($n$ = 7152, increased risk individuals – family history, ADH, LCIS, etc. – ~33% breast cancer (ER+) reduction in tamoxifen users, endometrial cancer increased by 2–3-fold), *NSABP-P1* ($n$ = 13,388, tamoxifen in high risk, including LCIS – risk reduction by ~50%). *Royal Marsden chemoprevention trial* (8 years of tamoxifen in family history positives – reduced ER+ breast cancer incidence at 20-year follow-up, but study had limitations).
- *STAR-NSABP-P2* (high risk individuals – tamoxifen vs. raloxifene), *MORE* (raloxifene trial for osteoporosis – reduced ER+ invasive breast cancer risk by ~90%). Same group – further follow-up – CORE study
- *IBIS-II* (prevention arm - anastrozole), MAP-2 (exemestane).

DCIS

*IBIS-II, SLOANE Project* (National DCIS Audit – 5-year period), *RTOG98-04, NSABP-B24* (tamoxifen beneficial), *NSABP-B06 and B17, and EORTC 10853* (radiotherapy decreases recurrence, but overall survival same), *UK-DCIS trial* (radiotherapy decreases recurrence, tamoxifen no benefit), *NSABP-B35* (tamoxifen vs. anastrazole in DCIS).

Surgical procedure

- NSABP-B04 (1971–1974; no significant difference in survival or DFS between radical mastectomy vs. simple mastectomy+ axillary, chest wall, supraclavicular and internal mammary RT in node +ves vs. simple mastectomy without RT), NSABP-B06 (1976–1984; mastectomy vs. lumpectomy vs. lumpectomy + RT (all including ANC) – no significant survival difference).

- **Milan trial** (mastectomy vs. QUART – quadrantectomy + ANC + RT) **NCI, EORTC 10801, DBCCG**-Danish (1983–1987) trials of mastectomy vs. lumpectomy + RT – all survival rates the same.

## Axillary management

**Sentinel node – ALMANAC** (1999–2003 SLN-515 pts, ANC-516 pts): positive SLN, followed by RT or ANC. Severe lymphoedema reduced from 13 to 5%, sensory loss 31 to 11%, axillary recurrence at 12 months – 4 vs. 1 patient in SLN group, 7 deaths each). **EORTC 10981 -AMAROS Trial, NSABP-B32** (ANC vs. SNB +/– ANC, SNB 90% sensitive). **IEO185 Trial** (ANC vs. SNB +/– ANC – both arms identical, 0% relapse at median 26 months follow-up for negative SNB cases. 96% overall accuracy). **ACOSOG-Z0010, 0011.**

## Endocrine treatment

- **AI studies:** in general DFS and DDFS are reduced (around 20%) compared with tamoxifen. Overall survival is the same, but longer-term results are awaited. ATAC (RCT – 5 years up-front anastrozole or tamoxifen alone or in combination – combination arm stopped, n = 9366, DFS 17% improvement over tamoxifen, 3.3% absolute improvement), BIG-I-98 (RCT – up-front letrozole later changed to switching trial), IES (RCT– exemestane switching trial), TEAM (upfront exemestane ), IMPACT (upfront anastrozole), ABCSG and ARNO95 (anastrozole switching), MA-17 (n = 5187. letrozole – 5 years after 5 years of tamoxifen – study terminated at 4 years due to improvement, 4.8% reduction in DFS, 7.5% absolute benefit in node positive patients, and 39% improvement in DDFS, but overall survival same – in node + OS improved), ITA Study.
- **NSABP B-24 and P-17:** tamoxifen in DCIS + lumpectomy + RT (tamoxifen reduced ipsilateral recurrence by 30%, tamoxifen + RT reduced by 66%), NSABP-B14 (tamoxifen – ER+, node negative cancer – no benefit in continuing beyond 5 years)
- ATTOM (>5 years tamoxifen in early breast cancer), ATLAS (>5 years tamoxifen) IBIS-II (DCIS arm – anastrozole vs. tamoxifen in DCIS), ATLAS, NSABP-B-35. ZEBRA trial (Zoladex–Goserelin study in early breast cancer, goserelin equivalent to CMF in ER+ pre/peri-menopausals), SOFEA (fulvestrant +/– anastrozole vs. exemestane – post-menopausal ER+ advanced cancer), TEXT (triptorelin), ABCSG12 (Goserelin+ tamoxifen vs. G+ anastrozole, +/- zoledronic acid), ABC-OAS trial, FASG-06 (tamoxifen+ triptorelin vs. FEC), SWOG-S0226 (anastrozole +/– fulvestrant as first line in metastatic disease).

## Radiotherapy

- **START, PRIME, SUPREMO** (post-mastectomy RT), **BASO-II**.
- **DBCCG 82b,c and British Columbia trial** (NEJM 1997) - recurrence rate and overall survival improved with post-mastectomy RT.
- **Value of RT following BCS in DCIS – NSABP-B17, EORTC10853, UK/ANZ trial** (all have significant reduction in ipsilateral recurrence, but no true survival advantage).
- **RTOG 9517** (brachytherapy – good control), **TARGIT, ELLIOT** (intraoperative radiotherapy), **NSABP-B39, RTOG0319,0413.**

Chemotherapy and other adjuvants

- *Trastuzumab trials: HERA, NSABP-B31 and NCCTG N9831* (87% DFS at 3 years in trastuzumab group vs. 75% in control, absolute survival- 94.3 vs. 91.7%), *BCIRG-006* (AC→T vs. AC→TH vs. TCH).
- *Neo-adjuvant chemotherapy: NSABP-B18* (no survival disadvantage, increased rate of breast conservation 68 vs. 60%).
- *TACT* (DNA polymerisms in prediction of response to taxane), *TOPIC, NEOTANGO* (paclitaxel and gemcitabine), *NSABP – B27, B28* (AC vs. AC→paclitaxel), *BCIRG001* (FAC vs. TAC - docetaxel), *BCIRG008* (TAC vs. TAC→capecitabine), *ECOG1199* (AC→ paclitaxel vs. docetaxel), *CALGB studies*.
- *MINDACT* (gene expression profiling, as a predictive factor to select node negative patients for chemotherapy).
- *AZURE* (zoledronic acid).

# Organization of breast cancer care and medicolegal aspects

Experience in the UK and other countries has shown the benefits of a structured re-organization of breast cancer services and its recognition as a separate specialty, resulting in a significant reduction in overall mortality and morbidity from breast cancer. One of the primary drivers for this change has been the introduction of breast screening.

The various factors needed to provide high quality breast cancer service include:
- Good quality Information: data collection on epidemiology and results of treatment.
- Introduction of screening in the appropriate age groups.
- Focus on risk reduction.
- Adequate funding/structure to improve early diagnosis and treatment
- Input into palliative care.
- Multidisciplinary team working and decision making.
- Breast care specialist nurse support.
- Patient access to information and communication.
- Robust audit process and quality control of all aspects of care.
- Research/trials with appropriate funding.
- Adequate administrative support.
- Manpower planning and continued training.
- Recognition of breast cancer care as a dedicated specialty.
- Good horizon scanning to plan for the future – changes in incidence, newer treatments, and health care cost projection.

## Breast cancer: medicolegal aspects
- Common reasons for litigation include:
  - delay in diagnosis and treatment;
  - poor informed consent process and inadequate discussion of options;
  - unnecessary over-aggressive/radical treatment (e.g. mastectomy where BCS was appropriate);
  - unrealistic patient cosmetic expectations and failure to warn about needing future procedures;
  - inappropriate management of complications;
  - breakdown/poor communication channels or access to information.
- For a claim to be sustained the care received should have fallen below established/accepted standards and a resulting direct tangible harm has occurred to the plaintiff ('causation'). Oncology teams must therefore continually update themselves to keep up with national standards.
- Steps to reduce litigation include:
  - robust informed consent and decision making process giving adequate time (generally more than one sitting) for decision making;
  - input and continued counselling from breast care nurses;
  - adequate documentation at all stages;
  - use of patient information leaflets and, where appropriate, audiovisual aids;
  - patient support groups;

- robust administrative process to avoid delays;
- frequent auditing of processes, patient feedback and continued staff education;
- multidisciplinary approach to decision making and care delivery;
- improved patient access for consultation/communication.

# Thyroid and parathyroid tumours

# Thyroid cancer

## Incidence

- Most common endocrine malignancy.
- Remains rare: 0.6% of all cancers diagnosed in UK in 2003.
- Overall incidence increasing.
- Age-standardized incidence is from 1.8 to 2.5 per 100 000.
- Population between 1995 and 2004 (UK): 1641 new cases diagnosed in UK in 2004 (350 deaths in UK each year).
- Female > male (ratio is 3:1) 3.5 per 100 000 in females ; 1.3 per 100 000 males (UK).
- Significant geographical variation.
- Highest rates in Malta (12.6 per 100 000 population).
- ↑ Incidence with age in males up to 75 years.
- Incidence remains constant in females aged 30–55 years, then ↓; peak at 35–39 years.
- 90% of thyroid cancers are well differentiated: papillary, follicular, and Hurthle cell tumours.
- 10% are poorly differentiated: anaplastic, medullary, and lymphomas.

## Prognostic factors

- Outcome for differentiated cancers treated effectively is favourable.
- Overall, 10-year survival for middle aged patients with differentiated cancers 80–90%.
- 5–20% develop local or regional recurrences.
- 10–15% develop distant metastases.
- 9% of patients die from their disease.

# Neck lumps: differential and clinical evaluation

## Definition

Any congenital or acquired mass arising in the anterior or posterior triangles of the neck, between clavicles inferiorly, the mandible superiorly, and base of skull posteriorly.

## Differential diagnosis

- Take careful history to include symptoms of systemic illness (malaise, fever, loss of appetite, or weight), and those specific to head and neck (pain, local infections, voice changes).
- Most are visible swellings – **site** of lump important in differential diagnosis.
- Multiple lumps are usually lymph nodes.
- Majority likely to be lymphadenopathy either due to primary or secondary disease.
- **Inflammatory:** acute infective lymphadenopathy, collar stud abscess, cystic hygroma, branchial cyst, parotitis.
- **Neoplasm:** metastatic carcinoma (2 years), 1 year lymphoma, salivary gland tumour, sternocleidomastoid tumour, carotid body tumour.
- **Congenital:** thyroglossal duct cyst, dermoid cyst, torticollis.
- **Vascular:** subclavian aneurysm, subclavian ectasia.
- **Thyroid:** goitre, cyst, solitary nodule.

## Clinical evaluation of thyroid

- Normal thyroid is impalpable.
- **Goitre:** diffuse enlargement of the thyroid gland (see Table 3.1).
- A discrete swelling (nodule) is in one lobe with no palpable abnormality elsewhere is a solitary nodule.
- Discrete swellings with evidence of abnormality elsewhere within the gland are termed dominant.

**Table 3.1** Useful classification of goitres in WHO grading system

| Grade | Features |
|---|---|
| 0 | No palpable or visible goitre, even with neck extended |
| 1 | Patients with palpable goitre: <br> 1A Goitre detected by palpation only <br> 1B Goitre visible and palpable with neck fully extended |
| 2 | Goitre visible with neck in the normal position |
| 3 | Very large goitre visible from considerable distance |

*Classification of thyroid swellings*

- **Simple goitre (euthyroid):** multinodular, diffuse hyperplastic (physiological, pubertal, pregnancy).
- **Toxic:** diffuse (Grave's disease), multinodular, toxic adenoma.
- **Neoplastic:** benign, malignant.
- **Inflammatory:** autoimmune (chronic lymphocytic thyroiditis, Hashimoto's disease), granulomatous (de Quervain's thyroiditis), fibrosing (Riedel's thyroiditis), infective (acute and chronic), amyloid.

## Diagnostic evaluation of thyroid

### Fine needle aspiration cytology

- Highly accurate and cost effective for discrete swellings.
- Cannot distinguish between benign follicular adenoma and follicular carcinoma.
- Few false positives with malignancy, but definite false negative rate.
- Less reliable in cystic than solid swellings (often yields only fluid).
- Fine needle non-aspiration cytology (FNNAC) is useful in assessment of vascular lesions found on FNAC.

### Diagnostic categories on FNAC

- **Thy 1:** non-diagnostic.
- **Thy 2:** non-neoplastic (including cysts, if benign epithelial cells present).
- **Thy 3:** follicular lesion/suspected follicular neoplasm.
- **Thy 4:** suspicious of malignancy.
- **Thy 5:** diagnostic of malignancy.

### Ultrasonography

- Formerly used as non-invasive supplement to clinical palpation.
- Limited use with nodules, but allows clear delineation of multinodularity.
- Of value for guidance of FNAC, reduces inadequate sampling rates.
- Useful to evaluate coexisting lymphadenopathy.

### Radioisotope studies

- Usually non-diagnostic of thyroid cancer, therefore of limited value.
- Used when toxicity associated with nodularity.

### MRI and CT scanning

- Indicated when the limits of the goitre cannot be clinically determined for fixed tumours and for patients with haemoptysis.
- Avoid use of iodinated contrast media with CT scanning as these can reduce subsequent radioiodine uptake by the gland.
- Gadolinium-enhanced MRI can be of use and does not compromise later radioiodine uptake.

### Serum calcitonin

- Useful if medullary thyroid cancer suspected.
- Not routinely used for all thyroid nodules.

# Thyroid status

The vast majority of thyroid nodules are benign (95%) and thyroid cancer is uncommon in euthyroid patients; therefore, assessment of patient's biochemical thyroid status is vital.

Serum thyroid hormone concentrations (thyroid function tests or TFTs) allows accurate evaluation of thyroid status to confirm the clinical diagnosis or to clarify a diagnostic problem.

## Thyroid hormones

T4 (thyroxine) and T3 (liothyronine)
- Stored in thyroid colloid bound to thyroglobulin (Tg).
- Control of synthesis and release is by thyroid stimulating hormone (TSH) released from anterior pituitary.
- Negative feedback system of TSH-release controlled by serum thyroid hormone concentrations.
- Thyrotrophin-releasing hormone (TRH) released from hypothalamus also influences TSH secretion.
- T3 and T4 bound in serum to thyroxine-binding globulin (TBG), thyroxine-binding pre-albumin (TBPA), and albumin.
- Only minute amounts of T3 and T4 are unbound; these produce the principal metabolic effects of thyroid hormones.

Precise assessment of thyroid function possible with assays for serum free T3, free T4, and TSH.

As a single test of thyroid function, serum TSH is the most sensitive, discriminating between hypothyroidism, hypothyroidism, and euthyroidism.

*Pitfalls:* hypopituitarism, with the 'sick euthyroid' syndrome and with dysthyroid eye disease – all may give false low results, implying hypothyroidism.

Carcinomas of the thyroid gland are autonomous and do not require TSH for growth, whereas benign lesions do.

When T3 and T4 feedback to the pituitary to decrease TSH production, thyroid nodules that continue to enlarge are likely to be malignant.

NB: measurement of serum Tg before thyroidectomy has no diagnostic or prognostic value, and therefore should not be undertaken.

# Solitary/dominant nodule

## Investigation

- A discrete swelling (nodule) in one lobe with no palpable abnormality elsewhere in a solitary nodule.
- Discrete swellings with evidence of abnormality elsewhere within the gland are termed dominant.
- Majority of thyroid nodules are benign, but solitary nodules pose the clinical problem of the distinction between benign and malignant diseases.
- **Thyroid nodules:** more common in 5–10% detected on palpation in 5; 2% in 4. Solitary nodule in 4 thought to carry a malignant risk.
- Rapidly growing, firm painful nodule in elderly likely to be anaplastic carcinoma.
- Young at risk of malignancy: solitary nodule in child under 14 years has 50% risk of malignancy

## Symptoms and signs that warrant investigation

### Patients with thyroid nodules who can be managed in primary care

- History of a nodule or goitre that has not changed for years, and has no other concerning features (i.e. adult, no history of neck irradiation, no family history of thyroid cancer, no palpable cervical lymphadenopathy).
- Impalpable, asymptomatic nodule <1 cm, discovered incidentally on neck imaging without other features of concern.

### Patients who should be referred non-urgently

- Nodule + abnormal TFTs – refer to endocrinologist. Cancer rare.
- Sudden onset of pain within thyroid lump (likely to have bled into benign thyroid cyst).
- New thyroid lump or lump increasing in size over months.

### Symptoms needing urgent referral

- Unexplained hoarseness or voice changes in presence of goitre.
- Nodule in a child.
- Nodule + cervical lymphadenopathy (usually deep cervical or supraclavicular).
- Rapidly enlarging, painless thyroid mass over period of weeks (rare presentation of cancer and usually associated with anaplastic thyroid cancer or thyroid lymphoma).

### Symptoms needing immediate referral

- Stridor + thyroid lump.

# Differentiated thyroid cancer

90% of thyroid cancers are well differentiated: papillary thyroid cancer (PTC), follicular thyroid cancer (FTC) and Hurthle cell tumours.

## Predisposing factors

FTC is more prevalent in iodine-deficient areas and associated with ↑ risk of anaplastic cancer. PTC accounts for 80% of tumours in iodine-replete areas. Ionizing radiation is significant risk factor and initiator of PTC. Exposure under age 10 years ↑↑ risk (peak age 4 years). External beam radiotherapy to head and neck for adult lymphomas or scattered radiation for breast cancer also ↑ risk.

## Genetic features

- Most well differentiated tumours are sporadic, but some have a genetic basis. *RET* proto-oncogene rearrangement demonstrated in 50% of tumours.
- Inherited predisposition includes:
  - relatives of those with PTC with no extrathyroid tumours;
  - Cowden syndrome – association of DTC, breast cancer and multiple hamartomas. Due to germline mutations in tumour suppressor gene *PTEN*.
  - familial adenomatous polyposis coli associated with germline mutations in *APC* gene with ↑↑ incidence of PTC.

## Prognostic scoring

Risk assessment important in patients with DTC using prognostic scoring system enables accurate prognosis provision and management planning.

- *Age* at time of diagnosis is consistently a prognostic factor:
  - risk of recurrence and death ↑ with age, particularly after age 40 years;
  - young children <10 years are at higher risk of recurrence.
- *Gender* independent risk factor in males.

### Histology

- Prognosis of PTC better than FTC.
- **PTC:** poorer prognosis with degree of cellular differentiation and vascular invasion and histological types 25–28.
- **FTC:** poorer prognosis with 'widely invasive' and vascular invasion features, as well as poorly differentiated carcinomas.
- *Tumour extent* prognostic factors:
  - size of 1 year tumour;
  - extrathyroidal invasion;
  - lymph node metastases;
  - distant metastases.

**Prognostic Scoring Classification**

### Table 3.2  Tumour, nodes, metastases (TNM) system

**Primary tumour**

| | | |
|---|---|---|
| pT1 | Intrathyroidal tumour | ≤1 cm greatest dimension |
| pT2 | Intrathyroidal tumour | >1–4 cm greatest dimension |
| PT3 | Intrathyroidal tumour | >4 cm in greatest dimension |
| pT4 | Extending beyond thyroid capsule | Tumour of any size |
| pTX | Primary tumour cannot be assessed | |

**Regional lymph nodes (cervical or upper mediastinal)**

| | |
|---|---|
| N0 | No nodes involved |
| N1 | Regional nodes involved. If possible, subdivide |
| N1a | Ipsilateral cervical nodes |
| N1b | Bilateral, midline or contralateral cervical nodes or mediastinal nodes |
| NX | Nodes cannot be assessed |

**Distant metastases**

| | |
|---|---|
| M0 | No distant metastases |
| M1 | Distant metastases |
| MX | Distant metastases cannot be assessed |

**Papillary or follicular carcinoma staging**

| | <45 years | > 45 years |
|---|---|---|
| Stage I | Any T, any N, M0 | pT1, N0, M0 |
| Stage II | Any T, any N, M1 | pT2, N0, M0<br>pT3, N0, M0 |
| Stage III | | pT4, N0, M0<br>Any pT, N1, M0 |
| Stage IV | | Any pT, any N, M1 |

## Papillary thyroid cancer (PTC)PTC)

Age at presentation is usually 30–50 years, 5 > 4.

### Pathology

- Commonest thyroid tumour.
- 1-year tumour can vary in size from tiny deposits to lesions >5 cm. Multiple foci can occur in same lobe as 1 year tumour or in both lobes (less common).
- Macroscopically solid, whitish, obviously invasive and 10% have complete capsule. Microscopically demonstrate true papillae (sometimes combined with follicles).
- Pathological diagnosis depends on specific nuclear features:
  - 'Orphan Annie' nuclei (*not* seen on frozen section as are an artefact of paraffin fixation);
  - nuclear pseudo-inclusions;
  - nuclear grooves (in oval or spindle nuclei);
  - psammoma bodies seen in 50% of cases (rounded calcified deposits).
- Spread to lymph nodes common, but blood-borne metastases unusual unless tumour is extrathyroidal, (when 1-year tumour has infiltrated through the capsule of the thyroid gland).
- 10-year survival rate is 95%

## Follicular thyroid cancer (FTC)

Accounts for 15–25% of thyroid cancers with greater incidence in iodine-deficient areas and patients with history of previous irradiation.

### Clinical features

- Age at presentation 50–60 years.
- Presents as discrete solitary thyroid nodule – increasing in size.
- Usually firm, but due to haemorrhage within lesion, can be softer.
- Cervical lymphadenopathy not usually present (only in 10%), but distal metastases may be (33%), as spreads via the bloodstream initially, with lymphatic spread being a late occurrence.

### Pathology

Malignant epithelial tumour with follicular cell differentiation.
Two main types, based on degree of invasiveness:

*Minimally invasive*

- Solid, encapsulated tumour (can look like simple adenoma).
- Thick, irregular capsule (unlike adenoma).
- Some foci of capsular invasion can be seen (often difficult to distinguish from traumatic rupture after FNAC).

*Widely invasive*

- Widespread infiltration of blood vessels, capsule and adjacent thyroid tissue.
- Capsule may be absent.
- Variable structural features, but follicular element will be present.
- Spreads via bloodstream to lungs, bones and brain (less common).
- Does not invade lymphatics.
- Tg on immunostaining usually positive.
- 10-year survival rates 70–95%.

## Hurthle cell tumours

- Represent 5% of thyroid cancers.
- High risk lesions with 5-year mortality ranging between 20 and 40%.
- Defined by presence of more than 75% of follicular cells.
- Macroscopically solid, well vascularized, and encapsulated.
- Microscopically can be follicular (most common), trabecular, solid or even papillary. Nuclei are pleomorphic with prominent nucleoli. Granular acidophilic cytoplasm is characteristic.
- Tg immunostaining positive (less so than FTC).
- May be more aggressive than other types of DTC, often associated with extrathyroidal extension, lymph node (25% at presentation), and distant metastases.
- Hurthle tumours tend not to concentrate $^{131}$I, therefore, total thyroidectomy should be considered.

# Medullary thyroid carcinoma and multiple endocrine neoplasia (MEN)

- Together these account for 5–10% of all thyroid cancers.
- 80% are sporadic and often present aged >50 years.
- 20% are familial medullary thyroid cancers and commonly present aged >40 years. There 3 main forms: familial non-MEN and multiple endocrine neoplasia (MEN) types IIA and IIB, all of which are due to mutations in the *RET* proto-oncogene. Associated endocrine abnormalities should be excluded in all patients and if a genetic defect is found, screen all family members.
- MTC is derived from the calcitonin-secreting parafollicular C cells
- Secretes a number of tumour markers, e.g. calcitonin.

## Three familial forms of MTC

### Familial medullary thyroid cancer

- Good prognosis.
- Slow growing course with no MEN features.
- Average age at diagnosis is >40 years.

### Multiple endocrine neoplasia type IIa

- Also have phaeochromocytomas – often bilateral and can be extra-adrenal.
- Hyperplastic thyroid glands are less common and usually unilateral.
- Rarely, patients can have amyloid deposits in upper back skin.

### Multiple endocrine neoplasia type IIb

- Typical phenotype in these patients with marfinoid characteristics (tall with high arched palates; neuromas on tongue and eyelids), but unlike true marfinoids they do not have cardiac lesions or ectopia lentis.
- Hyperparathyroidism is rare, but phaeochromocytomas are common.

## Clinical features

- Neck lump or lymph node metastases.
- Presentation of familial form as a phaochromocytoma is rare, but may occur. [All phaeochromocytomas should have MTC excluded by ensuring serum calcitonin is undetectable].
- Any bizarre thyroid mass or histology should have MTC excluded.

## Pathology

- MTC originates in the parafollicualr or C cells of thyroid gland, which secrete calcitonin.
- Calcitonin is antagonistic to parathyroid hormone (PTH) in the role of calcium metabolism.
- Bilateral C-cell hyperplasia is thought to precede MTC and is actually pre-invasive cancer, as lymph node mets can occur. True invasive C-cell hyperplasia is present when there are >50% C cells per low power field, or it is bilateral or extensive. (Therefore, can be distinguished from the occasional C cells in the normal thyroid.

*Histopathologically:*
- Ill-defined, non-encapsulated invasive mass.
- Composed of round, polygonal, or spindle-shaped cells with areas of tumour separated by fibrous bands.
- Elongated nuclei abundant with amyloid deposits.
- Positive immunostaining for calcitonin, carcinoembryonic antigen and amyloid is common, and aids diagnosis of MTC.

MTCs are indolent, but tend to metastasize early (commonly before tumour reaches 2 cm in diameter.

50% of patients will have regional mets at time of diagnosis (cervical and upper mediastinal).

10-year survival rates vary, depending on extent of disease at presentation:
- 90% when disease is confined to thyroid gland.
- 70% when cervical mets present.
- 20% when distant mets present..

70% of patients with MEN IIB have mets at the time of diagnosis with MTC (5-year survival in this group is <50%).

## Management
- The mainstay of treatment is to achieve loco-regional control surgically.
- There is no response to ablative radioactive iodine as C cells will not respond.
- For both sporadic and familial, diagnosis should be made by FNAC and serum calcitonin. Once diagnosis is established, all patients should undergo a total thyroidectomy and central compartment node dissection with the inferior limit of the dissection being the brachiocephalic vein (levels VI and VII).
- Patients with pT2–4 tumours, or palpable lymph nodes in the central or lateral compartment should in addition undergo bilateral selective neck dissection of levels IIa–Vb.
- The sternocleidonmastoid, internal jugular vein, and accessory nerve should be preserved unless directly invaded.
- Even in sporadic cases with disease presentation in one lobe, as >20% have intrathyroidal lymphatic spread.

# Anaplastic carcinoma

- Rare and very aggressive, accounts for <5% of thyroid cancers.
- Peak incidence between 60–70 years, female = male.
- At presentation, often inoperable and has very poor overall prognosis.
- Mutation of the *p53* gene is present in almost all anaplastic cancers, where it enhances the transformed phenotype. It is hoped that in the future, enzyme inhibitors that prevent tumour growth may be identified.
- Mutations in the *RAS* proto-oncogene initiate anaplastic cancer. Mucomycin blocks *RAS* by interfering with farnesylation of the RAS protein and, therefore, with tumour growth.

## Clinical features

- Rapidly growing neck mass.
- Tumour rapidly invades local structures – causing symptoms of dysphagia, dyspnoea, dysphonia, or threatened airway.
- Metastasizes via bloodstream and lymphatics.

## Pathology

- FNA specimens containing giant multinucleated and pleomorphic tumour cells, with high mitotic rate and vascularity.
- Due to common finding of foci of papillary or follicular carcinoma in anaplastic tumour, has been thought to originate in an unrecognized or untreated differentiated tumour.
- Non-encapsulated and often contain areas of necrosis.

## Management

- If FNAC has not confirmed the diagnosis, open, core biopsy may be useful.
- Any evidence of distal spread should indicate that surgery as a therapeutic treatment is not indicated. The aim of treatment is to optimize quality of life, maintaining the integrity of aero-digestive tract. In impending airway obstruction, central thyroid resection only should be performed, freeing the trachea +/– tracheostomy.
- In a very small number of cases chemotherapy/radiotherapy + surgery may achieve slightly prolonged survival.
- $^{131}$I ablation or therapy has no use in anaplastic cancer.
- External beam radiotherapy is the mainstay of treatment +/– chemotherapy.
- Rarely, if a patient is found to have no extrathyroidal spread, a total thyroidectomy and central neck dissection should be performed.

# Rare thyroid tumours: lymphomas, SCC, and secondaries

Thyroid lymphomas
- These represent 5% of all thyroid malignancies.
- More than 50% present at age <60 years, female > male   Prognosis is excellent.
- Primary lymphomas occur on a background of Hashimoto's thyroiditis in most cases (including those in which Hashimoto's is not diagnosed). Most are non-Hodgkin's B-cell lymphomas, but some are MALT (mucosa-associated lymphoid tissue). The confirmed diagnosis of Hashimoto's thyroiditis increases the risk of lymphoma 70-fold.
- Lymphomas can be associated with a previous history of thyroxine replacement therapy, and may present as hypothyroidism or even recurrent laryngeal nerve palsy.
- FNAC confirms diagnosis, with the addition of molecular techniques. In order to allow the full range of immunocytological tests a core biopsy may be needed. Most are of diffuse histiocytic type, varying from intermediate to high grade. Tumour cells appear monomorphic , non-cohesive and stain positive for lymphocyte markers like CD20.
- MALTomas rarely disseminate; therefore vital to differentiate from B-cell lymphomas.
- Extrathyroidal extension or metastases confer a worse prognosis.
- Staging should be performed with total body scanning and bone marrow biopsy.

Staging
- **IE:** localized to thyroid gland.
- **IIE:** thyroid involved and >1 lymph node on ipsilateral side of diaphragm.
- **IIIE:** Disease on both sides of the diaphragm.
- **IVE:** Disseminated disease.

Treatment
- Thyroidectomy is not indicated and mainstay of treatment is radiotherapy +/– chemotherapy.
- 30% of clinically localized tumours develop distant metastases, so chemotherapy provides the element of systemic treatment. Most centres use radiotherapy and chemotherapy for IE disease, with a 5-year survival rate of 80%. Chemotherapy regimes do vary, but usually use cyclophosphamide, doxorubicin, vincristine, and prednisolone.
- For MALTomas, treatment with radiotherapy gives a 5-year survival rate of 90%.
- It is vital to note that, in thyroid lymphoma, tracheal obstruction almost always responds to chemotherapy, negating the requirement for tracheostomy.
- Those with stage IVE disease have a 5-year survival rate of <35%.

## SCC

- Rare tumour, differing from the squamous metaplasia seen in papillary cancers.
- Aggressive disease course similar to anaplastic cancer. Most are unresectable giving a poor prognosis.

### Secondary disease of the thyroid

- Occasionally, the thyroid gland is the site of metastatic spread from other tumours, such as primary cancers of the breast and kidney.
- Clinical assessment should indicate the correct diagnosis, which can be confirmed by FNAC.
- If the primary disease is otherwise well controlled, resection of the thyroid gland is indicated.

# Indications for thyroid lobectomy and total thyroidectomy

- *Lobectomy:* complete removal of one thyroid lobe including isthmus.
- *Near-total lobectomy:* total lobectomy leaving only the smallest amount of thyroid tissue (to protect recurrent laryngeal nerves).
- *Near-total thyroidectomy:* complete removal of one lobe (lobectomy) with near-total lobectomy on contralateral side *or* bilateral near-total.
- *Total thyroidectomy:* removal of both lobes, isthmus, and pyramidal lobe.

Previously used terms 'subtotal lobectomy' and 'subtotal thyroidectomy' should be avoided due to their imprecise description.

### Recurrent laryngeal nerve

- This should be identified and preserved in almost all cases.
- Permanent damage to this nerve should not occur in >5% of operations for thyroid cancer. Bilateral injuries are rare and rates of injury are greater in re-operations. In malignant disease, tumours can infiltrate the nerve, contributing to nerve palsy rates.
- In small cancers and benign disease, where no infiltration of the nerve has occurred, total thyroidectomy is not associated with any greater risk of nerve palsy, compared with lesser operative procedures, *if* the nerves are identified.

### External branch of the superior laryngeal nerve

This should be preserved by ligation of the superior thyroid vessels close to the thyroid capsule. Damage to this nerve is associated with morbidity, particularly in changes to voice quality.

### Parathyroid glands

Attempts should be made to identify and preserve these glands. If there is compromise to their blood supply, they should be excised and re-implanted into muscle. Level VI, central neck compartment dissection for lymph nodes is associated with a greater risk of post-operative hypoparathyroidism.

### Indications for surgery: papillary cancer

Node negative cancer <1 cm should be treated by lobectomy + levothyroxine therapy.

In most patients a total thyroidectomy is indicated, including those with:
- Tumours >1 cm tumours.
- Multifocal disease.
- Extrathyroidal spread.
- Familial disease.
- Clinically involved nodes.
- History of neck irradiation in childhood.

If diagnosis is made post-lobectomy, completion thyroidectomy is indicated and should be offered as soon as possible.

Tumours >1 cm, but in whom risk of recurrence is thought to be low by the MDT, lobectomy can be performed.

High risk patients include:
• Males.
• Age >45 years.
• Tumours >4 cm in diameter.
• Extracapsular or extrathyroidal disease.

Patients who have any of the high risk features and clinically uninvolved lymph nodes, should undergo total thyroidectomy + level VI node dissection.

At surgery, if palpable nodes are discovered in level VI, these should be dissected.

If suspicious nodes are found pre-/intraoperatively in the lateral neck, disease can be confirmed by FNAC or frozen section and a selective block dissection (IIa–Vb) should be performed, preserving sternocleidomastoid muscle, internal jugular vein, and accessory nerve.

### Indications for surgery: follicular cancer

• As FNAC cannot distinguish between benign or malignant follicular cells, Thy 3 result requires lobectomy.
• If histopathologically after lobectomy, follicular adenoma or an hyperplastic nodule are identified, no further treatment is necessary.
• Follicular carcinoma <1 cm + minimally invasive features should be treated by lobectomy.
• If evidence of vascular invasion is present, total thyroidectomy should be performed.
• Follicular carcinoma >4 cm should be treated with near-total or total thyroidectomy.
• In low risk patients (Females, <45 years) with tumours <2 cm may be managed by lobectomy alone and levothyroxine therapy following MDT discussion.
• If the diagnosis of thyroid cancer has been made after thyroid lobectomy and completion (contralateral) thyroid lobectomy is required.
• Palpable/suspicious cervical lymph nodes are dealt with in similar way to papillary cancer (see 'Indications for surgery: papillary cancer', p. 192).
• Low risk patients with tumours 2–4 cm, with minimal capsular invasion should be discussed locally in the MDT.

### Indications for surgery: oncocytic follicular (Hurthle cell) cancer

Due to their aggressive nature compared with other types of DTC and because they do not concentrate $^{131}$I, total thyroidectomy should be offered.

### Indications for surgery: follicular and papillary microcarcinoma

Patients with DTC <1cm can be treated with lobectomy if:
- The tumour is not extracapsular.
- There is no evidence of vascular invasion, multifocality, metastases, or contralateral disease.

### Indications for surgery: medullary cancer

- All patients with confirmed MTC should undergo total thyroidectomy and central compartment node dissection levels VI and VII.
- In those with pT2–4 tumours or palpable lymph nodes in the central or lateral neck compartment should undergo bilateral selective neck dissection of levels IIa–Vb.
- The sternocleidonmastoid, internal jugular vein, and accessory nerve should be preserved unless directly invaded.
- Dissection of levels I, IIb, and Va should only be considered if there are palpable or suspicious nodes at these sites.
- In the presence of metastatic disease, surgery in the form of a total thyroidectomy and central neck dissection of lymph nodes should be offered, in order to prevent future compromise of the trachea, oesophagus, and recurrent laryngeal nerves.
- Patients who have been identified by the genetic screening programmes and who are disease free, but carry the germ line RET mutations, should be offered prophylactic surgery. These patients would be expected to have C-cell hyperplasia at time of presentation, but the transition to MTC may already have occurred. It is important to distinguish the need for therapeutic or prophylactic surgery, depending on the genotype, age of the patient, and the baseline calcitonin.
- In children with MEN2A should undergo total thyroidectomy before the age of 5 years. In these children, those older than 10 years (7 those with MEN2B) should have central compartment neck dissection of lymph nodes. Ideally, children with MEN2B should undergo total thyroidectomy within the first year of life.
- Gene carriers who are related to those with familial MTC should undergo prophylactic surgery after age 10 years, but lymph node dissection should not be offered until age 20 years.

# Pre-operative assessment: thyroidectomy

Written, informed consent, normally obtained by the operating surgeon, should be obtained from patients after full discussion of risks, complications, and benefits of surgery.

Specific complications relating to thyroid surgery, in addition to those pertaining to any surgical procedure should be clearly documented in the notes.

These include:
- Recurrent laryngeal nerve injury.
- External superior laryngeal nerve injury.
- Hypoparathyroidism.
- Laryngeal oedema – airway obstruction.
- Bleeding.
- Hypo- and hyperthyroidism.
- Wound infection.
- Keloid scar formation.

Thromboprophylaxis should be considered in the form of thromboembolic deterrent stockings, but prophylactic heparin preparations are not routinely required.

Assessment of vocal cord function is recommended prior to thyroid surgery, particularly in those with suspected cancer.

USS assessment of the neck can be helpful in the planning of surgery, but if there is vocal cord paralysis or bulky disease, CT or MRI imaging is indicated.

# Surgical anatomy of thyroids and parathyroids

Thyroid anatomy
- Thyroid gland consists of two lobes joined by an isthmus.
- Total weight ~15-25g depending on the iodine content in the diet.
- Each lobe is of conical shape, measuring ~ 5 × 3 × 2 cm.
- Midline structure, with isthmus crossing 2nd and 3rd tracheal rings.
- Gland is enveloped by its own capsule and deep cervical fascia, and is attached firmly to the trachea by the ligament of Berry.
- Medial aspect of each lobe lies against the trachea and larynx.
- Superior pole lies against the inferior constrictor muscle 7 posterior aspect of the cricothyroid muscle.
- Inferior pole flanks the trachea at level of 4th and 5th tracheal rings.
- Oesophagus lies posteromedially.
- Posterolaterally, each lobe abuts the carotid sheath.
- Sternohyoid and sternothyroid muscles lie anteriorly over each lobe.
- A pyramidal lobe extending superiorly from the isthmus on the trachea can sometimes be present and represents a vestige of the embryonic thyroglossal duct.
- The relations of the isthmus:
  - anastamosis between superior thyroid arteries;
  - tributaries of the inferior thyroid veins.

*Blood supply*
Each lobe derives blood supply from 2 main arteries:
- **Superior thyroid artery** (branch of external carotid artery): descends downwards and medially, entering the superior pole of the gland on the anterior surface.
- **Inferior thyroid artery:** from thyrocervical branch of the subclavian artery. Passes superiorly behind the carotid artery and jugular vein. At the level of the thyroid, it loops downwards and enters the middle aspect of each lobe, laterally – not the inferior pole.
The thyroidea IMA artery is present in ~3% of the population. It is a branch of the brachiocephalic artery, right common carotid or can originate directly from the arch of the aorta.

*Venous drainage*
- This can be variable, but is usually 3-fold and paired.
- **Superior thyroid vein:** drains into internal jugular or facial vein, and run with the superior thyroid artery.
- **Middle thyroid veins** (can vary in number): pass from the lateral borders of the lobes and drain directly into the internal jugular vein.
- **Inferior thyroid plexus:** these veins form a plexus within the inferior pole of the gland, are separate from the inferior thyroid arteries and drain into the brachiocephalic veins.

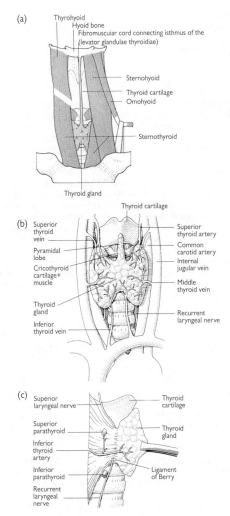

**Fig. 3.1** Operative anatomy: thyroid and parathyroid. From Rogers (1992) *Textbook of Anatomy*. With kind permission of Elsevier.

*Lymphatic drainage*

- **Upper poles:** drain to the anterior-superior group of deep cervical lymph nodes.
- **Lower poles:** drain to the posterior-inferior group of deep cervical lymph nodes.

*Nerves*

*Recurrent laryngeal nerve*

- **On the right:** arises from the vagus nerve, loops posteriorly around the subclavian artery and ascends behind the right lobe of the thyroid. It enters the larynx behind the cricothyroid muscle and the inferior cornu of the thyroid cartilage, innervating all the intrinsic laryngeal muscles except the cricothyroid. They are also sensory to the larynx below the vocal folds.
- **On the left:** arises from the left vagus nerve, loops posteriorly around the arch of the aorta, and ascends in the tracheoesophageal groove posterior to the left lobe of the thyroid, where it enters the larynx and innervates the musculature in a similar fashion as the right nerve.
- **Recurrent laryngeal nerves(s)** must be identified and preserved during surgery in all cases. Incidence of permanent damage to the nerve should occur in less than 5% of patients undergoing surgery for cancer, although rates are higher after reoperation.
- **Malignant disease** can lead to infiltration of the nerve by the tumour leading to nerve palsy, whereas in benign disease and small cancers, there is no increased risk of nerve injury during total thyroidectomy if the nerves are identified.

*Non-recurrent laryngeal nerve*

- Occurs on the right side (0.6%) more than on the left (0.04%). Is associated with vascular anomalies, e.g. aberrant take-off of the right subclavian artery from the descending aorta (on the right) or a right-sided aortic arch (on the left). In these abnormal positions, each nerve is at greater risk of being divided.
- The recurrent nerve is not always in the tracheoesophageal groove. It is often posterior or anterior to this position or may even be surrounded by thyroid parenchyma. The nerve is therefore vulnerable to injury if it is not visualized and traced up to the larynx during thyroidectomy.
- The nerve often passes anterior, posterior, or through the branches of the inferior thyroid artery. Medial traction of the lobe often lifts the nerve anteriorly, thereby making it more vulnerable. Similarly, ligation of this artery can be dangerous if the nerve is not identified first.
- Large thyroid tumours can displace the nerves from their usual anatomical locations and may even be found lying anterior to the thyroid.

## Parathyroid anatomy

These are small brownish coloured glands located in the space around the thyroid gland. Due to the longer embryological descent, the inferior parathyroids have a greater variability of location compared with the superior glands.

Four glands are usually present, 2 on each side, but 3–6 glands have been found. Each gland normally weighs 30–40 mg. In ~80% of cases, the superior and inferior glands have a symmetrical position, compared with those on the contralateral side.

Superior parathyroids usually found immediately superior to the junction of the recurrent laryngeal nerve and the inferior thyroid artery. ~50% of inferior parathyroids are found in the vicinity of the lower pole and ~30% are in the thyrothymic ligament.

Blood supply is from the inferior thyroid artery in ~80% of cases.

Because of their small size, delicate blood supply, and their usual anatomic position adjacent to the thyroid, these glands are at risk of being accidentally removed, traumatized, or devascularized during thyroidectomy.

### Further reading

Rogers AW (ed.) (1992) *Textbook of Anatomy*. Churchill Livingstone.

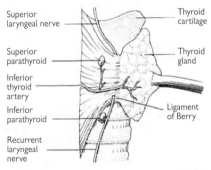

**Fig. 3.2** Parathyroid anatomy. Taken from McLatchie & Leaper (2006). Reproduced with permission of Oxford University Press © 2006.

# Operative technique: FNA thyroid lump

Fine needle aspiration cytology (FNAC) or fine needle non-aspiration cytology (FNNAC) should be performed on all significant thyroid nodules.

*Important aspects of FNAC technique*
- Aspirate different sites of the nodule or multinodular goitre.
- Aspirate obvious malignant nodules.
- With cystic lesions, perform biopsy of the cyst wall under USS guidance. If cystic fluid is clear, send for PTH and culture.
- Biopsy even if thyroid nodule is 'hot' on scanning (could be malignant).
  The thyroid gland should be palpated carefully and the nodule(s) to be biopsied identified. The procedure should be explained carefully to the patient and all the patient's questions should be answered completely – gaining verbal informed consent.

Inform the patient that local anaesthetic is not used, that the biopsy will take several minutes, that 2–4 aspirations are made and that we expect no serious complications, but there will be slight pain with minor haematoma or swelling at the biopsy site(s).

The patient is placed supine with the neck hyperextended to expose the thyroid; for support, a pillow can be placed under the shoulders. The patient is asked not to swallow, talk, or move during the procedure. It is best to talk to the patient and keep them informed of the progress of the biopsy.
- Clean the overlying skin with an alcoholic skin wipe.
- Use a 10-ml plastic syringe in one hand and firmly grasp the thyroid nodule to be biopsied with 2 fingers of the other hand.
- The needle is then rapidly inserted through the skin and into the nodule.
- Once the needle tip is in the nodule, gentle suction is applied while the needle is moved in and out within the nodule vertically.
- This manoeuvre allows the dislodging of cellular material and easy suction into the needle. During this period of 5–10 s, suction is maintained, and as soon as fluid or aspirate appears in the hub of the needle, the suction is released and the needle is withdrawn. The appearance of fluid suggests that the nodule is cystic.
- Suction is maintained and all the fluid aspirated.
- It is important to release the syringe plunger and remove the vacuum before withdrawing the needle; this allows the aspirate to remain in the needle and not be sucked into the syringe.
- Then detach the needle from the syringe and draw ~5 ml of air into the syringe.
- Reattached the needle to the syringe, and with the bevel facing down, 1 drop of aspirated material is forced onto each of several glass slides.
- Smears are prepared by using a second glass slide in a manner similar to that of making blood smears.

- The slides for wet-fixation should be placed immediately in 95% alcohol for staining with the Papanicolaou stain. For Giemsa staining, air-dried smears are necessary, and prepared slides are left unfixed and transported to the laboratory.

Usually 4–6 aspirations should be made, and these should be obtained from the peripheral areas and different parts of the nodule, sequentially, in order to gain representative sampling.

For larger nodules, the deep centre of the mass should be avoided, as it is more likely to contain degeneration and fluid, decreasing the chance of a diagnostic specimen.

For cystic lesions, the fluid should be completely aspirated and FNA attempted on residual tissue. Aspirated fluid should be placed in a sterile pot for cytological evaluation.

# Operative technique: total thyroidectomy

### Patient position

Supine with the neck extended (e.g. with a pillow or fluid-filled bag between the shoulders, and the headpiece of the table lowered), so that the thyroid is pulled superiorly and anteriorly.

### Incision

3–4 cm above the suprasternal notch and, in most cases, lie within the medial borders of the sternocleidomastoid muscles. Curve of the incision should lie symmetrically across the neck.

### Procedure

- The incision should include skin, subcutaneous tissues and platysma.
- Develop a plane between platysma and the underlying tissues, by holding the superior aspect of the incision with tissue forceps, dissecting laterally (where platysma is thicker and therefore easier to develop this plane) and superiorly, to the level of the thyroid cartilage notch. The central area can then be dissected more easily under direct vision.
- The lower flap of the wound should then be dissected free down to the level of the suprasternal notch, with minimal bleeding if in the correct plane.
- A self-retaining retractor can then be used to hold the wound open at the superior and inferior skin edges.
- The strap muscles are separated exposing the thyroid gland. The deep fascia is divided in the midline between the suprasternal and thyroid notches. This should be done lower down the neck, where the strap muscles diverge.
- Picking up the edges of sternohyoid, form a plane between this muscle and the sternothyroid below, by blunt dissection and then extending this plane laterally to the descendens hypoglossi nerve. The sternothyroid is then dissected off the thyroid fascia, exposing the lateral aspect of the thyroid gland.
- The larger lobe is resected first, allowing for an easier mobilization of the smaller, contralateral lobe.
- By retracting the strap muscles laterally, the gland is further exposed by pushing the surrounding fascia away from the thyroid capsule. The middle thyroid vein may be met laterally and should be ligated and divided, enabling the delivery of the lobe out of the neck.
- The recurrent laryngeal nerve is identified low in the neck, following its course to the entry into the larynx. It should be preserved in almost all cases.
- In order to then mobilize the superior pole, the plane between this structure and cricothyroid muscle is opened, and each superior pole vessel dissected out before ligating and dividing close to the capsule of the gland. This is done to ensure that the external branch of the superior laryngeal nerve is protected.

- The terminal branches of the inferior thyroid artery are divided separately, distal to the parathyroid glands that they supply, at the thyroid capsule. Identification of the parathyroid glands should allow the m[Q9] to be separated from the thyroid capsule on their vascular pedicle. If vascular supply to the glands is thought to be compromised, the affected gland should be excised and re-implanted into muscle.
- The lower pole can now be lifted up and freed from the lateral aspect of the trachea.
- In order to dissect the isthmus free, the bloodless plane anterior to the trachea is opened directly on the surface of the trachea – dividing the ligament of Berry below the cricothyroid muscle.

## Closure

Ensure haemostasis, place a drain in the thyroid bed and approximate strap muscles in the midline. By now changing the position of the patient's neck to the flexed position, tension-free closure of the superficial layers is possible. Platysma and subcutaneous tissues are approximated and skin closed.

## Lymph node surgery

**Table 3.3** Compartments of the neck

| Lateral | Level I | Submental and submandibular nodes |
|---|---|---|
| | Level II | Deep cervical chain from skull base to hyoid and divided according to relation to accessory nerve: IIa medial and IIb lateral |
| | Level III | Deep cervical chain from hyoid to cricoid |
| | Level IV | Deep cervical chain from cricoid to suprasternal notch |
| | Level V | Posterior triangle, divided according to relation to omohyoid muscle: Va above and Vb below |
| Central | Level VI | Pretracheal and paratracheal nodes from hyoid to sternal notch and carotids laterally |
| Mediastinal | Level VII | Superior mediastinal (as far as superior part of brachiocephalic vein) |

### Selective neck dissection

Any dissection involving less than level I–V, where spinal accessory nerve, internal jugular vein, and sternocleidomastoid muscle are preserved. The level of the node dissection should be recorded clearly in the operation note.

### Radical neck dissection

- Very rarely indicated.
- Removes all lymphatic tissue level I-V, including spinal accessory nerve, internal jugular vein and sternocleidomastoid muscle.
- Extended neck dissection is the removal of one or more of the additional lymph node groups, e.g. superior mediastinal, parapharangeal and paratracheal nodes +/– non-lymphatic structures, (skin, digastric muscle).

- *Modified neck dissection* is removal of the lymph nodes level I-V but preserving one or more of the non-lymphatic structures.
  - Type I: spinal accessory nerve preserved.
  - Type II: spinal accessory nerve and internal jugular vein preserved.
  - Type III: spinal accessory nerve, internal jugular vein, and sternocleidomastoid preserved.

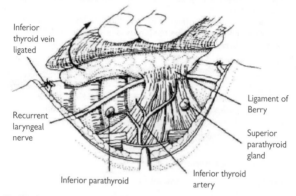

**Fig. 3.3** Anterior dislocation of the left thyroid lobe to show recurrent laryngeal nerve and parathyroids. Taken from McLatchie & Leaper (2006). Reproduced with permission of Oxford University Press © 2006.

# Post-thryoidectomy: emergencies and complications

### Early post-surgical management

- After total or near-total thyroidectomy, start patients on liothyronine (T3). Normal dose for adults is 20 µg TDS. This should be stopped for 2 weeks before a radioiodine scan or [131]I ablation of the thyroid remnant.
- Check serum calcium within 24 h of surgery.
- A baseline postoperative Tg should be checked within 6 weeks of surgery.

### Management of hypocalcaemia

- If the serum calcium is low within 24 h of surgery, it should be rechecked daily until it normalizes.
- Treatment should be initiated with calcium supplementation, with an initial dose of 500 mg calcium tds – adjusting the dose as indicated by the response.
- Monitor closely in order to avoid hypercalcaemia. If the serum calcium does not improve with oral supplementation, alfacalcidol should be added to treatment.
- Intravenous calcium is only occasionally indicated. Mild, asymptomatic hypocalcaemia does not require supplementation, but should be monitored closely.
- After total thyroidectomy, 30% will require calcium +/– alfacalcidol supplementation, but by 3 months only 10% will require continued treatment.

### Voice dysfunction

If external laryngeal nerve +/– recurrent laryngeal nerve injury has occurred during surgery, voice dysfunction may be present. This must be investigated if symptoms persist >2 weeks after surgery, as most injuries are a transient neuropraxia. Assessment should be by direct +/– indirect larngoscopy.

### Long-term suppression of serum thyrotrophin

Levothyroxine should be used and the dose adjusted by 25 µg every 6 weeks until the serum TSH is <0.1 mIU/L. (Most patients will require 175–200 µg OD).

### Airway obstruction

- Although mortality from thyroid surgery is very rare, airway obstruction remains the most potentially dangerous complication. Historically, it was thought that postoperative haemorrhage caused airway obstruction due to the pressure of the expanding haematoma on the trachea. However, this is now not thought to be the case, except in the rare condition of tracheomalacia.
- It is now thought that subglottic and laryngeal mucosal oedema leading to venous and lymphatic obstruction that occludes the airway. This can

occur if there is intraoperative manipulation of the trachea without the presence of any haemorrhage deep to the strap muscles.
- Recognition of the early signs of airway obstruction is vital and immediate removal of wound sutures should be performed.
- Conservative measures, such as provision of humidified oxygen +/− helium with IV steroids, should be started if symptoms are mild.
- It is prudent to seek the assessment of a senior anaesthetist at the earliest opportunity, as intubation may be required if airway obstruction is imminent.

# Adjuvant treatment: radioiodine therapy and radiotherapy

## Radioiodine therapy

- Following total or near-total thryoidectomy, some radioiodine uptake is exhibited by the thyroid bed. Radioiodine 'remnant ablation' is the term given to iodine-induced destruction of the residual thyroid tissue. 'Radioiodine therapy' refers to the administration of $^{131}$I with the intention to treat recurrent or metastatic disease.
- In preparation for $^{131}$I ablation or therapy, patients should adopt a low iodine diet for 2 weeks prior to treatment.
- If $^{131}$I is to be administered within 4 weeks of thyroidectomy, then levothyroxine is not required during this interim period. This would allow the TSH to be >30mL/U/L at the time of the ablation. If the interval is likely to be >4weeks, patients should be started on liothyronine (T3) 20μg TDS following surgery, stopping it 2 weeks prior to ablation, allowing the TSH to rise to >30mL/U/L.
- Pre-ablation scans of the thyroid remnant are not routinely used, but can be performed in order to assess the remnant size. If large remnants are revealed, further surgery should be considered.
- Pregnancy is a contraindication to $^{131}$I therapy or ablation. Breast-feeding should be stopped 4–8 weeks prior to treatment and must not be resumed.

## Post-operative $^{131}$I ablation

- There are no randomized trials recommending indications for $^{131}$I ablation and there seem to be no adverse effects with regard to second malignancies after treatment.
- In the USA, treatment is also given to children. It is recommended that all treatments are discussed locally and are individualized to the patient.
- Considerations should be made to size of tumour, presence of metastatic disease, completeness of surgery, age of patient, degree on invasion of tumour, and associated patient co-morbidity.

### Benefits of 131I ablation

- Eradication of all thyroid cells (including the destruction of postoperative microscopic disease) thereby reducing risk of tumour recurrence.
- Patient reassurance if iodine scan is negative and serum Tg undetectable.
- Possible prolonged survival.
- ↑ Monitoring sensitivity with serum Tg and, thus, potentially earlier detection of recurrent or metastatic disease.

### Administration

The recommended dose for ablation therapy is being assessed in trials, but is currently 3.7GBq in the UK. However, in patients with known metastases, 5–7.4GBq is used.

Three days after this treatment, the patient should then be given carbimazole 10mg TDS for 1 month. This has the benefit of counteracting the effects of thyroid hormone release, potentially precipitating a thyroid crisis.

### Indications for 131i ablation
#### *Definite indications*
- Distant metastases.
- Incomplete tumour resection.
- Complete tumour resection, but ↑ risk of recurrence or mortality (extracapsular spread of tumour, or >10 involved lymph nodes, or extracapsular spread + >3 lymph nodes).

#### *Probable indications*
- Less than total thyroidectomy (thyroid remnant present).
- Lymph node status not assessed at operation.
- Tumour size is 1–4cm in diameter.
- Tumours <1cm diameter + unfavourable histology (widely invasive and poorly differentiated follicular cancers or tall-cell, columnar-cell or diffuse sclerosing papillary cancers).
- Multifocal tumours <1cm.

#### *No indication*
Low risk of recurrence or cancer-specific mortality. Patients need to satisfy all of the below criteria in order for ablation therapy to be omitted:
- Complete surgery.
- Favourable histology.
- Tumour is unifocal, 1cm or less diameter, N0, M0, or minimally invasive FTC, or <2cm tumour diameter without vascular invasion.
- No extracapsular spread of tumour.

A post-ablation scan should be performed 3–10 days after the ablation. The patient should then be assessed 2–3 months after therapy to adjust the levothyroxine dose in order to suppress TSH 7 to make arrangements for Tg follow-up measurements and scanning.

### External beam radiotherapy
The main indications for adjuvant radiotherapy are:
- Gross evidence of localized tumour invasion at time of operation or the patient is presumed to have significant residual disease, especially if the tumour fails to concentrate radioiodine.
- Extensive pT4 disease in patients >60 years with extensive extranodal spread after surgery, (even in the absence of obvious residual disease). High dose radiotherapy as part of primary treatment is indicated for:
- Unresectable bulky tumours in combination with radioactive iodine treatment.
- Unresectable tumours that do not concentrate radioactive iodine.

# Surveillance and management of recurrence

Most recurrences of well-differentiated thyroid cancers occur within the first 5 years, especially with FTC. However, recurrences can occur many years later. Early detection of recurrence improves long-term survival, especially if disease is operable or takes up radioactive iodine.

Patients with DTC who have undergone ablation, should be seen every 3–6 months for the first 2 years, 6–8 months for 3 years with annual review thereafter. This allows for early pick up of recurrent disease, adequate TSH suppression and management of hypocalcaemia.

Commonest sites for metastases are: lungs, bone, brain, liver, adrenal glands, and soft tissues; lung mets commoner in the young and bone mets more common in the older patients.

Lifelong follow up is vital because:
- Late side effects of $^{131}$I can develop (e.g. leukaemia).
- DTC has a long natural history.
- Late recurrences may develop and if detected early, can be treated improving survival.
- Levothyroxine replacement requires monitoring.

Due to the varied presentation of recurrent disease, all follow-ups should include:
- Thorough clinical examination.
- Blood tests:
  - TSH and T4 to check adequate suppression and possible effects of Thyrotoxicosis;
  - serum thyroglobulin (Tg) – a sensitive marker of disease recurrence (TgAb should also be measured, as many patients will have these antibodies, giving a falsely low Tg result);
  - calcium – in those with hypoparathyroidism.
- USS neck (sensitive method of detection of recurrent disease in the thyroid bed and lymphadenopathy).
- CXR annually +/– CT scan without contrast (for micrometastases).

Detection of an abnormal mass should be assessed with FNAC, in the usual manner.

### Neck recurrence

Ideally, reoperation is required + $^{131}$I treatment. If this does not control disease, palliative high-dose radiotherapy should be given (50–66Gy – as patients are likely to survive for many years).

### Metastatic disease

#### Lung/soft tissue

Treatment is with $^{131}$I, as these sites are not amenable to surgery and can often confer significant survival. Repeated doses are usually given: 5.5GBq every 4–6 months until no further $^{131}$I is taken up.

If disease is persistent, continued radioactive treatment may be required. No maximum dose. FBC/U&E should be checked prior to administration.

Whole body scanning 3–10 days after treatment can be used to assess response to treatment.

### Bone metastases
Radiotherapy may be needed in addition to $^{131}$I in extensive disease, especially in the management of spinal cord compression due to vertebral metastases.

### Cerebral metastases
- Surgical excision if appropriate or palliative radiotherapy.
- In the surveillance for other cancers of the thyroid, there is no indication for Tg measurements.
- Follow-up for medullary cancer is with measurement of calcitonin or pentagastrin-stimulated calcitonin levels. Anaplastic cancer and lymphoma require regular follow up with thorough clinical examination +/− radiological investigations.

# Parathyroid cancer: clinical evaluation and staging

- Very rare malignancy, often diagnosed retrospectively after malignant disease presents.
- Cause of hyperparathyroidism in ~ 1–4% of cases.
- Incidence in 5 = 4
- Usually presents aged 50–60 years.
- ~50% develop local recurrence and distal metastases to regional lymph nodes and lungs. Development of the secondary deposits is accompanied by worsening hyperparathyroidism. In addition to histopathological confirmation, the only definitive criterion for a malignancy is metastasis disease.
- 5-year survival is 69% (death usually due to metabolic sequelae of hypercalcaemia.
- Some association with familial hyperparathyroidism – MEN syndrome.
- Primary hyperparathyroidism: 80% solitary adenomas, 12% diffuse hyperplasia, 2% multiple adenomas, and 1 % cancer.

## Presentation

- 95% are functional.
- 20% are entirely asymptomatic.

Signs and symptoms of the hyperparathyroid state associated with parathyroid cancer that may be found at diagnosis include:

- Subcortical bone resorption.
- Bone pain.
- Pathological fractures.
- Palpable neck mass.
- Renal calculi, renal disease, ureteric colic
- Peptic ulcer.
- Recurrent pancreatitis.
- Fatigue.
- Muscle weakness.
- Weight loss.
- Anorexia.
- Polyuria.
- Polydipsia.
- Dehydration.
- Anorexia.
- Nausea and vomiting.
  Parathyroid carcinoma should be suspected clinically if:
- Hypercalcaemia > 14mg/dL.
- Serum PTH >twice normal.
- Palpable neck mass in an hypercalcaemic patient.
- Hypercalcaemia + unilateral vocal cord paralysis (<10% have involvement of recurrent laryngeal nerve).
- Concomitant renal and skeletal diseases are observed in a patient with a markedly elevated serum PTH.

## Clinical diagnosis

- Clinical suspicion in patients with palpable neck mass and raised serum calcium (>14 mg/dL).
- FNAC contraindicated as risk of seeding in tract of biopsy.
- CT indicated to define local and metastatic extent.

### Sestamibi parathyroid scan

- Nuclear medicine procedure identifies parathyroid adenoma. Sestamibi (methoxy-isobutyl-isonitrile)is bound to $^{99m}$Tc. $^{99m}$Tc-sestamibi is taken up by thyroid and parathyroid gland (also enlarged thymus or neck lymph nodes).
- $^{99m}$Tc-sestamibi absorbed at a greater rate in a hyperfunctioning parathyroid gland.
- Correlates with mitochondrial activity within the parathyroid cells, oxyphil parathyroid adenomas: very high avidity for sestamibi, while chief cell adenomas moderate affinity, and clear cell adenomas minimal activity.
- 60% of parathyroid adenomas imaged by sestamibi scanning.
- Imaging unreliable in multiglandular parathyroid disease.
- Determination of hyperactive adenoma may take 3–4/24 when thyroid and normal parathyroid glands activity fades; the abnormal parathyroid gland retains its activity.
- In MNG or functioning thyroid Ca nodules increased uptake may make parathyroid localization unreliable.

**Staging:** As parathyroid cancers are so rare, currently there is no international staging system that can be used. Also, tumour size and lymph node involvement do not appear to be important in the prognosis. Patients are considered to have either localized or metastatic disease.

**Localized parathyroid cancer:** disease that involves the parathyroid gland with or without invasion of adjacent tissues.

**Metastatic parathyroid cancer:** disease that spreads beyond the tissues adjacent to the involved parathyroid gland(s). Mets to regional lymph nodes and lungs, and other distant sites e.g. liver, bone, pleura, pericardium, and pancreas.

## Treatment

Surgery with en bloc resection of tumour is the only effective therapy with pre-operative medical management of hypercalcaemia and other metabolic disturbances due to hyperparathyroidism.

# Management of deranged serum calcium

Treatment is based on aggressive rehydration/volume resuscitation, causing ↑ renal excretion of calcium, ↓ calcium release from bone.

- 200–500mL/h IV normal saline in order to maintain urine output >100mL/h.
- Then give loop diuretic, e.g. furosemide, to enhance calciuresis by inhibiting calcium resorption in the loop of Henle.
- During this resuscitation phase, monitor patient closely for electrolyte abnormalities (hyperkalaemia, hypomagnesaemia) and fluid overload.
- In acute hypercalcaemic crisis, the above measures will not normally alone normalize the serum calcium. Next line of treatment is the use of pharmacological agents, which inhibit bone resorption:
  - IV bisphosphonates 60–90mg slow IV infusion of disodium pamidronate, followed by continued oral, or repeated intravenous bisphosphonates to prevent relapse.
  - calcitonin (4–8U/kg) in conjunction with bisphosphonates, due to its short duration of action. Has rapid effect.
- IV phosphate e.g. sodium or potassium phosphate (Initial: 8mmol IV qds (32mmol/24h) aggressive: 15mmol IV over 6h) also has a place in the emergency management of severe hypercalcaemia, but is reserved for patients in whom other less toxic therapies have failed.

# Operative technique: parathyroidectomy/exploration

Intraoperative recognition of the cancer vital for a favourable outcome and reduction of risk of recurrence, with *en bloc* excision of the tumour avoiding rupture of the capsule. Such a procedure may involve ipsilateral thyroid lobectomy; resection of the recurrent laryngeal nerve (at risk from invasion by any residual tumour). Cervical lymph node dissection is performed for enlarged or firm nodes, especially those in levels III, IV, and VI.

### Incision

Should be made 3–4cm above the suprasternal notch and, in most cases, lie within the medial borders of the sternocleidomastoid muscles. Curve of the incision should lie symmetrically across the neck.

### Procedure

- The incision should include skin, subcutaneous tissues, and platysma.
- Develop a plane between platysma and the underlying tissues, by holding the superior aspect of the incision with tissue forceps, dissecting laterally (where platysma is thicker and, therefore, easier to develop this plane) and superiorly to the level of the thyroid cartilage notch. The central area can then be dissected more easily under direct vision.
- The lower flap of the wound should then be dissected free down to the level of the suprasternal notch, with minimal bleeding if in the correct plane.
- A self-retaining retractor can then be used to hold the wound open at the superior and inferior skin edges.
- The strap muscles are separated exposing the thyroid gland. The deep fascia is divided in the midline between the suprasternal and thyroid notches. This should be done lower down the neck, where the strap muscles diverge.
- Picking up the edges of sternohyoid, form a plane between this muscle and the sternothyroid below, by blunt dissection, then extending this plane laterally to the descendens hypoglossi nerve. The sternothyroid is then dissected off the thyroid fascia, exposing the lateral aspect of the thyroid lobe.
- By retracting the strap muscles laterally, the gland is further exposed by pushing the surrounding fascia away from the thyroid capsule. The middle thyroid vein may be met laterally and should be ligated and divided.
- Identify the recurrent laryngeal nerve (may need to be sacrificed).
- Look for upper parathyroids (1cm above the junction of the inferior thyroid artery and the recurrent laryngeal nerve). Look in the tracheo-oesophageal groove, retro-oesophageal, and retropharyngeal spaces.
- Look for the lower parathyroids (inferior pole of the thyroid gland to thyrothymic ligament).

- Perform transcervical thymectomy.
- Look in the carotid sheath.
- Perform thyroid lobectomy.
- Lymph node dissection is performed for enlarged or firm nodes, especially those in levels III, IV, and VI.

## Closure

Ensure haemostasis, place a drain in the thyroid bed and approximate strap muscles in the midline. By now changing the position of the patient's neck to the flexed position, tension-free closure of the superficial layers is possible. Platysma and subcutaneous tissues are approximated and skin closed.

## Adjuvant therapy and recurrence

- Due to rarity of this tumour, there are no large studies published to allow the systematic evaluation of adjuvant therapies.
- No chemotherapeutic agents have been found to be effective against parathyroid tumour growth or secretion of PTH.
- The appearance of recurrent or metastatic tumour can be the first sign of malignancy. 40–60% of patients experience a post-surgical recurrence, usually 2–5 years after the initial resection.
- These tumours are slow growing, so repeated resection of local recurrences +/– distant metastases can result in significant palliation.
- Recurrence is regional in two-thirds of cases, either in the tissues of the neck or in cervical lymph nodes.
- Local recurrences in the neck are difficult to identify as may be small, multifocal and may involve scar tissue from a previous surgery.
- If recurrence is hard to detect, USS neck, sestamibi-thallium scan +/– PET scan may be helpful.

# Oesophageal cancer

# Epidemiology, presentation, and clinical evaluation

## Epidemiology

- Variable incidence depending on worldwide location:
  - highest rates in Ethiopia, China, Japan, Iran;
  - in UK, 12.6 men/5.9 Women per 100 000 population;
  - increasing incidence in Western world – particularly adenocarcinomas near oesophagogastric junction.
- 9th most common cancer in UK (comprises 3% all UK cancers).
- 7000 new diagnoses/6700 deaths per year (UK).
- 5-year survival rates 8% overall (UK).
- 1-year survival rate 30% men/27% women (UK).
- Mean age 65–70 years/very rare under 40 years.
- 2/3 of those diagnosed >65 years age
- Male > female.
- Epidemiology of both oesophageal and gastric tumours changed – now concentrating adjacent to oesophagogastric junction.

## Presentation

Elderly male with short history of dysphagia is commonest:
- Progressive dysphagia – solids initially, then liquids.
- Site identified by patient as area of blockage, is usually above actual site.
- 25% of all presenting with true dysphagia will have oesophageal cancer.

### Other history

- PMH/ongoing Hx of symptomatic reflux.
- Regurgitation of food and saliva.
- Weight loss, anorexia, and emaciation – usually rapid onset.

### Occasional symptoms

- Odynophagia (painful swallowing).
- Hoarse voice/bovine cough – laryngeal irritation and invasion of recurrent laryngeal nerve.
- Chest pain – bolus food impaction and local infiltration.
- Respiratory symptoms – overspill symptoms or rarely.
- Tracheo-oesophageal fistula.
- Halitosis – residual food or bronchial involvement.

## Clinical evaluation

Often absent clinical signs:
- Weight loss/cachexia.
- Anaemia.
- Cervical lymphadenopathy.
- Jaundice/hepatomegaly – metastatic disease.
- Chest signs – overspill/fistula/metastatic disease.

## Referral guidelines for suspected upper GI cancer

- Dysphagia.
- Dyspepsia combined with weight loss, anaemia, recurrent vomiting, GI blood loss, or anorexia.
- Dyspepsia in a patient aged over 55 years with onset of dyspepsia less than a year ago, or continuous symptoms since onset
- Dyspepsia combined with at least 1 of the following risk factors – FHx of upper GI cancer in more than 1 first-degree relative, Barrett's metaplasia, pernicious anaemia, peptic ulcer surgery over 20 years ago, known dysplasia, atrophic gastritis, intestinal metaplasia.
- Jaundice.
- Upper abdominal mass.

All patients referred should be seen within 2 weeks by a team specializing in the management of upper GI cancer.

- Patients diagnosed with oesophageal cancer should be offered written information with a named contact on the multi-disciplinary team.
- All results should be confirmed by a second pathologist in cases where radical intervention is contemplated based upon histology.

# Barrett's oesophagus

- Pre-malignant condition referring to glandular epithelium cephalad to the gastro-oesophageal junction.
- Can lead to dysplasia and malignant change to adenocarcinoma.
- Usually secondary to GORD (oesophageal epithelium undergoes metaplasia from squamous to columnar epithelium following chronic reflux), but can be due to ectopic mucosa.
- Usually acquired, but possible genetic import – family clusters.
- 10% with GORD will develop Barrett's – bile reflux appears to be of greatest significance.
- 1% per year will progress to carcinoma (30× increased risk).

## Presentation

- Typical patient:
  - obese;
  - male;
  - >45 years;
  - poor lifestyle – heavy smoker/poor diet;
  - symptomatic reflux for over 10 years – heartburn/indigestion/ nausea and vomiting;
  - FHx of oesophageal/gastric cancer.
- Barrett's *per se* is usually asymptomatic – may have dysphagia or odynophagia.
- Usually nil to find on clinical examination.

## Diagnosis

By upper GI endoscopy:

- Irregular edge of pink mucosa (metaplastic gastric mucosa) seen extending more than 3cm above gastro-oesophageal junction.
- Long segments (8-10cm) – increased risk carcinoma.
- Significance of short segments (<3cm) unknown and often missed on endoscopy anyway.
- Ultra short segments (intestinal metaplasia at the cardia only detectable histologically) – much lower malignant risk – likely related to *H. pylori* rather than GORD.
- Structured biopsy protocol – multiple biopsies from all 4 quadrants, at 2cm intervals throughout the length of the oesophagus (+/– cytological brushings) and biopsy any visible lesion or ulcer (can develop in Barrett's).
- If dysplasia – more biopsies can be taken for accurate assessment

## Histology

- 3 types of glandular epithelium can be seen:
  - gastric fundal type epithelium with mucous secreting cells;
  - gastric junctional type epithelium with mucous secreting cells;
  - specialized columnar epithelium with mucous secreting goblet cells, amounting to intestinal metaplasia.
- 10–20% with Barrett's develop dysplasia (low to high grade, as per revised Vienna classification).
- Dysplasia most commonly occurs in intestinal type mucosa.

- 40% with dysplasia have carcinoma focus within dysplastic area.
- Low-grade dysplasia can convert to high grade and then cancer, but can undergo spontaneous regression.
- Those more likely to progress to malignancy are:
  - male;
  - >60 years;
  - endoscopy signs – ulceration and severe oesophagitis, nodularity, stricture, or dysplasia.

## Treatment

- High-grade dysplasia is indication for resection – re-evaluation demonstrates malignant change in up to 40%.
- If malignancy is ruled out, those with high-grade dysplasia should undergo endoscopic treatment (endoscopic mucosal resection/ablation)
- Oesophagectomy for dysplasia has excellent prognosis (80% 5-year survival) and is necessary in longer segments.
- Also:
  - lifestyle changes – lose weight/stop smoking/drink less alcohol/small, regular meals/avoid foods aggravating symptoms/raise head of bed to help reflux;
  - life-long acid suppression – PPI/H2 receptor blocker (little evidence this leads to regression of metaplasia);
  - also – photodynamic therapy/cold coagulation/argon plasma coagulation/radiofrequency ablation/multipolar electro coagulation endoscopic placation;
  - reduction of risk of progression to adenocarcinoma is not an indication for anti-reflux surgery.

## Follow-up

3-month to 3-year endoscopies will detect dysplasia before progression to carcinoma (interval depends on degree of dysplasia and hospital protocol).

Therefore, oesophageal cancers diagnosed in Barrett's patients tend to be early and have a good prognosis.

However, studies have reported a large number of endoscopies with little overall effect upon diagnosis and survival.

# Adenocarcinoma

- Comprise approx 50% all oesophageal carcinomas.
- Increasing in incidence.
- More common in Western Europe/USA and now more prevalent than squamous cell carcinoma.
- There are a number of risk factors (Table 4.1).

**Table 4.1** Risk factors

| | |
|---|---|
| Proven strong association | Barrett's oesophagus |
| | Male gender (M:F – 5–10:1) |
| | Symptomatic GORD – leads to: Barrett's metaplasia, obesity and high BMI, previous mediastinal radiotherapy [e.g. breast Ca (2× risk)], Hodgkin's |
| Proven weak association | Heavy smoking and alcohol (weaker association than squamous cell carcinoma) |
| | Poor diet – low in fruit and vegetables |
| | Achalasia/scleroderma/caustic or chemical injury to oesophagus- associated with metaplasia antimuscarinics/β-agonists/ aminophyllines – relax lower oesophageal sphincter and increase reflux |
| Possible association | Trichloroethylene (dry-cleaning) |
| | Silica dust |

## Protective factors

- **Regular NSAIDs/aspirin use:** weaker association than squamous cell carcinoma.
- **Helicobacter pylori:** may protect against reflux effects.

## Diagnosis

- History and clinical examination
- **Barium/Gastrografin® swallow:** irregular filling defect identified, but will miss a proportion of early cancers and can lead to confusion with other conditions that may mimic cancer.
- **Rapid access endoscopy and biopsy:** principal method of diagnosis – can take biopsies and evaluate small lesions more accurately than radiological techniques
  - *site* – predominantly lower 1/3 of oesophagus or gastro-oesophageal junction;
  - *appearance* – papilliferous mass/annular stricture/ulcer;
  - *biopsy* – multiple biopsies to confirm histology and grade.

## Treatment

Treatment should be arranged and planned by a multi-disciplinary team
- Surgery +/– neo-adjuvant chemotherapy.
- Chemoradiotherapy (if not fit for or refused surgery), although adenocarcinoma tends to be resistant to radiotherapy.
- Palliative procedures in metastatic or advanced disease.

## Oesophagogastric junction tumours

- Evidence shows they should be classified as a separate entity.
- True O-G junction tumours behave more aggressively than oesophageal tumours.
- It is also argued that these tumours should undergo different surgical approaches to ensure clear surgical margins.
- There are three types.

### Tumour types

- *Type I:* distal oesophageal (centre of tumour lies 1–5cm above anatomical cardia).
- *Type II:* cardia of stomach (centre of tumour from 1cm above to 2cm below anatomical cardia).
- *Type III:* proximal stomach (centre of tumour from 2–5cm below anatomical cardia).

# Squamous cell carcinoma

- Comprise roughly 50% of oesophageal malignancies, but is likely to decrease as adenocarcinoma incidence increases.
- More common in China, Japan, parts of Africa, Iran, where there is a very high incidence.
- No strong gender link (unlike adenocarcinoma).

## Risk factors

- *Heavy alcohol intake:* acts synergistically with tobacco.
- *Tobacco:* chewing or smoking increases risk 9-fold (much stronger association than adenocarcinoma).
- *Diet:* low in fruit and vegetables/high in pickled, smoked, and salted foods/high in nitrosamines/trace element and vitamin deficiencies/mycotoxins and aflatoxins.
- *Previous mediastinal radiotherapy:* e.g. breast Ca (2× risk), Hodgkin's
- *Achalasia:* cardiac sphincter malfunction (16× increased risk).
- *Coeliac disease:* gluten sensitivity, malabsorption.
- *Tylosis:* autosomal dominant condition with palmoplantar keratosis.
- *Paterson–Kelly–Plummer–Vinson syndrome:* Fe-deficiency anaemia, glossitis, and oesophageal web.
- *Human papillomavirus (types 16 + 18:* 15% malignancies analysed +ve for HPV DNA.

## Protective factors

Aspirin.

## Diagnosis

- History and clinical examination.
- *Barium/Gastrografin® swallow:* irregular filling defect identified, but will miss a proportion of early cancers and can lead to confusion with other conditions that may mimic cancer.
- *Rapid access endoscopy and biopsy:* principal method of diagnosis – can take biopsies and evaluate small lesions more accurately than radiological techniques:
  - site – predominantly middle or upper 1/3 of oesophagus;
  - appearance – papilliferous mass/annular stricture/ulcer;
  - biopsy – multiple biopsies to confirm histology and grade.

## Treatment

Treatment should be arranged and planned by a multi-disciplinary team
- Surgery +/– neo-adjuvant chemotherapy.
- Chemoradiotherapy alone (if not fit for or refused surgery).
- Palliative procedures in metastatic disease.

## Other oesophageal tumours

Other tumours of the oesophagus are rare.

## Other tumours of the oesophagus

*Benign*
- **Leiomyoma:** commonest benign tumour, usually asymptomatic + discovered incidentally.
- **GIST:** gastrointestinal stromal tumour.

*Malignant*
- **Leiomyosarcoma**.
- **GIST**.
- **Secondary:** direct invasion from stomach/lung.

# Staging classification

Staging needs to be accurate and thorough so that therapeutic strategies can be planned appropriately and potentially curative therapy can be targeted to those likely to benefit

## Modes of spread

Both squamous cell and adenocarcinomas spread in a similar fashion. Longitudinal submucosal spread is indicative of all types of oesophageal cancer and accounts for a high rate of resection margin positivity:

- **Direct:** circumferentially/longitudinally within mucosa (intra-epithelial), submucosa and muscle layer (intramucosal).
- **Local:** to adjacent structures, e.g. trachea, bronchi, pleura, aorta, pericardium, thoracic duct, recurrent laryngeal nerves.
- **Lymphatic:** intramural lymphatic permeation and embolization to para-oesophageal, tracheobronchial, supraclavicular, and sub-diaphragmatic nodes.
- **Blood:** to liver, lung, and bone.

## Staging

American joint committee (AJCC) on cancer designated staging by the TNM classification.

### TNM classification

*T: primary tumour*
- **Tx:** primary tumour cannot be assessed.
- **T0:** no evidence of primary tumour.
- **Tis:** carcinoma *in situ*.
- **T1:** tumour invading lamina propria or submucosa.
- **T2:** tumour invading muscularis propria.
- **T3:** tumour invading adventitia.
- **T4:** tumour invading adjacent structures.

*N: regional lymph nodes*
- **N0:** no regional lymph node metastasis.
- **N1:** 1–6 regional lymph node metastases.
- **N2:** 7–15 regional lymph node metastases.
- **N3:** >15 regional lymph node metastases.

*M: distant metastasis*
- **M0:** no distant metastasis.
- **M1:** presence of distant metastases – depends on site of primary tumour:
  - upper oesophagus M1a – mets in cervical nodes;
  - upper oesophagus M1b – other distant metastases;
  - middle oesophagus M1a – not used (same prognosis as distant nodes);
  - middle oesophagus M1b – non-regional nodes +/– other distant mets;
  - lower oesophagus M1a – mets in coeliac lymph nodes;
  - lower oesophagus M1b – other distant metastases.

## AJCC stage groupings

- *Stage 0:* Tis/N0/M0.
- *Stage I:* T1/N0/M0.
- *Stage IIa:* T2 or 3/N0/M0.
- *Stage IIb:* T1 or 2/N1/M0.
- *Stage III:* T3/N1/M0 or T4/any N/M0.
- *Stage IVa:* any T/any N/M1a.
- *Stage IVb:* any T/any N/M1b.

- *Regional or coeliac nodes:* should not be considered as having unresectable disease; should undergo resection of primary tumour and lymphadenectomy where appropriate
- *Distant metastases or lymph nodes in 3 compartments* (neck, thorax and abdomen): not candidates for curative therapy. 50% stage IV patients have distant spread, amenable to palliation only.

## Reasons for poor survival

- *Present late:* once symptoms are present, tumour has usually invaded muscularis propria or beyond.
- Often elderly with multiple co-morbidities.

# Staging and pre-operative preparation

Patients who should undergo staging
- Patients diagnosed with malignancy.
- Patients diagnosed with high-grade dysplasia (to exclude co-existing malignancy or focus of malignancy).
- Patients that have undergone neo-adjuvant therapy should always be re-staged.

Diagnosis by endoscopic biopsy
- Site and size of tumour.
- Biopsy for histological grade.
- Assess suitability of oesophageal replacement (stomach/colon/jejunum)
- Minimum 8 biopsies should be taken to diagnose malignancy.
- Routine use of chromoendoscopy is not advised, but may be of use in those patients at high risk of oesophageal cancer.
- **Barium swallow:** irregular filling defect, often long tortuous stricture with variable amount of dilatation above, but will miss a proportion of smaller tumours.

Staging: mandatory

*History and clinical examination*
- **CXR:** presence of mets/oesophageal invasion of lung/effects of respiratory complications/co-morbid disease assessment.
- **CT thorax/abdomen:** to assess local spread and exclude distant, unresectable disease. Spiral, IV contrast-enhanced scans with thin (5mm) collimation, and gastric distension with water or oral contrast. The liver should be imaged in the portal venous phase. CT cannot delineate the different layers of the oesophageal wall and can therefore not differentiate T1 and T2 tumours, and also cannot detect microscopic invasion in T3 tumours. Predicts mediastinal invasion in over 80% cases and involvement of aorta, tracheobronchial tree, and crura are usually easily identified.
- **Endoscopic USS:** all patients with oesophageal or oesophagogastric cancer who are candidates for curative resection should have EUS +/– FNA. Can assess tumour size, depth of invasion and local lymphadenopathy. Able to distinguish the component layers of the oesophageal wall and is therefore superior to CT for local tumour staging, as well as assessment of lymphadenopathy (see p. 22)
- **PET-CT** (with radio-labelled FDG)/bone scintigraphy.

Staging: adjuncts
- **Abdominal USS:** assess hepatic and peritoneal deposits.
- **Laparoscopy:** if suspicion of peritoneal spread. Consider in all oesophageal tumours with a gastric component to assess lymphadenopathy.
- **MRI:** reserve for those who cannot undergo CT or use for additional investigation following CT/EUS.
- **Bronchoscopy +/– USS:** if imaging evidence of tracheobronchial invasion.

- *Thoracoscopy:* if there is evidence of suspicious nodes that are not amenable to biopsy or assessment by CT, or other image-guided techniques.
- *Neck imaging:* EUS or CT in patients with cervical tumours.

Pre-operative assessments
- *Bloods:* FBC/U&E/LFT/Clot/G&S
- *Arterial blood gas and lung function tests:* assess lung function in terms of tumour effects and co-morbid disease.
- *ECG +/– exercise test:* assessment of cardiac status.
- *Respiratory or cardiology review*
- *Anaesthetic review:* suitability for single-lung anaesthesia and thoracic epidural. Only patients with an ASA score of 3 or less should be considered for surgery.

Pre-operative preparation
- *Nutrition assessment +/– hyperalimentation:* using a validated nutritional risk tool. At-risk patients are offered advice and considered for pre-operative nutrition. Those with BMI <18.5 or >20% weight loss – increased risk of post-surgical complications. Obesity also carries an increased risk of complications, but is rare in these patients.
- *Psychological preparation:* counsel patients about treatment options and supply detailed description of peri-operative period. Psychological counselling should be available if needed.
- *Smoking cessation.*
- *Dental treatment.*
- *Thromboembolic prophylaxis:* anti-thromboembolic stockings, low molecular weight heparin and per-operative pneumatic calf compression.
- *IV broad-spectrum antibiotics:* immediately pre-operatively or at induction (cefuroxime/co-amoxiclav).
- *X-match 4 units blood:* avoid use if possible due to risks associated with transfusion.
- *HDU or ITU bed available.*
- *Colon prepared:* if required as conduit (Picolax®/Fleet phospho-soda®/ Klean-Prep®).
- *Epidural placement:* for post-operative analgesia.

# Management algorithms

Resectability criteria (Table 4.2)

**Table 4.2** Resectability criteria

| | |
|---|---|
| Resectable | Patient fit |
| | >5cm from cricopharyngeus |
| | T1a endoscopic mucosal resection |
| | T1–T3 ± N1 |
| | T4 if diaphragm, pleura or pericardium involved only |
| | Lower oesophageal Stage IVa – any T/any N/M1a coeliac nodes <1.5cm and no major arterial or other organ involvement |
| | Salvage oesophagectomy following primary chemoradiation if conditions above met and no distant metastases |
| Unresectable | Patient unfit |
| | Systemic metastases or non-regional nodes |
| | Stage IVa involving major arteries or other organs or coeliac nodes >1.5cm |
| | T4 heart, great vessels or contiguous organs invaded |

Metastatic disease (Table 4.3)

**Table 4.3** Metastatic disease

| | | |
|---|---|---|
| Metastatic disease | Good performance status: ECOG<2, Karnofsky >60 | Chemotherapy: |
| | | 5-FU based |
| | | Oxaliplatin based |
| | | Cisplatin based |
| | | Irinotecan based |
| | | Taxane based |
| | | Up to second line then palliative support |
| | Poor performance status | Palliative support |

Palliative support (Table 4.4)

**Table 4.4** Palliative support

| Pain | DXT and/or analgesics |
|---|---|
| Obstruction | Dilation, stenting, argon beam laser, photodynamic therapy |
| Bleeding | Endoscopic Rx, DXT |
| Nutrition | Oral support, gastrostomy, jejunostomy |

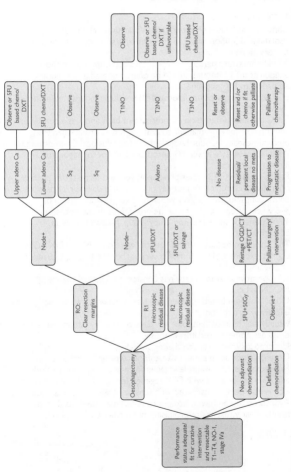

**Fig. 4.1** Oesophageal cancer management algorithm, based on NCCN guidelines.

# Neo-adjuvant therapy

## General

- Not everyone will benefit from neo-adjuvant therapy.
- Rationale is to downgrade tumour prior to surgery – all patients should therefore be re-staged following treatment.
- Pre-operative radiotherapy or chemoradiotherapy should not be offered unless in the context of clinical trials.
- Current standard of care under debate.

## Chemotherapy

- Controversial evidence shows that neo-adjuvant chemotherapy with cisplatin and 5-fluorouracil (5-FU) improves short-term survival over surgery alone.
- All patients with operable oesophageal cancer, apart form those with unequivocal T1 tumours, should be offered neo-adjuvant therapy according to UK guidelines.
- ECF (epirubicin, cisplatin, fluorouracil) are the standard treatments in the UK.
- E + C are administered on an intermittent basis and F as a continuous infusion – require permanent central line (PICC or Hickman line).
- Medical Research Council Adjuvant Gastric Infusional Chemotherapy (MAGIC) trial: 26% lower 1/3 oesophagus and oesophagogastric junction tumours.
- Pre-operative ECF: 3 cycles pre-operatively and three cycles post-operatively. Epirubicin IV first day of cycle 5-FU daily for 21 days as continuous infusion. Surgery within 6/52 surgery-only group or 3–6 weeks after completion of the pre-operative chemotherapy cycles in the peri-operative chemotherapy group. Median follow-up 50 months.
- Trial criticized because 10% of patients were off protocol DXT, Chinese cohort excluded. Slim 3.5-month survival benefit 16.8 vs. 13.5 months at 2 years.
- Pre-operative chemotherapy not considered standard of care by NCCN in US.
- Other platinum-based regimens, such as oxaliplatin, can be used just as effectively as cisplatin.
- Usually stay as in-patient for a few days, or as a day-patient, while the drugs are administered intravenously.
- Undergo 2 cycles – repeated after 3 weeks.
- Dose depends upon patient size, tumour type and renal function.
- Fluorouracil is now available in tablet form as capecitabine (Xeloda®) and trials are ongoing with ECX regimen (epirubicin, cisplatin, Xeloda®).
- ECF is also being investigated with sensitizing agents, such as paclitaxel.
- Also some research with taxanes (taxotere/paclitaxel) as therapeutic agents – early results are promising, but further trials are necessary.

Radiotherapy
*Oesophageal Cancer Collaborative Group meta-analysis:* no survival benefit from pre-operative radiation alone.

Chemoradiotherapy
- There is some evidence that pre-operative chemoradiotherapy may improve long-term survival, but most trials so far can be criticized (utilizing inadequate dosages or not giving the treatments concurrently).
- A recent meta-analysis showed reduced 3-year mortality and locoregional recurrence, but increased early post-operative mortality for resectable cancer.
- CALGB 9781 trial tri-modality vs. surgery alone for Stage I–III disease (cisplatin/5-FU) median survival 4.5 vs. 1.8 years.
- Neo-adjuvant chemoradiation vs. surgery alone for locally advanced disease: no significant difference.
- Ongoing trials include development of more effective combination regimens with newer therapeutic agents, such as taxanes, administering continuous low doses of cytotoxic agents throughout radiotherapy and delivering radiotherapy in hyperfractionated twice daily schedules.

# Primary chemoradiotherapy

Non-surgical treatment with curative intent.

## Indications
- Chemoradiation should be considered in patients with locally advanced disease not amenable to surgery, those unfit for surgery, or those who refuse surgery.
- In those unsuitable for surgery and intolerant to chemoradiation, single modality radiotherapy can be used with curative intent in localized disease.
- Should be offered as part of a clinical trial.

## Radiotherapy
- Given in a similar fashion to adjuvant therapy.
- Can be internal or external.

## Chemoradiotherapy

### Localized squamous cell carcinoma of the proximal oesophagus <5cm from cricopharyngeus
- Chemoradiation is the definitive treatment of choice for these patients (Table 4.5).
- Squamous cell cancers are more common proximally, present a greater surgical challenge and also often present later.
- In this situation, the survival figures are similar to those for surgery.

### Other patients
- Median survival is maximally 18months with primary chemoradiotherapy.
- Objective response rates are between 30 and 50%.
- Commonly used regimens include platinum-based combination regimens with fluorouracil (ECF), a taxane or a topoisomerase inhibitor.
- Pearson (1977) in Edinburgh showed 19% 5-year survival with chemoradiotherapy alone.
- *RTOG 85-01 trial:* SCC – DXT 64Gy vs. 4 cycles 5-FU and cisplatin + concurrent DXT 50Gy at 2Gy/day. Chemoradiation arm: median survival: 14 vs. 9 months. 8-year survival: 22% vs. 0%.
- *INT 0123 trial:* 85% SCC, 15% adenocarcinoma 50.4 and 64.8Gy DXT otherwise same regime as RTOG 85-01. Higher dose radiation gives no significant improvement in survival or local/regional control/recurrence.
- Recent trials have assessed paclitaxel, docetaxel, oxaliplatin, and irinotecan. Results remain inconclusive.

**Table 4.5** Primary chemoradiation

| Patient unfit for surgery or tumour unresectable or patient choice, but fit for chemoradiation | DXT 50–50.4Gy + 5-FU +- cisplatin-based chemotherapy or palliative support/intervention |
| --- | --- |
| Unsuitable for surgery and unfit for chemoradiation | Palliative support/intervention |

## Further reading

Pearson JG. The present status and future potential of radiotherapy in the management of esophageal cancer. *Cancer* 1977; **39(2 Suppl)**: 882–90.

RTOG 85–01 : *JAMA* 1999; **281(17)**: 1623–1627

INT 0123: Phase III trial of combined-modality therapy for oesophageal cancer : high dose vs standard dose radiation therapy.

JCO 2002 : **20(5)** 1167–1174.

# Operative considerations

## Operative settings

- All patients should be discussed in a multi-disciplinary setting and surgery only undertaken if it is the general consensus of the team. Surgical decisions should be taken based upon the predicted prognosis and the effect of intervention upon quality of life.
- Surgery should only take place in high volume centres with sufficient surgical and anaesthetic experience.
- Laparoscopic and thoracoscopic techniques should only take place in specialist centres, by experienced surgeons, with full informed consent and local clinical governance committee support.

## Operative indications

- *Malignancy:* fit patients with early lesions should undergo resection with curative intent (T1–3/N0/M0).
- High grade dysplasia in a long Barrett's segment (consider endoscopic treatments in short segments).
- Surgery has no place when haematogenous spread has occurred.
- Where radical surgery is based upon histology alone, the results should be confirmed by a second pathologist particularly relevant for Barrett's oesophagus with severe dysplasia.

## Operative rationale

Radical surgery and lymphadenectomy should aim for R0 resection – proximal, distal, and circumferential margin clearance. Treatment should aim to:
- Achieve optimal staging.
- Control local disease.
- Improve cure rates.

## Operative results

- Surgery is the only treatment modality that has consistently been shown to prolong survival, albeit only in approx. 20% cases.
- Excellent results for early squamous and adenotumours – 5-year survival >80% when tumour confined to mucosa and 50% when submucosa involved.
- Overall surgical treatment gives 5-year survival of 5–20%.
- In-hospital mortality should be <10%.
- Clinical anastomotic leak rates should be <5%.
- Curative resection rates (R0) should exceed 30%.

## Choice of operative procedure

- Type of surgical procedure is determined by:
  - site and type of tumour;
  - extent of lymphadenectomy needed;
  - surgeons expertise – type of reconstruction and use of pyloric drainage procedures should depend on surgical preference.
- *Upper 1/3 tumours:* require a cervical incision – transhiatal or 3-stage oesophagectomy.
- *Carcinoma above diaphragm:* requires thoracotomy for lymph node dissection – Ivor–Lewis procedure. 3rd cervical stage can be added to improve clearance and anastomosis performed in the neck.

- *Tumours below diaphragm:* require radical excision of lower thoracic oesophagus and gastric cardia/entire stomach – left thoraco-laparotomy.
- *In 2-stage/2-incision procedures:* possible with careful positioning to have 2 teams working simultaneously.
- There is no evidence favouring 1 type of resection over another.

## Resection margins

- Extensive studies show resection margins should be 10cm proximal to macroscopic tumour and 5cm distal (when oesophagus is in natural state).
- Adenocarcinoma of lower oesophagus commonly invades gastric cardia, fundus and lesser curve – some degree of gastric excision essential for adequate resection and lymphadenectomy in the abdomen.
- Adequate radial margins also need to be considered and contiguous excision of the crura, and diaphragm needs to be considered particularly for junctional tumours.

## Resection specimen

As a minimum, the pathology report should include:
- Type of tumour.
- Grade of tumour.
- Depth of invasion.
- Involvement of resection margins.
- Vascular invasion.
- Presence of Barrett's metaplasia.
- Number of nodes resected and the number containing metastatic tumour.

## Lymphadenectomy

Aims of lymphadenectomy include:
- Improve staging: minimum 15 LN excised.
- Reduce loco-regional recurrence.
- Increase the number of patients undergoing R0 resection – improve 5-year survival rate.

The majority undergoing surgery have lymph node metastases at presentation and the extent to which lymphadenectomy reduces local recurrence is unknown. The existing evidence that thorough lymphadenectomy improves survival may simply represent more adequate staging

In squamous cells, the number of lymph nodes involved are of prognostic significance, as is the ratio of invaded to resected lymph nodes

- *Abdominal single field dissection:* dissection of right and left cardiac nodes, nodes along lesser curve, left gastric, hepatic, and splenic artery territories.
- *2-field dissection:* involves thoracic lymph nodes, including para-aortic nodes (with thoracic duct), para-oesophageal nodes, right and left pulmonary hilar nodes, and tracheal bifurcation nodes.
  In Japan – extended superiorly to include paratracheal nodes, including those along left recurrent laryngeal nerve.

- **3-field dissection:** advocated in Japan and extends lymphadenectomy to the neck, including brachiocephalic, deep lateral and external cervical nodes, and deep anterior cervical nodes adjacent to recurrent laryngeal nerve chains in neck. 3-field operation is advocated in Japan for squamous cell tumours, but its benefits may simply reflect decreases in staging error as nearly 25% of all Japanese patients will have cervical lymph nodes. No evidence that 3-field lymphadenectomy improves outcome for adenocarcinoma and it is associated with a higher incidence of poor outcome

### Guidelines

- Studies show that 2-field dissection is associated with no increase in operative mortality or morbidity.
- In UK, 2-field lymphadenectomy should not be extended into the superior mediastinum or neck.

### Other treatment options

- Superficial cancer limited to the mucosa should be treated by endoscopic mucosal resection (EMR) – endoscope injects fluid below the tumour to make it more prominent and tumour is then removed with an endoscopic snare. Can be combined with other therapies e.g. post-procedure photodynamic therapy. Commonest side-effects are bleeding and stricture.
- Mucosal ablative techniques such as photodynamic therapy, argon plasma coagulation or laser, should be reserved for the management of residual disease following EMR, and not for initial management in patients with invasive cancer that are fit for surgery.

# Surgical anatomy of the oesophagus

The course of the oesophagus (Table 4.6)

- The oesophagus is a hollow muscular tube, 25cm in length.
- Extends from cricopharyngeal sphincter (C6) to cardia of stomach.
- Passes through lower part of neck, passing slightly to left and then returns to midline at T5.
- Then passes down and forwards through superior and posterior mediastinum, before piercing diaphragm through an elliptical opening in the right crus (oesophageal hiatus) at T10.
- Last 4cm lies below the diaphragm and is retroperitoneal with peritoneum covering anterior and lateral borders only.
- Terminates at gastro-oesophageal junction to left of midline at T11-junction marked by abrupt change from oesophageal (bluish) to gastric columnar (florid pink) mucosa – the 'Z-line'.

**Table 4.6** Course of the oesophagus

| | |
|---|---|
| Cervical oesophagus | Lower border of cricoid cartilage to jugular notch |
| Upper oesophagus | Jugular notch to tracheal bifurcation |
| Middle oesophagus | Tracheal bifurcation to midpoint of carina and gastro-oesophageal junction |
| Lower/abdominal oesophagus | Midpoint of carina and gastro-oesophageal junction downwards – includes the lower thoracic and abdominal oesophagus |

*3 Anatomical narrowings*: strictures (benign or malignant) commonest at these sites (measured from the incisors).
*15cm*: cricopharyngeal sphincter.
*25cm*: aortic arch and bronchial bifurcation.
*40cm*: diaphragmatic hiatus.

Layers of the oesophageal wall

- **Mucosa:** non-keratinizing stratified squamous epithelium. May have gastric-type columnar epithelium in lower 3–4 cm (non-acid secreting cells). If columnar epithelium higher up – Barrett's metaplasia has taken place. Mucosa is thick and thrown into multiple folds in collapsed state.
- **Submucosa:** contains sparse mucous glands (mainly upper + lower 1/3).
- **Musculature:** striated in upper 1/3 + smooth muscle in lower 2/3 – internal circular layer + external longitudinal layer.
- **Areolar tissue:** thin external covering.
- **Serosa:** no serosa except for short abdominal segment (last 4cm).

### Relations

- **Anterior:** trachea in neck/trachea, L bronchus and L atrium in thorax.
- **Posterior:** cervical vertebrae in neck/aorta in thorax – starts on left and then moves posteriorly.
- **Right and left:** in neck, carotid artery and thyroid/subclavian artery and thoracic duct also on left at root of neck/in thorax – pleura and lung. Vagus nerves closely associated on right and left. Crossed only by azygos vein and right vagus on the right – least hazardous surgical approach.

### Arterial supply

Requires varied sources of vascular supply and drainage due to its length.
- **Upper 1/3:** inferior thyroid artery.
- **Middle 1/3:** oesophageal branches of thoracic aorta and bronchial arteries.
- **Lower 1/3:** oesophageal branches from left gastric (from coeliac axis) and also from left inferior phrenic artery.

### Venous drainage

- **Upper 1/3:** inferior thyroid and brachiocephalic veins.
- **Middle 1/3:** azygos system.
- **Lower 1/3:** azygos system (systemic) and left gastric vein (portal)– provides a site of porto-systemic anastomosis.

### Lymphatic drainage

- **Lymph channels** exist within the oesophageal walls – allows lymph to pass for long distances before draining out to nodes. Drainage from one area does not necessarily follow a particular pattern.
- **Cervical/upper oesophagus:** peri-oesophageal lymph plexus drains to deep cervical nodes, then thoracic nodes, tracheobronchial, and finally posterior mediastinal nodes.
- **Lower/abdominal oesophagus:** peri-oesophageal lymph plexus drains to nodes around left gastric and then to coeliac nodes.

### Nerve supply

- **Parasympathetic:** vagus nerves form intrinsic and extrinsic nerve plexuses on the oesophageal surface. Anterior and posterior vagal trunks contribute to plexus – anterior trunk mainly left vagal fibres and posterior trunk mainly right vagal fibres (but both are mixed).
- **Sympathetic:** upper part from middle cervical ganglia running with inferior thyroid arteries, middle and lower parts from thoracic sympathetic trunks, and greater splanchnic nerves.

# Operative technique: left thoracolaparotomy and subtotal oesophagectomy

## General

- Used for tumours of lower and middle third oesophagus if Ivor-Lewis is not preferred.
- Contra-indicated for malignancy above aortic arch – due to poor access.
- Gives good access to lower thoracic oesophagus and upper stomach.
- Gives poor access to abdomen, nodes and thoracic duct.

## Preparation

- With the patient on their right side, left leg extended, right leg flexed at knee and hip, arms flexed with forearms before face.
- Fix hips with encircling band and support left shoulder with padded post.
- Double lumen ET tube allows exclusion of 1 lung.
- Prophylactic antibiotics.
- DVT prophylaxis.

## Incision

- Incise midway between xiphisternum and umbilicus, and continue obliquely up and left.
- At this stage perform laparotomy to assess fixity and nodal involvement (ensure no unresectable disease).
- If resection possible – extend incision across costal margin to continue along line of 6th/7th intercostal space to rib neck.
- In the elderly or those with fixed ribs it is sometimes necessary to excise a few cm of bone near the rib neck to allow access to chest.
- Deepen the incision by dividing thoracic wall muscles with diathermy and open pleura at upper border of rib.
- Divide costal margin and incise diaphragm radially 10–25cm towards oesophageal hiatus or peripherally parallel to chest wall (phrenic nerve sparing).
- Insert self-retaining rib retractor.
- Use double lumen tube to collapse lung and anchor incised edge of diaphragm to skin to prevent lung prolapsing into operative field.
- Divide peritoneum from rectus sheath to costal margin.

## Abdominal phase

- Assess tumour – if stomach largely involved, plan for total gastrectomy.
- Open lesser sac, dissect greater omentum from transverse colon, and divide avascular portion of lesser omentum.
- Divide gastrohepatic, gastrosplenic, and gastrocolic ligaments (preserve right gastric and right gastro-epiploic vessels if proximal gastrectomy being performed).
- Ligate and divide each vascular pedicle of the stomach, and even if they appear to be uninvolved, left gastric area and root of left gastric artery should be removed – ligate and divide left gastric artery and vein separately.
- Perform pyloroplasty and kocherize duodenum (for length).

- Divide stomach (proximal gastrectomy) or duodenal bulb (total gastrectomy) with linear stapler.
- Remove diaphragmatic anchor stitch and pass a tape through oesophageal hiatus.
- Pull tape downwards to gain good exposure to left thoracic cavity.

## Thoracic phase

- Divide pulmonary ligament to free lower lobe of left lung (take care to preserve pulmonary vein).
- Incise mediastinal pleura anterior to lower thoracic aorta and dissect to expose oesophageal vessels.
- Ligate and divide aortic oesophageal vessels.
- Elevate and pull forward lower lobe of left lung to expose posterior mediastinum and incise mediastinal pleura posterior to pericardium.
- Oesophagus can now be gently mobilized by blunt dissection (take care not to injure thoracic duct or azygos vein).
- Mobilize oesophagus from hiatus upwards to level of 1st rib (as necessary).
- Take care to preserve left recurrent laryngeal nerve, while mobilizing at level of aortic arch.
- Tape can be passed around oesophagus to aid retraction and dissection up into root of neck.
- Transect oesophagus and perform intrathoracic oesophagogastric anastomosis or jejunal interposition if total gastrectomy performed (see later).

## Closure

- Close diaphragm and costal margin with continuous, strong, absorbable suture, e.g. 1 nylon.
- Insert apical and basal underwater seal chest drains.
- Re-expand collapsed lung.
- Re-approximate ribs with interrupted, strong, absorbable suture, e.g. 0 vicryl.
- Close muscle in layers with 1 PDS and clips to skin.
- Insert feeding jejunostomy via Witzel tunnel.
- Close abdomen with routine mass closure.

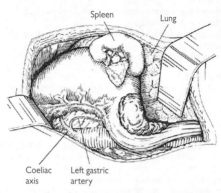

**Fig. 4.2** Thoraco-abdominal approach for lower-third oesophageal carcinoma. Taken from McLatchie & Leaper (2006). Reproduced with permission of Oxford University Press ©2006.

# Operative technique: Ivor–Lewis oesophagectomy

## General

- **The most widely practiced approach:** initial laparotomy and formation of a gastric tube, then right thoracotomy to excise tumour and form anastomosis at apex of mediastinum.
- **Classic procedure for mid-oesophageal tumours,** but can also be used for lower third tumours.
- Also known as **Lewis–Tanner** or **abdominal and right thoracic subtotal oesophagectomy.**

## Preparation

- The patient should be supine for the abdominal phase and in left lateral position for thoracic phase.
- Prophylactic antibiotics.
- DVT prophylaxis.
- Double lumen ET tube for 1 lung exclusion.

## Abdominal phase

- Upper midline incision to xiphisternum.
- Peritoneum opened to left of falciform ligament.
- Assess fixity and nodal involvement (assess suitability for resection).
- If resection possible – ligate and divide ligamentum teres and falciform ligament.
- Assistant elevates liver with flat-bladed retractor and draws down stomach to enable oesophagus to be palpated through oesophageal hiatus.
- Can divide left triangular ligament and remove xiphoid process to improve exposure if necessary.
- Mobilize stomach, but preserve right gastric and gastro-epiploic vessels.
- Transversely incise peritoneum and fascia over abdominal oesophagus to expose lower thoracic oesophagus, while preserving anterior vagal trunk.
- Incise diaphragmatic crus to enlarge the hiatus and mobilize lower oesophagus up into thorax by blunt and finger dissection.

## Thoracic phase

- Right thoracotomy at level of 5th or 6th rib.
- Divide intercostal muscles and muscles of thoracic wall with diathermy, and excise neck of lower rib for better exposure.
- Control intercostal vessels and diathermize intercostal nerve (better post-operative pain control).
- Collapse right lung.
- Pull lung down and forward to expose and incise mediastinal pleura.
- Mobilize, divide, and doubly ligate azygos vein, as it arches over lung root (2/0 vicryl).
- Divide right pulmonary ligament until inferior pulmonary vein can be seen.
- Excision thoracic duct and para-aortic lymph nodes en bloc.

- Incise mediastinal pleura over anterior border of aorta and ligate oesophageal aortic branches.
- Oesophagus is now exposed and can be mobilized by blunt dissection from lung hilum and pericardium, taking all lymph nodes *en bloc* – a tape can be passed around the oesophagus to aid retraction and dissection.
- Excise carinal, bronchial, para-aortic and paratracheal lymph nodes *en bloc* – take care not to damage fragile posterior membranous aspect of the trachea.
- Ligate and divide thoracic duct just above the diaphragm (prevent s chylothorax).
- Continue thoracic oesophageal mobilization until it meets abdominal mobilization.
- Divide all pleural attachments to allow stomach to pass into thorax.
- Withdraw NGT, place proximal oesophageal stay sutures and transect oesophagus at level of apex of thorax.
- Divide stomach along lesser curve with linear stapler and remove specimen with lymph nodes *en bloc*.
- Perform gastro-oesophageal anastomosis within thorax.

## Closure

- Insert basal, apical, and left pleural underwater seal chest drains.
- Re-approximate ribs with strong, absorbable, interrupted sutures, e.g. 0 vicryl.
- Re-expand lung.
- Close muscles in layers with 1 PDS and clips to skin.
- Close incision in crus and diaphragm.
- Insert feeding jejunostomy via Witzel tunnel.
- Close abdomen with mass closure as routine.

# Operative technique: transhiatal oesophagectomy

## General

- Fewer pulmonary complications than transthoracic routes, but often achieve sub-optimal lymphadenectomy – some report higher rates of local recurrence.
- Similar mortality figures to other approaches.
- Oesophagus resected by blunt dissection with anastomosis of conduit (stomach/jejunum/colon) via neck incision.
- Modern retractors allow resection and anastomosis to be performed under direct vision in the neck – technique often used for benign disease.
- Can have major blood loss due to surrounding structures.

## Preparation

- Supine with neck extended and head turned to opposite side.
- Prophylactic antibiotics.
- DVT prophylaxis.

## Abdominal phase

- Upper midline incision to xiphisternum.
- Assess fixity of stomach and lymphadenopathy (exclude distant or unresectable disease).
- Routine gastric or colonic mobilization (depending on conduit) – to facilitate tension-free passage to the neck.
- Perform pyloroplasty and kocherize duodenum.

## Mediastinal phase

- Mobilize lower 1/3 to 1/2 of oesophagus by combination of blunt and finger dissection.
- Divide anterior connections to tracheobronchial tree, posterior connection to aorta, and lateral connections to pleura and lung.

## Cervical phase

- Right-sided approach is preferable as left sided approach endangers thoracic duct.
- 5–8cm incision along anterior border of sternocleidomastoid – centred at level of cricoid cartilage.
- Incise through platysma, cervical fascia, and omohyoid muscle.
- Ligate and divide middle thyroid vein.
- Enter space between oesophagus, larynx, trachea, and thyroid medially and sternocleidomastoid and carotid sheath laterally, by retracting the medial and lateral structures.
- Inferior thyroid artery crosses this space and can be divided if necessary (leave intact if possible).
- Identify recurrent laryngeal nerve in tracheo-oesophageal groove – even small retractors cause damage. Nerve on the opposite side cannot be seen and is at risk.

- Rotating the medial structures (oesophagus, trachea, larynx, thyroid) to opposite side exposes the posterior surface of the oesophagus and the tracheo-oesophageal groove.
- Separate the oesophagus from the trachea with blunt forceps (e.g. Lahey's).
- Pass a tape around the oesophagus and into the jaws of the forceps to form a sling.
- The sling can now be used for retraction and the oesophageal blunt dissection continued down the cervical and thoracic oesophagus to the level of the carina.
- Insert tube thoracostomy with underwater seal.
- Divide proximal oesophagus in the neck.
- Suture a drain to the distal cut end and bring it out in the abdomen.
- Excise specimen at the appropriate level.
- Prepare conduit – stomach/colon/jejunum and suture it to a drain and pass it up into the neck.
- Anchor conduit to pre-vertebral fascia in the neck and perform anastomosis to proximal severed end (see later).

## Closure

- Leave drain close to anastomosis and bring out near cervical wound.
- Re-approximate platysma (2-0 vicryl) and close skin with clips.
- Insert feeding jejunostomy via Witzel tunnel.
- Close abdomen with routine mass closure.

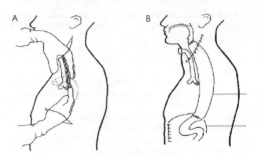

**Fig. 4.3** Transhiatal mobilization of oesophagus. Taken from McLatchie & Leaper (2006). Reproduced with permission of Oxford University Press ©2006.

OXFORD MEDICAL PUBLICATIONS

# Surgical Oncology

Published and forthcoming Oxford Specialist Handbooks

**General Oxford Specialist Handbooks**
A Resuscitation Room Guide
Addiction Medicine
Perioperative Medicine,
second edition
Post-Operative Complications,
second edition

**Oxford Specialist Handbooks in Anaesthesia**
Cardiac Anaesthesia
General Thoracic Anaesthesia
Neuroanaesthesia
Obstetric Anaesthesia
Paediatric Anaesthesia
Regional Anaesthesia, Stimulation and
Ultrasound Techniques

**Oxford Specialist Handbooks in Cardiology**
Adult Congenital Heart Disease
Cardiac Catheterization and
Coronary Intervention
Echocardiography
Fetal Cardiology
Heart Failure
Hypertension
Nuclear Cardiology
Pacemakers and ICDs

**Oxford Specialist Handbooks in Critical Care**
Advanced Respiratory Critical Care

**Oxford Specialist Handbooks in End of Life Care**
End of Life Care in Cardiology
End of Life Care in Dementia
End of Life Care in Nephrology
End of Life Care in Respiratory
Disease
End of Life in the Intensive Care Unit

**Oxford Specialist Handbooks in Neurology**
Epilepsy
Parkinson's Disease and Other
Movement Disorders
Stroke Medicine

**Oxford Specialist Handbooks in Paediatrics**
Paediatric Endocrinology and
Diabetes
Paediatric Dermatology
Paediatric Gastroenterology,
Hepatology, and Nutrition
Paediatric Haematology and
Oncology
Paediatric Nephrology
Paediatric Neurology
Paediatric Radiology
Paediatric Respiratory Medicine

**Oxford Specialist Handbooks in Psychiatry**
Child and Adolescent Psychiatry
Old Age Psychiatry

**Oxford Specialist Handbooks in Radiology**
Interventional Radiology
Musculoskeletal Imaging

**Oxford Specialist Handbooks in Surgery**
Cardiothoracic Surgery
Hand Surgery
Hepato-pancreatobiliary Surgery
Oral and Maxillofacial Surgery
Neurosurgery
Operative Surgery, second edition
Otolaryngology and Head and Neck
Surgery
Paediatric Surgery
Plastic and Reconstructive Surgery
Surgical Oncology
Urological Surgery
Vascular Surgery

# Operative technique: further techniques

### 3-stage oesophagectomy

- Also known as McKeown oesophagectomy.
- Same abdominal and thoracic phases as Ivor–Lewis technique with addition of cervical phase (as per transhiatal technique) for neck anastomosis.
- Used for proximal tumours where slightly more dissection and resection required to achieve safe proximal margin.
- Some use as they prefer to expose, divide, or anastomose the oesophagus in the neck.

### Radical curative surgery (Akiyama technique)

- Performed in Japan.
- Initial Ivor–Lewis abdominal and thoracic phases, and then bilateral cervical incision with extensive lymphadenectomy in neck, mediastiunm, and abdomen.
- Not used in west – less incidence of lymphadenopathy (higher incidence of squamous in Japan, whereas higher incidence of adeno in west) and additional morbidity, such as recurrent laryngeal nerve injury.
- Need reliable pre-operative assessment by conventional methods.
- Operative survival is similar to western figures and 5-year survival over 50% in those undergoing curative resection.

### Pharyngolaryngo-oesophagectomy

- For carcinoma of the upper cervical oesophagus or hypopharynx.
- Usually performed by head and neck surgeons.
- Usually use free jejunal graft as interposition.

# Laparoscopic oesophagectomy

Thoracoscopically-assisted oesophagectomy. Consists of two stages:
- Collapse lung on operative side, perform thoracoscopy with 4 ports, and mobilize and transect thoracic oesophagus.
- Oesophagogastric anastomosis performed open or laparoscopically.

Usually slower and not suitable for all tumours, but often less painful and shorter in-hospital stay. May require open conversion.

## NICE guidelines

- Effective enough to be available on NHS, but only if surgeon has sufficient experience and training.
- Needs full informed consent and local clinical governance committee support.
- Convincing data in terms of long-term outcome and comparisons with other techniques needed.

# Operative technique: anastomosis

### Aims
- Tension-free.
- Good vascular supply (note colour and temperature) – blood supply tenuous when oesophagus is mobilized so care must be taken to maintain as much as possible.
- Close apposition of epithelial margins.

### General advice
- Can be hand-sewn or stapled.
- Can be sited in neck or thorax – no evidence for 1 being preferable in outcome or functionality.
- Ensure 2 ends to be anastomosed are not twisted.
- Avoid trauma from non-crushing clamps.
- Advance NGT through anastomosis at end of procedure.
- Ensure drain (24 Fr Robinson) placed close to anastomosis, prior to closure.

### Stapled
- Circular stapling devices usually quicker and can be used in difficult positions, e.g. under aortic arch/high in abdomen or thorax.
- Can use with any type of conduit, in neck or thorax, and can perform end-end or end-side anastomoses.
- If stapler fails – usually difficult to hand-sew and often requires higher transection of conduit, as well as causing crushing effect on tissues.
- Withdraw NGT from proximal oesophageal remnant while aspirating.
- Hold oesophageal lumen open with sponge forceps to pass a test head or measuring device – choose largest that fits.
- Hold oesophageal lumen open with stay sutures and place purse-string suture to proximal oesophageal remnant at 5mm intervals and 5mm depth (2/0 prolene on small round-bodied needle).
- Insert correct size head of stapling gun into proximal oesophagus and tighten purse-string around its neck – insert second purse-string if oesophagus not drawn tight to neck.
- Open stapling device so that gun spike passes through distal conduit (stomach/colon/jejunum) and secure around neck of gun with a purse-string suture.
- Reattach head to body of stapling device.
- Ensure there is nothing interposed between the 2 ends, release the safety catch and fire the gun.
- Inspect completeness of toroidal oesophageal and viscous remnants (doughnuts) – ensure they contain all layers of the wall.
- Separate jaws of instrument and carefully rotate it to withdraw it.
- Some oversew with 2/0 PDS.

### Sutured
- Often preferable in the neck as often insufficient distal conduit to place gun through.
- Many different techniques – key to success is care with which they are applied.

- Oesophageal wall largely composed of longitudinal muscle – longitudinal sutures can cut out, particularly as longitudinal muscle leads to shortening of oesophagus after anastomosis – this must be allowed for.
- Oesophagus has large lumen when relaxed and action of circular muscle makes the lumen appear smaller – unless lumen is dilated, closely spaced sutures will be widely spaced when the muscle relaxes and lead to leaks.
- Withdraw NGT, while aspirating.
- Lie two ends together and ensure hole in the distal conduit matches the size of oesophageal lumen after dilatation.
- Insert traction sutures through all coats of both conduits and slightly posteriorly to the lateral angles.
- Draw traction sutures apart to tauten posterior walls and keep them in apposition, while leaving anterior walls slack.
- Place traction suture in the middle of the anterior walls and draw them apart so that posterior walls can still be seen.
- Carefully place sutures at 2–3mm intervals and with 2–3mm bites – include all layers of the wall, and take mucosa on both sides. Sutures cut easily through longitudinal muscle so suture strength depends largely on submucosa and partly mucosa.
- Use fine 4/0 or 5/0 sutures on a small, round-bodied needle, in a continuous or interrupted fashion. Use absorbable or non-absorbable suture (many use PDS or vicryl).
- Start posteriorly and work anteriorly so that last few stitches to be placed are in centre of anterior wall.
- Knots are placed internally on the posterior aspect of the anastomosis and then externally on the anterior aspect.
- Sutures can be placed and tied, or placed, left loose, and oesophagus parachuted down, with all knots tied sequentially.
- When nearly complete, do not tighten last few stitches until sutures inspected to ensure they pass through all layers – cut stitches out, rather than place rescue sutures.
- Do not tie sutures too tight – oesophagus swells post-operatively and will cut out.
- Gently rotate to inspect anastomosis at end.

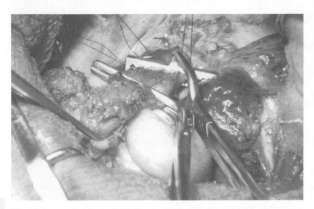

**Fig. 4.4** Purse string clamp across the oesophagus 5–6 cm proximal to the tumour. Taken from McLatchie & Leaper (2006). Reproduced with permission of Oxford University Press ©2006.

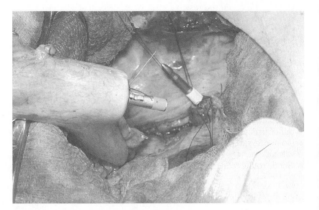

**Fig. 4.5** Staple gun in the gastric conduit with the staple head in the proximal cut end at the oesophagus. Taken from McLatchie & Leaper (2006). Reproduced with permission of Oxford University Press ©2006.

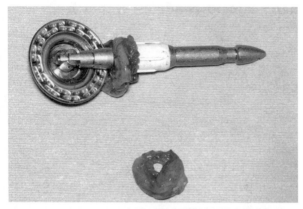

**Fig. 4.6** Gastric and oesophageal donuts with the staple head. Taken from McLatchie & Leaper (2006). Reproduced with permission of Oxford University Press ©2006.

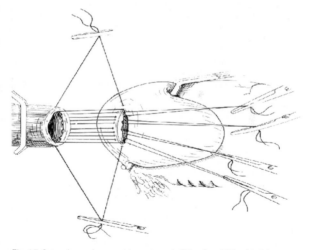

**Fig. 4.7** Sutured oesophago-gastric anastomosis. Taken from McLatchie & Leaper (2006). Reproduced with permission of Oxford University Press ©2006.

# Replacement conduits: stomach

### General

First choice of conduit, when available, should be:
- Well-vascularized.
- Only one anastomosis required.
- Simple to mobilize into thorax or neck.
- Good functional results.
- Posterior mediastinal/pre-vertebral route to pass stomach up to anastomosis site.
- Anterior mediastinal (retrosternal) and subcutaneous (presternal) routes can be used but longer and non-anatomical.

### Procedure

- Supine position.
- Upper midline incision.
- Exclude distant or unresectable disease.
- Use 3/0 or 2/0 vicryl to tie vessels.
- Divide greater omentum from transverse colon and gastro-colic omentum below right gastro-epiploic vessels to enter lesser sac.
- Dissect towards gastric fundus and left gastro-epiploic vessels.
- Divide crossover vessel to middle colic vein.
- Dissect inferiorly to origin of right gastro-epiploic vein.
- Dissect hepatic flexure from duodenum and kocherize duodenum to the midline to provide maximum gastric length.
- Divide lesser omentum close to liver, preserving right gastric artery as it emerges from common hepatic inferiorly.
- Divide hepatic branch of the vagus as it can have a large associated vessel (preserve other aberrant hepatic vessels).
- Divide gastro-splenic ligament and ligate short gastric arteries to free fundus.
- Divide lesser sac adhesions from pancreas and lift stomach.
- Divide and tie left gastric artery and vein separately.
- Perform lymphadenectomy of left gastric, common hepatic, splenic artery and coeliac territories, and skeletonize abdominal aorta up to diaphragmatic hiatus.
- Stomach is now completely mobile.
- Perform pyloroplasty and skeletonize lesser curve by dividing lesser omentum and left gastric tissue above right gastric pedicle (the necessary vagotomy can produce gastric paresis – pyloroplasty morbidity is low so should be performed where possible)
- Once specimen removed, draw fundus superiorly to neck or apex of thorax.
- Excise a portion of lesser curve and proximal stomach (depending upon extent of gastric involvement) with linear stapler to form gastric tube.
- Perform hand-sewn or stapled anastomosis with oversew (2/0 PDS).

- Anastomosis should be performed in posterior fundus at high point of stomach and well away from resection line (to ensure no vascular compromise) – if stapling device to be used, ensure that spike of the gun passes through fundus at least 2cm from suture or staple line.
- Place feeding jejunostomy via Witzel tunnel.
- Close abdomen as routine.

# Replacement conduits: colon

## General

- Second most common conduit following stomach.
- Most favoured pre-vertebral route for reconstruction.
- Used only in certain situations:
  - absent or damaged stomach, e.g. caustic injury, ischaemia;
  - where site and size of tumour requires total gastrectomy;
  - for extra-anatomical bypass where extra length needed e.g. anterior mediastinal or subcutaneous routes;
  - surgical preference;
  - vagal preserving procedures.

## Pre-operatively

- *Colonoscopy:* rule out significant disease, e.g. inflammatory bowel disease, severe diverticulosis, multiple polyps, malignancy.
- *Mesenteric angiogram:* assess pattern and sufficiency of blood supply and identify part of colon to be used (usually iso-peristaltic left colonic segment based upon left colic vessels).
- *Colonic preparation:* Picolax/Fleet phosphosoda/Klean-prep.

## Procedure

- Supine position.
- Long midline incision.
- Exclude distant or unresectable disease.
- Dissect greater omentum from transverse colon.
- Mobilize hepatic and splenic flexures, ascending and descending colon so that whole colon is mobile on its mesentery.
- Bring apex of left colonic loop identified up to xiphisternum and mark with a suture.
- Measure distance from xiphisternum to mandible and mark the length proximal to previous marking suture – usually in area of splenic flexure.
- Divide marginal vessels and middle colic pedicle below its bifurcation (to preserve any arcade).
- Divide transverse mesocolon and then divide right colon with a linear stapler.
- Draw left colon carefully up to the anastomotic site (usually within a bowel bag or other atraumatic device), once specimen has been removed.
- Ensure colon not twisted and anchor it to diaphragm.
- Perform hand-sewn or stapled proximal anastomosis.
- Divide distal colon 10cm below diaphragm with a linear stapler.
- If vagotomy performed, better functional outcome achieved by additional proximal 2/3 gastrectomy and end-end cologastric anastomosis to the antrum (2/0PDS), with pyloroplasty.
- If vagal-preserving procedure performed, stomach can be retained with posterior end-side cologastric anastomosis, using circular stapling device through a small anterior gastrotomy.

- Insert NGT and pass through proximal anastomosis.
- Restore colonic continuity with end-end colocolic anastomosis (2 layers of 2/0 PDS).
- Place feeding jejunostomy via Witzel tunnel.
- Close abdomen as routine.

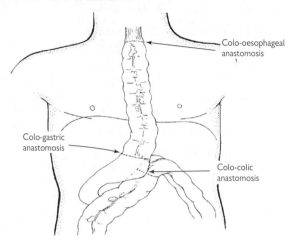

**Fig. 4.8** Right colonic interposition from cervical oesophagus to antrum with colo-colic anastomosis. Taken from McLatchie & Leaper (2006). Reproduced with permission of Oxford University Press ©2006.

# Replacement conduits: jejunum

## General
- Jejunum rarely used as a conduit.
- Can be used after pharyngolaryngo-oesophagectomy for tumours in proximal cervical oesophagus and hypopharynx.
- Usually passed retrocolically.
- Can perform anastomosis in neck or apex of thorax.
- Can be hand-sewn or stapled anastomosis.

## Procedure
- Supine position.
- Long midline incision.
- Isolate a long jejunal segment based upon second or third jejunal artery.
- Divide the jejunal segment with a linear stapler to form free conduit.
- Draw the divided end superiorly through the oesophageal diaphragmatic hiatus to the site of anastomosis.
- Perform gastrojejunal anastomosis by stapling or suturing the caudal end of the jejunal segment to the gastric remnant.
- Restore jejunal continuity by performing jejo-jejunal anastomosis.

# Post-operative care and complications

## Post-operative care

- **Intensive care or high dependency unit:** meticulous fluid balance and respiratory support as necessary.
- **Pain relief:** epidural or PCA. Can also assist with respiration.
- **Nausea and vomiting:** regular antiemetics often required.
- **Nasogastric tube:** monitor output amount and type.
- **Nutritional support:** early enteral nutrition is important and feeding via jejunostomy can be commenced on the first or second post-operative day. Ongoing nutritional support is often required until the patient is eating normally. Patients may continue to lose weight initially and should be advised that this will settle once they recommence a normal diet.
- **Chest drains:** monitor output amount and type.
- **Physiotherapy support:** respiratory (particularly following thoracotomy) and mobility support are crucial (early mobilization is key to prevent DVT and PE).
- **Mouth care and washes:** patients often complain of a bad taste in their mouth and good care also allows earlier feeding.
- **Bowel disturbances:** constipation and diarrhoea are both common.
- **Depression:** may require emotional and/or psychological support.

## Complications

### Early

- **Haemorrhage.**
- **Recurrent laryngeal nerve injury:** more common during dissection of the cervical and upper oesophagus. The majority are unilateral and transient. Left nerve is at risk during mediastinal lymphadenectomy, and if cervical anastomosis to take place at the same time – perform it on the left side so that both nerves are not at risk. Injury impairs the ability to cough and protect the airway in the early post-operative period – can be an important contributor to pulmonary morbidity. In most patients there will be adequate compensation from the contralateral side, but if not, tracheostomy should be considered to protect the airway and improve pulmonary toilet. Thyroplasty or vocal cord injections are rarely required.
- **Atelectasis:** very common, secondary to pain, and can lead to pneumonia and respiratory failure.
- **Pneumonia.**
- **Acute pulmonary oedema:** secondary to extensive pulmonary lymphadenectomy and poor lymphatic drainage of the alveoli.
- **ARDS.**
- **Pleural effusions.**
- **Pneumothorax.**
- **Chylothorax:** occurs in 2–3% of thoracic oesophagectomies and may be higher with transhiatal techniques. Recognized by thick, creamy stuff passing through chest drain. Prolonged conservative treatment has high mortality due to hypoalbuminaemia and leucocyte depletion. If chyle production >10ml/kg/day on the fifth post-operative day, indication for re-operation and ligation of the thoracic duct.

- *Thrombo-embolism:* DVT and PE.
- *Anastomotic leak:* most bowel has serosa that forms fibrinous adhesions and seals small leaks, but oesophagus has no serosa except upon anterior aspect of abdominal segment. If leak occurs within 72 h, usually represents technical failure – if general condition of the patient is good, exploration and repair is advisable. Majority of leaks occur at 2 weeks and probably represent anastomotic tension +/– local ischaemia. Diagnosed by clinical suspicion and confirmation with water-soluble contrast studies (can miss some leaks). Majority of leaks are minor and can be managed conservatively with nasogastric suction, local drainage, antibiotics and jejunal feeding. Major thoracic leaks require early recognition and exploration for a good outcome. Overall, leak rate should not exceed 5%, and no evidence for difference in leak rates between hand-sewn and stapled anastomoses. Neck leaks are more common than thoracic, but have less severe consequences.
- *Gastric outlet obstruction:* particularly if no pyloroplasty.
- *Mortality* (in-hospital <10%).

*Late*

- *Anastomotic stricture:* particularly with small, circular stapling devices and cervical anastomoses. Benign strictures can occur in first few months and usually relate to post-operative fibrosis. Later strictures are often due to reflux – differentiating from recurrence is difficult and endoscopic assessment, and biopsy is therefore required. Early strictures are easily treated by endoscopic dilatation although multiple sessions may be required.
- *Reflux.*
- *Dumping syndrome.*
- *Post-vagotomy diarrhoea.*
- *Post-thoracotomy pain.*
- *Cancer recurrence:* loco-regional, metastatic or both.

# Adjuvant therapy

## General
- The rationale is to attempt to prevent local recurrence.
- Should be considered for T2 tumours and above.
- Patients with advanced tumours (T3/N1) should be considered for randomized controlled studies to assess the role of novel multimodal therapies in conjunction with surgery.
- The majority of clinical studies evaluating the effectiveness of adjuvant therapy have dealt with squamous cell carcinoma, which is slowly being overtaken by adenocarcinoma as the commonest tumour, data therefore becoming less relevant.
- Surgical excision remains the standard treatment and the effectiveness of adjuvant therapies are still under evaluation.
- Oesophageal adenocarcinoma tends to be radio-resistant.
- Oesophagogastric junction tumours should generally be considered as gastric tumours, and there is little evidence to support the role of adjuvant or neo adjuvant therapies.

## Radiotherapy
Should be considered in squamous cell carcinoma, particularly when the proximal level of the tumour is high.

### External
- Given as short daily sessions.
- Length of course depends upon type and size of cancer.
- Skin is initially tattooed/marked to indicate direction of therapy.
- Often require PEG insertion prior to treatment as radiotherapy can make swallowing very painful and also leads to decreased saliva production.
- Often need antiemetics for nausea and vomiting.
- Other side-effects include depression, lethargy, and hair loss.

### Internal
- Brachytherapy – insertion of a radioactive metal rod, as a source of radiotherapy, into the oesophagus.
- Radioactive source contained within protective tubing.
- Inserted by upper GI endoscopy or via NGT, which is left *in situ* with the source inside it.
- Removed via endoscopy or by removing NGT.
- Left for between 30 min to a few days depending upon amount of radiation required.
- Provides more focused treatment within a shorter time.
- Causes dysphagia so often need PEG and liquid analgesics.
- Leads to less systemic side-effects, such as nausea, lethargy, hair loss.
- Often remain in hospital during their period of treatment.

## Chemotherapy
- The use of post-operative chemotherapy is complicated in oesophagectomy by the prolonged recovery period and conflicts with the aims of adjuvant therapy.

- Trials usually include variations of the ECF regimen (epirubicin/cisplatin/fluorouracil).
- Side-effects include decreased resistance to infection, bone marrow suppression, bruising or bleeding, anaemia, nausea, mouth sores and ulcers, hair loss, diarrhoea, lethargy, and soreness of hands and feet

## Chemoradiotherapy

- Only used in the context of clinical trials.
- McDonald (2001): 556 patients surgery or surgery +FU/FA.
- Median overall survival 27 vs. 36 months.
- 3-year relapse-free survival 48 vs. 31%.

**Table 4.7** Treatment stages and options for treatment

| Treatment stage | Options currently in use |
|---|---|
| Neo-adjuvant chemotherapy | 5-FU/Cisplatin |
| | Taxane |
| Neo-adjuvant or definitive chemoradiation | 5-FU/Cisplatin |
| | Taxane based |
| | Irinotecan based |
| Adjuvant chemoradiation | 5-FU/FA |
| | 5-FU/Cisplatin |
| Adjuvant chemotherapy | Eprubicin/cisplatin/5-FU |
| | Taxane based |
| Advanced metastatic disease | 5-FU based |
| | Oxaliplatin based |
| | Cisplatin based |
| | Irinotecan based |
| | Taxane based |

## Further reading

Macdonald JS, Smalley SR, Benedetti J, Hundahl SA, Estes NC, Stemmermann GN, et al. Chemoradiotherapy after surgery compared with surgery alone for adenocarcinoma of the stomach or gastroesophageal junction. N Engl J Med 2001; **345(10)**:725–30.

# Follow-up and surveillance protocols

## General
- Usefulness of surveillance is still largely unknown – rapid disease progression means the majority are having active treatment with only a minority attending for symptomatic review.
- The development of clinical nurse specialist roles in follow-up should be encouraged – they have a crucial role to play in the continuity of care between primary and secondary care and their role should include follow-up to reduce the need for medical review.

## Aims
- Detection of functional disorders related to complications of treatment.
- Detection of recurrence at the earliest opportunity.
- Assessment and management of nutritional requirements.
- Provision of psychosocial support to patients and carers, including liaison with palliative care where appropriate.
- Facilitation of treatment and outcome audit.

## Format
- There is no evidence that intensive follow-up improves the speed of detection of recurrence. Subsequently, there is no consensus for the mode, duration, or intensity of follow-up.
- The process of follow-up should reflect the Calman–Hine report in to the provision of services for those with cancer.
- Local protocols should be agreed upon. Follow-up may be in the hospital or primary care setting. However, the first follow-up should always be in the hospital setting with MDT input, and the patient then consulted and their wishes respected.
- When follow-up occurs in the hospital, it must be in a multi-disciplinary setting to avoid investigation duplication, and wasting time and money.
- General practices taking part in follow-up should do so according to protocols and should be able to communicate effectively with hospital teams. They should take part in joint audit protocols and should be guaranteed access to specialist services when necessary.
- Patients should be able to access services between appointments as and when necessary, and a named member of the MDT as contact helps to facilitate this.
- Nutritional support is crucial following radical treatment and palliative therapy, and all patients should be offered dietary advice.

**Table 4.8** Algorithm for post oesophagectomy recurrence

|  | Progression | Management |
|---|---|---|
| 3–6 months OPD follow-up, FBC, OGD/CT according to symptoms | Local or regional recurrence post surgery + no previous chemo or DXT | Chemoradiation with 5-FU based agent as tolerated or palliative support<br>Palliative chemotherapy on further progression |
|  | Local recurrence following primary chemoradiation | Surgery if meets resectability criteria and fit<br>Palliative chemotherapy or support in other cases |
|  | Metastatic progression | Palliative chemotherapy if fit and palliative support |

# Chemotherapy for metastatic disease

- No major overall survival benefit proven.
- Improves quality of life in many cases.
- SCC more radio-, chemo-, and chemoradiosensitive than adenocarcinoma, but no survival advantage by any modality.
- 5-FU, cisplatin, mitomycin, bleomycin, methotrexate, and doxorubicin all traditionally used. Newer drugs include epirubicin paclitaxel, docetaxel, and oxaliplatin used with 5-FU and irinotecan. Tyrosine kinase inhibitors gefinitib and erlotinib show some activity.
- Cisplatin 20% response rate as single agent. 5-FU + *cis*- 20–50%.
- Irinotecan + cisplatin may be particularly good for SCC, but very low power studies.
- *South-west oncology group (US) phase II trial:* gemcitabine + cisplatin: 64 patients with a median survival rate of 7.2 months. RR 45% in similar trials. Docetaxel, Irinotecan, Cisplatin RR 64% low power trial n=16.
- Adequately powered Phase III RCTs rare.
- *REAL II trial:* multicentre randomized phase III trial for advanced oesophagogastric cancer. 30% oesophageal.
- Adenocarcinoma, SCC, undifferentiated all included.
- Regimes epirubicin, cisplatin, 5-FU (ECF), epirubicin, oxaliplatin, 5-FU (EOF), epirubicin, cisplatin, capecitabine (ECX), and epirubicin, oxaliplatin, capecitabine (EOX).
- Median follow-up 17.1 month. Response rate 41–48% for regimes no significant difference. No survival advantage, but improved quality of life.

# Palliative therapy

## General

- High proportion of patients present with late disease – highlights the importance of palliative care.
- Same principles also apply to those who are unfit for surgery.
- Consider for advanced tumours the spread beyond the submucosa locally and spread to distant organs.
- If tumour is inoperable, average life expectancy is 3–4 months (max. 1 year).
- Aim to relieve dysphagia and other symptoms, and improve quality of life, with as little morbidity as possible – studies show that relief of dysphagia correlates strongly with quality of life.
- Multi-disciplinary team planning with direct involvement of the palliative care team, and the clinical nurse specialist.
- Needs to be close association and liaison between primary and secondary care.
- The most commonly utilized are intubation and laser, but the complimentary use of all modalities results in a better quality of swallow than either alone.
- Best results occur by individualizing therapy and different modalities may be appropriate at different stages – palliation should occur in centres that can offer all treatments.

## Endoscopic dilatation

- Improves dysphagia in 70% when a guide wire can be passed.
- Needs repeat in 2–4 weeks – most clinicians reserve it for patients with very short life expectancy (<4 weeks) and unable to swallow saliva, or as short-term measure while more definitive treatment is planned.
- Similar success rate with different dilators such as balloon, Maloney and Savary-Gillard dilators.
- Can be performed alone or be followed by stent insertion.
- Complications – haemorrhage/perforation in 2.5–10%.

## Oesophageal intubation

- Endoscopic/radiological placement of stents most common, whereas open oesophageal intubation are now obsolete.
- Stents are usually plastic/metal wire or mesh.
- Treatment of choice for firm stenosing tumours, capable of retaining an endoprosthesis and sited more than 2cm from cricopharyngeus (not used in cervical tumours).
- Effective at relieving dysphagia as a single procedure – dysphagia improved in >90% cases.
- Only a small proportion (usually plastic tubes) are able to eat solids, with the remainder on a semi-liquid or liquid diet.
- Can be inserted under general or local anaesthetic.
- Can be inserted after surgery and also useful following radiotherapy – particularly in presence of tight, fibrotic strictures.
- Endoscopic insertion of Atkinson tube is the commonest – requires serial prior dilatation (risk of perforation).

- Rigid and semi-rigid plastic tubes (Atkinson, Wilson–Cook, Celestin) are less expensive than self-expanding metal stents (Gianturco Z-stent, Wall stent, ultraflex stent, oesophacoil).
- Expandable metal stents generally have lower complication rates (require no dilatation/narrow insertion instruments/wider lumen) and shorter hospital stays, although there is no difference in terms of late complications or re-procedure rate.
- Covered expandable metal stents are effective in malignant tracheo-oesophageal fistula or perforation following dilatation.
- Need to watch diet to help prevent blockage – carbonated drinks can help keep lumen open.
- **Complications:** displacement/migration, perforation, incomplete stent expansion, blockage due to tumour over-growth/in-growth, food bolus obstruction, aspiration pneumonia, haemorrhage and persistent pain – overall complication rates 4–15% for all types, but previous chemo or radiotherapy tends to increase the post-procedure complications.
- Tumour in-growth/overgrowth (10%) can be treated by laser (take care not to damage stent), diathermy, or stent replacement (this narrows lumen further).

Laser therapy
- Effective in tumours with an exophytic component (2/3 patients) and can be repeated as many times as possible.
- Less effective with tumours crossing the cardia, but use prior to stenting may prevent stent failure.
- Useful for cervical tumours that are too close to cricopharyngeus for intubation.
- Can also be used to control bleeding from tumours.
- Recanalization of the lumen and initial relief of dysphagia in 85–96% of patients, in a mean of 2 sessions.
- 33–36% of patients can tolerate any food, whereas 37–59% tolerate solids or semi-solids for the duration of their illness.
- Mean dysphagia free interval is 4–16 weeks (due to tumour regrowth) – 50% will be palliated by initial laser treatment for the duration of their illness/rest may need 4–6 weekly repeat.
- Effects can be often be significantly prolonged by the use of brachytherapy or external beam radiotherapy.
- Oesophagus is dilated to pass an endoscope to the distal border of the tumour and laser therapy applied retrogradely.
- NdYag endoscopic lasers destroy tumour by photocoagulation.
- Done as day-case with local anaesthetic and sedation – takes approx 15 min, but usually require 2–3 treatments.
- Oesophagus often swells following treatment – swallowing may initially paradoxically worsen following treatment.
- Contra-indicated in patients with tracheo-oesophageal fistula or perforation.
- **Complications:** perforation (0–5%) often associated with initial dilatation, tracheo-oesophageal fistula (0–6%) is more common when treatment associated with radiotherapy.
- Overall 30-day mortality is 0–5%.

**Electrocautery**
- Endoscopic diathermy to destroy tumour and relieve bleeding.
- Not as effective as laser – not often used.

**Alcohol injections**
- Endoscopic injection of small amounts of ethanol leads to local tumour necrosis (0.5–1mL aliquots of 100% ethanol).
- Can take a few days to be effective and often need >1 session.
- Useful for eccentric or soft exophytic tumours unsuitable for endoscopic intubation (too close to cricopharyngeus) or for tumour overgrowth at the ends of a prosthesis.
- Can also be used for control of malignant bleeding.
- 80–100% success rate in alleviating dysphagia, but may need 4–6 weekly repeat treatments.
- Recurrence, and need for >1 treatment means it is generally reserved for patients where intubation not possible.
- *Complications:* tracheo-oesophageal fistula and mediastinitis (2%), particularly with large doses of sclerosant. Also post-procedure pain, oesophageal ulcers, and transient AF have all been reported.

**Surgery**
- Open tumour debulking to relieve dysphagia.
- Bypass (usually retrosternal) using stomach, colon, or jejunum as conduit, but substernal bypass should be avoided.
- Oesophagectomy for palliation and exploratory laparotomy should be avoided if possible.
- Possibility of reduced quality of life after surgery should be considered, when considering surgery for non-curative intent.

**Radiotherapy**
- Can be used with or without intraluminal intubation/dilatation and can be used to prolong the effects of laser therapy.
- Can be internal (brachytherapy) or external beam.
- Improves dysphagia in 50–85% of patients and also provides pain relief – the rest are often unable to complete treatment due to progressive disease.
- Time to onset of improvement is slow (mean 2 months) – may be better in mild dysphagia. Time to improvement can be quickened by combining brachytherapy and external beam, but increases complications.
- *Complications:* fibrotic stricture, fistula, systemic complications (often unsatisfactory as reduce quality of life significantly).

**Chemotherapy**
- In locally advanced/metastatic cancer, and good performance status cisplatin and infusional 5-fluorouracil should be considered according to UK guidelines. Multiple other agents used (see above).
- Modest non-statistically significant survival benefit and potential symptomatic improvement, but toxicity and side-effects – should have the opportunity to discuss with an oncologist prior to treatment.

- Slow to palliate dysphagia.
- ***Complications:*** systemic effects can reduce quality of life.

## Photodynamic therapy
- An IV photo-sensitizing agent is administered, then activated by exposing the tumour to light, usually a low-power laser introduced endoscopically.
- The sensitizing agent absorbs energy from the light and forms reactive oxygen radicals/molecules that destroy tumour cells.
- Usually performed under sedation as a day case.
- Recent studies suggest significantly higher response rates than laser ablation at 1 month, as well as lower risk of perforation.
- Studies show relief of dysphagia and improved swallowing within 4–5 days, with repeat treatment needed in 1–3 months.
- Tumour regrows at a similar rate to those treated with laser.
- Only offered in certain specialist centres.
- Commonest complication is skin sensitivity and sunburn – can occur in a prolonged fashion and reduce quality of life.

## Argon plasma coagulation
- Experimental treatment at present.
- May have a future role in treating tumour over- and in-growth of stents.
- Its efficacy has not been effectively studied so far.

## Other treatments
- Coeliac plexus block should be considered in patients with upper abdominal pain not amenable to other treatments.
- Corticosteroids or megestrol acetate should be considered for patients with advanced cancer who are anorexic.
- Octreotide and corticosteroids should be considered for patients with bowel obstruction caused by malignancy, where interventional therapy is not possible or not appropriate.
- Blood transfusion should take place in symptomatic anaemia and erythropoietin considered according to guidelines

## Recurrence
- Presents difficult problems for palliation.
- All of the above can be used together with supportive care as necessary.

# Oesophageal cancer and the future

## Causative agents

- **HPV 16 + 18:** increased incidence of squamous cell carcinoma associated with these strains. Studies to look at the mechanism and the possibility of vaccination.
- **Barrett's:** studies to investigate genetic clusters and foci.

## Drugs and therapies

- **Aspirin:** certain studies in the USA have shown a decreased incidence of squamous cell carcinoma in those patients taking aspirin regularly. Ongoing studies to look at the mechanism.
- **Curcumin:** small trials ongoing to see if it is helpful in Barrett's.
- **Thalidomide:** small trials ongoing to investigate whether it can slow or prevent weight loss in advanced disease.
- **Vaccines:** against HPV and CEA.
- **Growth factor blockers:**
  - *gefitinib* – blocks epidermal growth factor receptor;
  - *tyrosine kinase inhibitor* – blocks growth factor enzyme tyrosine kinase.
- **Monoclonal antibodies:** proteins made from a single copy of a human antibody. Trials currently ongoing in Manchester.
- **Photodynamic therapy:** Can be used for Barrett's or carcinoma. NICE undecided whether it should be considered as a novel treatment or an established treatment. Studies ongoing with stage 1 cancer and Barrett's.

## Microarray genetic classification

- DNA microarrays and bioinformatics using new technology may be capable of providing a more complete grading classification to explain why tumours of similar staging sometimes act very differently.
- They may be important in the classification of Barrett's, and oesophageal malignant and pre-malignant diseases, as well as responses to treatment.
- Studies are still ongoing.

# Gastric cancer

# Epidemiology

### Incidence

- 6th commonest cancer in males and 9th in females in the UK.
- 8000 new cases each year.
- Male to female ratio 5:3.
- Occurs mainly in elderly. Less than 8% of cases below age 55.
- Steadily increases with age and peaks 8th decade.
- Major geographical difference: Incidence high in Japan and some parts of Asia.
- Incidence halved in UK over last 20 years.

### Risk factors

Wide international variations in incidence and the dramatic falls seen across the developed world suggest that environmental factors are very important in gastric carcinogenesis

#### H. pylori *infection, gastric atrophy, and gastritis*

- *H. pylori* is the most important risk factor in gastric cancer.
- Most cases of gastric cancer are associated with the presence of *H. pylori* in the stomach.
- *H. pylori* infection is a common bacterial infection with a high prevalence in the developing world. Poor hygiene, crowded living conditions and low socio-economic status are all associated with high rates of *H. pylori* infection.
- *H. pylori* infection doubles the risk of non-cardiac gastric cancer and the risk is even higher in those with the cagA-positive strain.
- The precancerous lesion severe chronic atrophic gastritis can be induced by *H. pylori* infection. This is a premalignant condition that increases the risk of gastric cardia cancer by 11-fold and gastric non-cardia by 3-fold.
- Risk increases with the severity of gastric atrophy such that those with multifocal gastric atrophy have more than 90 times increased risk of gastric cancer.

#### Nutritional

- Low fat/protein diet, salted meat or fish, high nitrate consumption, high complex-carbohydrate consumption.
- High fruit and vegetable intake is associated with a reduced risk of gastric cancer in several studies.
- High salt intake increases risk of gastric cancer in those with *H. pylori* and atrophic gastritis. Risk is three times higher in those with a daily salt intake of 16g/day or higher.
- Heavily salted foods are high in N-nitroso compounds, which increase the risk of non-cardia stomach cancer in those with *H. pylori* infection
- Vegetables are a major source of nitrates and together with fruit have a protective effect against stomach cancer. The antioxidants of fruit and vegetables inhibit the formation of N-nitroso compounds.
- Processed meat (especially bacon, ham, and sausages) are associated with increased risk of gastric cancer.
- Frying and grilling food leads to the formation of chemicals, such as heterolytic amines which are carcinogenic.

*Smoking and alcohol*
- Smokers have double the risk of gastric cancer and the risk remains higher for 10–20 years after giving up.
- Nitrosamines are present in tobacco smoke and they are known to be carcinogenic.
- Smoking tobacco is now accepted to be a causal factor for gastric cancer.
- Heavy alcohol consumption is associated with increased risk of gastric cancer in particular in those who are heavy tobacco smokers.

*Medical conditions*
- **Obesity:** 2-fold increase in risk of gastric cancer.
- **Pernicious anaemia:** an autoimmune condition which causes severe gastric atrophy is associated with 2–3 times increased risk of gastric cancer.
- Previous gastric surgery is associated with increased risk of gastric cancer.

# Pathology

## Histological types
- Adenocarcinoma >90% of cases.
- Other types: squamous cell carcinoma, adenocanthoma, carcinoid tumours, gastrointestinal stromal tumours (GIST) and lymphoma.

## Borrmann's classification
- Developed in 1926.
- Divides gastric cancer into five types based on macroscopic appearance of the lesion:
  - Type 1: polypoid or fungating lesion;
  - Type 2: ulcerated lesion surrounded by raised borders;
  - Type 3: ulcerated lesion with infiltration to the gastric wall;
  - Type 4: diffusely infiltrating lesion (Linitis *plastica* when it involves whole stomach);
  - Type 5: lesions that do not fit to any of the above.

## Histological classifications
- Many classification systems proposed.
- No global consensus on the best method and none of them offer the complete answer.

### Borders' classification
- Developed in 1942 and is the original classification.
- Classifies gastric carcinoma on the degree of cellular differentiation independent of morphology.
- Ranges from type 1 (well differentiated) to type 4 (anaplastic).

### Lauren classification 1965
- Most useful and widely used.
- Separates gastric adenocarcinoma into intestinal or diffuse type based on histology.
- **The intestinal type:** typically arises in the presence of a precancerous condition such as gastric atrophy or intestinal metaplasia, more common in men than in women, incidence increases with age, dominant type in areas in which gastric cancer is epidemic, usually well differentiated and tends to spread haematogenously to distant organs.
- **The diffuse type:** poorly differentiated, lacks gland formation, composed of signet ring cells. Clusters of small uniform cells, tends to spread submucosally and metastasizes early by transmural extension and via lymphatics. Poor prognosis. More common in women and younger age groups. Associated with blood type A and familial cases suggesting genetic aetiology.

*WHO classification 1990*
- Based on morphological features and divides gastric cancer into five types.
- Adenocarcinoma, adenosquamous cell carcinoma, squamous cell carcinoma, undifferentiated carcinoma and unclassified carcinoma.
- Adenocarcinoma subdivided into 4 types according to growth pattern: papillary, tubular, mucinous and signet ring. Each type further subdivided by degree of differentiation.
- Widely used system, but offers little in terms of patient management.

# Clinical presentation

## Symptoms
- Gastric adenocarcinoma lacks specific symptoms early in its course.
- Vague symptoms of epigastric discomfort and indigestion – often ignored by patients mistaking it for gastritis.
- Pain tends to be constant and unrelieved by food or antacid therapy.
- More advanced cancer presents with weight loss, dysphagia, odynophagia, loss of appetite, early satiety, or vomiting.

### British Society for Gastroenterology guidelines for referral of suspected gastric cancer
#### Dysphagia
Dyspepsia combined with one or more of these alarm symptoms: weight loss, anaemia, and anorexia.

Dyspepsia in a patient aged 55 years or more with at least one of the following 'high risk' features:
- Onset of dyspepsia less than 1 year ago.
- Continuous symptoms since onset.
- Dyspepsia combined with at least one of the following known risk factors:
  - family history of upper gastrointestinal cancer in more than one first degree relative;
  - Barrett's oesophagus;
  - pernicious anaemia;
  - peptic ulcer surgery over 20 years ago;
  - known dysplasia;
  - atrophic gastritis;
  - intestinal metaplasia;
  - jaundice;
  - upper abdominal mass.

## Physical signs
- Develop late.
- Most commonly associated with locally advanced or metastatic disease.
- Findings may include: palpable abdominal mass, palpable supraclavicular (Virchow's) or peri-umbicular (sister Mary Joseph's) nodule, jaundice, ascites, and cachexia.
- Succussion splash on examination.
- **Acanthosis nigricans:** velvety skin changes around axilla associated with plantar tylosis.

# Clinical evaluation and staging

## Diagnosis and pre-operative staging

### Flexible upper endoscopy
- Modality of choice once gastric cancer is suspected.
- Multiple biopsies (seven or more required) from ulcer edges.
- Avoid biopsying ulcer crater (may reveal necrotic debris only).
- Note the size, location, and morphology of the tumour.

### Blood test should be carried out once gastric cancer is confirmed
- **Full blood count:** may reveal anaemia.
- **Liver function test:** abnormal in advanced disease and sign of liver metastasis.
- **Coagulation:** abnormal in advanced disease.

### Double-contrast barium swallow
- Cost effective and 90% diagnostic accuracy.
- However, unable to distinguish benign from malignant lesions.
- Endoscopy preferable.

### Endoscopic ultrasound scan (EUS)
- Can assess the extent of gastric wall invasion and nodal status.
- Better accuracy for T1 and T3 lesions, but poor for T2 (cannot assess invasion of the muscularis propria).
- Superior to CT for T1 and T3 tumours.
- Cannot reliably distinguish tumour from fibrosis, thus not suitable for evaluating response to therapy.
- Good for evaluating lymph nodes and have added advantage of fine-needle aspiration.
- Overall staging accuracy is about 80%.
- Complimentary to CT and not a replacement.

### CT (computed tomography)
- Chest, abdomen, and pelvis should be scanned.
- Stomach should be well distended to increase accuracy.
- Cannot distinguish T1 and T2 tumour (i.e. early gastric cancers that may be suitable for endoscopic mucosal resections).
- Cannot detect small (<5mm) metastasis in the liver or on peritoneal disease.
- Nodal detection relies on size and is a poor predictor of involvement particularly in the chest.
- **PET-CT** may improve the detection of distant metastasis. Not a routine exam in the UK. Mainly used in follow-up and where there is a suspicion of progression.
- Overall accuracy of 80–85%.

### Diagnostic laparoscopy
- Due to the inherent inaccuracies of CT and EUS, laparoscopy indicated for evaluation of patients with locoregional disease.
- Can detect metastatic disease in 30% of patients who are judged to be resectable on CT and EUS.

- Addition of laparoscopic ultrasound may improve detection of liver and peritoneal metastasis, though highly operator dependent.
- **Cytology** of peritoneal fluid obtained at laparoscopy may reveal the presence of free intraperitoneal gastric cells, but errors in reporting (false positive and false negative) decrease sensitivity of this method.
- **Immunostaining** of peritoneal fluid and reverse transcriptase polymerase chain reaction for carcino-embryonic antigen messenger RNA may provide better and more accurate detection in the future.

Staging systems
- TNM classification of carcinoma of the stomach (see Table 5.1).
- Most widely used.
- Based on the depth of invasion of the gastric wall, the number of involved lymph nodes and the presence or absence of distant metastasis (Fig. 5.1).
- Can accurately stratify patients into distinct groups with different risks for tumour-related death.
- Minimum 15 nodes must be evaluated for accurate staging.
- **pN1:** 1–6 positive nodes; **pN2:** 7–15 positive nodes; **pN3:** more than 15 nodes.

### Tumour staging systems
Tumour (T)
- **TX:** primary tumour cannot be assesses.
- **T0:** no evidence of primary tumour.
- **Tis:** carcinoma in situ (intraepithelial tumour without invasion of the lamina propria.
- **T1:** tumour invades lamina propria or submucosa.
- **T2:** invades muscularis propria or subserosa.
- **T2a:** invades muscularis propria.
- **T2b:** invades subserosa.
- **T3:** penetrates serosa without invasion of surrounding structures.
- **T4:** invades adjacent structures.

Regional lymph nodes (N)
- **NX:** nodes cannot be assessed.
- **N0:** no lymph node metastasis.
- **N1:** 1–6 positive nodes.
- **N2:** 7–15 positive nodes.
- **N3:** more than 15 positive nodes.

Distant metastasis (M)
- **Mx:** distant metastasis cannot be assessed.
- **M0:** no distant metastasis.
- **M1:** established distant metastasis.

**Table 5.1** Stage grouping

| Stage 0 | Tis, N0, M0 |
|---|---|
| Stage 1A | T1, N0, M0 |
| Stage 1B | T1, N1, M0 |
| | T2a/b, N0, M0 |
| Stage II | T1, N2, M0 |
| | T2a/b, N1, M0 |
| | T3, N0, M0 |
| Stage IIIA | T2a/b, N2, M0 |
| | T3, N1, M0 |
| | T4, N0, M0 |
| Stage IIIB | T3, N2, M0 |
| Stage IV | T4, N1–3, M0 |
| | T1–3, N3, M0 |
| | Any T, any N, M1 |

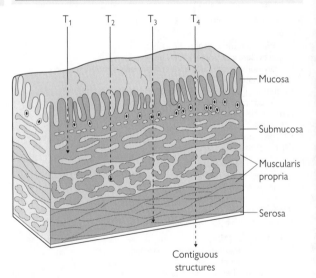

**Fig. 5.1** Cross-section of gastric wall.

*The R status*
- Used to describe the tumour status after resection.
- R0: microscopically negative margin.
- R1: microscopically positive margin.
- R2: gross residual disease.

## Japanese classification of gastric carcinoma

- Designed to describe the anatomic locations of nodes removed during gastrectomy (Fig. 5.2).
- 16 distinct anatomic stations of lymph nodes.
- Grouped into 3 groups (N1, N2, and N3).
- Nodal basin dissection dependent on the location of the primary.
- Not used in Europe and in America.

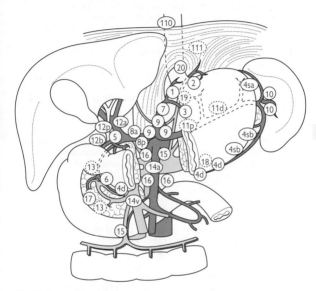

**Fig. 5.2** Anatomic lymph node groupings.

# Neoadjuvant treatment

### Chemotherapy
- Good evidence that peri-operative chemotherapy improves survival in operable gastric cancer.
- MRC trial 2006 (MAGIC trial):
  - Phase III trial for peri-operative chemotherapy;
  - patients randomized to either peri-operative chemotherapy (pre-operative and post-operative chemotherapy with epirubicin, cisplatin and 5-FU [ECF]) and surgery (250 patients) or surgery alone (253).
  - 5-year survival was 36% in chemotherapy group and 23% in the surgery alone group.
  - Peri-operative chemotherapy improves survival in patients with operable gastric cancer.
- This is the standard adjuvant regime for operable gastric cancer in the UK.

### Chemoradiation
- Non-randomized studies have shown substantial pathological response (i.e. downstaging of tumour) to pre-operative chemoradiation.
- Currently trials are underway to assess the usefulness of this regime.
- In the UK this is only available as part of a trial.

### Radiotherapy alone
- Recent randomized trials from China revealed a survival benefit with pre-operative radiotherapy (30 vs. 20%).
- Currently trials under way in the west to try and replicate this.
- In the UK pre-operative radiotherapy is not standard.

## Radiotherapy stages

### Initial work up
- History and physical examination.
- Direct gastroscopy.
- Blood test: FBC, U&E, LFT, coagulation.
- CT chest, abdomen, and pelvis.
- EUS if available.
- PET/CT if distant metastasis is suspected.
- MDT discussion.

### Staging
- **Stage IV disease (M1):** palliation therapy.
- All other stages if medically fit consider for diagnostic laparoscopy for further staging.

### After laparoscopy
- Stage M1 palliation only.
- Stage M0, but medically unfit either palliation only or radiotherapy and 5-FU radiosensitization.
- Stage M0 and medically fit, T1 or less. For surgery.
- Stage M0 and medically fit, T2 or higher. Neoadjuvant chemotherapy with ECF (MAGIC trial protocol) followed by surgery.

# Surgical anatomy of the stomach

**Gross anatomy (Fig. 5.3)**
- Originates as a dilatation in the tubular embryonic foregut during the fifth week of gestation.
- By the 7th week it descends, rotates, and comes to rest in its normal anatomical position.
- The stomach is fixed at the gastro-oesophageal junction and at the pylorus, its large mid-portion is mobile.
- Most of the stomach resides within the left upper quadrant of the abdominal cavity.
- Relations of the stomach:
  - anteriorly – left lobe of the liver;
  - superiorly – the diaphragm;
  - medially – the liver;
  - laterally – spleen;
  - inferiorly – transverse mesocolon, caudate lobe of liver, crura of the diaphragm, and retroperitoneal nerves and vessels.

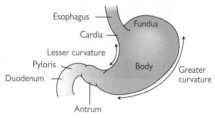

**Fig. 5.3** Regions of the stomach.

**Blood supply**
- Most of the blood supply is from the coeliac artery (Fig. 5.4).
- Four main arteries:
  - left and right gastric arteries along the lesser curvature of stomach;
  - left and right gastro-epiploic arteries along the greater curvature of the stomach;
  - proximal stomach receives substantial amount of blood from the inferior phrenic arteries and the short gastric arteries from the spleen;
  - in general the veins of the stomach parallel the arteries.

**Lymphatic drainage (Fig. 5.5)**
- The lymphatic drainage of the stomach parallels the vasculature.
- Drains into four zones of lymph nodes as shown below.
- All four zones drain into the coeliac group and the thoracic duct.
- Gastric cancer can metastasize to any of the four nodal groups regardless of the cancer location.
- The extensive submucosal plexus of the lymphatics accounts for the fact that there is frequently microscopic evidence of malignant cells several centimetres away from the resection margin of gross disease.

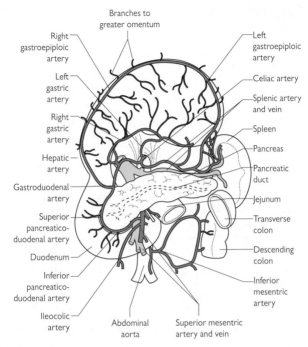

**Fig. 5.4** Gastric anatomy and relations.

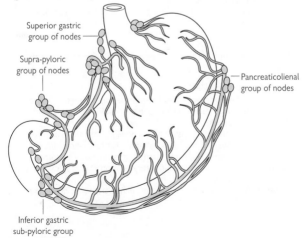

**Fig. 5.5** Lymphatic drainage of the stomach.

# Surgical management

- Primary treatment for gastric carcinoma.
- Less than 50% of patients at presentation currently are resectable.
- Most present with advanced disease and so extensive curative surgery is not an option.
- Over the past 20 years the anatomical location of gastric cancer has shifted from predominantly distal stomach to proximal stomach, such as cardia or gastro-oesophageal junction. As a result the type of gastrectomy has changed.
- In the UK about half of gastric cancer patients have surgery, but only 20% of cases have curative surgery.

## Principles of surgery

- Extent of gastric resection is determined by the need to obtain R0 margin.
- 6cm clearance from edge tumour is required in order to decrease risk of local recurrence. Proximal tumours are more advanced at presentation than distal tumours, so curative resections are rare.

### Proximal tumours

- Either total gastrectomy or proximal gastric resection.
- No evidence that one operation is better than the other for tumour removal.
- Abundant evidence that proximal gastric resection results in higher morbidity and mortality than total gastrectomy. In the Norwegian Stomach Cancer Trial 1988, incidence of morbidity and mortality following proximal gastric resections was 52% and 16%, respectively, compared to 38% and 8% for total gastrectomy.
- Therefore, total gastrectomy operation of choice for proximal tumours.

### Distal tumours

- About 35% of gastric cancer cases.
- No difference in 5-year survival for total gastrectomy or subtotal gastrectomy.
- Therefore, subtotal gastrectomy operation of choice for distal tumours.
- 5–6cm margin is required.
- Frozen section must be carried at operation in order to achieve this clearance.

## Lymph node dissection

- The extent of lymph node dissection remains controversial.
- The Japanese classification system is used to define extent lymphatic dissection performed.
- *Group 1 nodes (N1):* perigastric lymph node stations along the lesser curvature (stations 1, 3, and 5) and greater curvature (stations 2, 4, and 6).
- *Group 2 (N2):* nodes along left gastric artery (station 7), common hepatic artery (station 8), coeliac artery (station 9), and splenic artery (stations 10 and 11).
- *Group 3 (N3):* more distant nodes including para-aortic nodes are regarded as distant metastasis.

### D1 resection
- Removal of group 1 nodes plus the greater and lesser omenta.
- Either subtotal or total gastrectomy.

### D2 resection
Removal of group 1 and 2 nodes.

### D3 resection
- D2 resection plus removal of para-aortic lymph nodes.
- In Japan, this is achieved by performing splenectomy and partial pancreatectomy.
- In the West, the spleen and pancreas is only resected if there is a direct invasion because of the morbidity associated with this.

### D1 vs. D2
- Higher morbidity and mortality for D2 compared to D1 gastrectomy.
- No difference in overall survival between D1 and D2.
- **The Dutch Cancer Group Trial 1999:** long-term survival data comparing D1 and D2 resection: 711 patients randomized to D1 or D2. Morbidity D1 vs. D2 (25 vs. 43%); mortality D1 vs. D2 (4 vs. 10%). No difference in overall survival (30 vs. 35%).
- The Medical Research Council trial on lymphadenectomy of gastric cancer 2004 has shown similar results to the Dutch trial.
- Splenectomy, pancreatectomy, and age older than 70 years are risk factors for higher morbidity and mortality in the MRC trial.
- A phase II study of D2 dissection by the Italian Gastric Cancer Study Group 2004 has demonstrated a morbidity of 20.9% and a post-operatively mortality of 3%. This is comparable to D1 dissection in the Dutch and MRC trial results.
- One reason for the Italian Group results is the lack of routine pancreatectomy, except when warranted by direct invasion.
- However, Japanese studies have consistently showed survival benefit for D2 over D1 without increased morbidity or mortality.
- A surgical option that may decrease morbidity and mortality is an 'over-D1' (i.e. D1+) lymphadenectomy with preservation of the pancreatic tail and without splenectomy.

## Endoscopic techniques
### Endoscopic mucosal resection (EMR)
- Technique of resecting early gastric cancer (T1, mucosal and submucosal).
- Node negative T1 tumours have greater than 90% 5-year survival in open surgery, hence interest for EMR.
- Most experience with EMR is in Japan where there is a higher incidence of early gastric cancer and an active screening programme.
- Indications for EMR include well or moderately differentiated histology, tumour size less than 30mm, absence of ulceration, and no evidence of invasive findings.

*Laparoscopic gastric resection (Table 5.2)*
- Involves wedge resection of the stomach.
- **Indications:** potentially node negative T1 tumours or early gastric cancer (where EMR is not available or amenable), GIST (gastrointestinal stromal tumours) and symptom control (such as bleeding from the cancer) of medically unfit patient or for palliation.
- Currently not recommended for potentially resectable cases because of the technical difficulties of achieving nodal and mucosal clearance.

**Table 5.2** Gastric resection stages

| Aim | R0 resection |
| --- | --- |
| Stage carefully | CT +/− EUS and laparoscopy and PET-CT if needed |
| Unresectable | If level 3 or 4 lymph nodes involved, invasion, or encasement of major vascular structures, distant metastasis, or peritoneal seedings |
| Total gastrectomy | Gastro-oesophageal junction/cardia tumours |
| Subtotal gastrectomy | If mucosal clearance of at least 6cm to achieve R0 resection possible: less morbidity and mortality compared with total gastrectomy and survival is the same |
| Nodes | Perform D1 Lymphadenectomy aim >15 nodes |
| Splenectomy/ pancreatectomy | Not indicated unless direct invasion |
| Feeding | Jejunostomy recommended at time of operation |

# Operative techniques: total gastrectomy with Roux-en-Y reconstruction

## Indication
Proximal gastric tumours and linitis plastica.

## Pre-operative management
Thorough assessment of cardiorespiratory function and nutritional status.

## Operative procedure
- Access via upper midline or a roof top incision.
- Left thoraco-abdominal incision may be required for radical resection of gastro-oesophageal junction tumours.
- Goligher type retractors or Omnitract system improves access.
- On entering abdomen full examination of all structures is performed to look for metastatic disease.
- Frozen-section is carried out of any suspicious lesion on the liver or peritoneal lining.
- The first steps are to mobilize the splenic and hepatic colonic flexures.
- Kocherize the duodenum (i.e. mobilize the second and third part of the duodenum.
- Detach the greater omentum from the transverse colon avoiding opening the lesser sac.
- Continue to dissect to the right and towards the right gastro-epiploic vessels.
- Ligate and divide these vessels at their origin and sweep lymph nodes upwards with the stomach to be resected.
- Dissect over the surface of the pancreas to the left hand side.
- Ligate and divide the short gastric vessels.
- Retract liver to expose the gastro-hepatic ligament.
- Dissect from the oesophageal hiatus to the common bile duct, lifting nodes encountered.
- Expose the portal triad and resect portal nodes (station 12 lymph nodes) in continuity with the main specimen.
- Dissect the common hepatic artery and identify the right gastric artery, which arises from the common hepatic artery.
- Ligate the right gastric vessels at its origin.
- Kocherize the duodenum fully and dissect the retropancreatic and hepatoduodenal regions. This should expose the inferior vena cava, and the aorta allowing retrieval of right para-aortic and retropancreatic lymph nodes.
- Divide the duodenum with a linear stapler or alternatively between two crushing clamps and close the duodenum with 3/0 continuous absorbable suture.
- Dividing the duodenum reveals retropyloric nodes which are retrieved.
- Retract the stomach upwards and dissect towards the celiac axis.
- Ligate and divide the left gastric artery at its origin. Left gastric vessels should also be divided over the pancreas.

- Retrieve lymph nodes around the celiac trunk.
- Ligate the remaining the short gastric vessels and retrieve parasplenic lymph nodes as far and as safe as possible. In Japan splenectomy and distal pancreatectomy is performed to harvest these nodes.
- Divide remaining adhesions and make sure stomach is fully mobilized.
- Put two stay sutures on the oesophagus.
- Divide the oesophagus with straight scissors or scalpel making sure a cuff of oesophagus and diaphragm is included with the resection margin.
- Next prepare for the reconstruction stage.
- Divide the jejunum at a convenient point with a linear stapler.
- Bring up the distal end of the divided jejunum to the oesophagus to form an end to side anastomosis.
- The anastmosis can either be carried out by a single layer of interrupted monofilament sutures or by the use of a circular stapler.
- Next join the proximal end of the divided jejunum with the distal jejunum at a point 40–50cm away from the oesophageal anastomosis.
- Finally (optional) form a feeding jejunostomy.
- Close the abdomen.

# Operative technique: subtotal gastrectomy

## Indications
Distal gastric tumours.

## Operative technique
- Steps similar to total gastrectomy up to the point of dividing the remaining short gastric vessels.
- The most lateral short gastric vessels are left behind to be the sole blood supply to the gastric remnant.
- Divide the stomach to leave a small remnant.
- Reconstruction is usually by Roux-en-Y as above or can be by Bilroth I technique.
- In Bilroth I the gastric remnant is anastomosed with the duodenum either hand sewn or using circular stapler which is more common.
- Feeding jejunostomy optional.
- Close abdomen.

## Gastrojejunostomy

### Indication
- Palliation of gastric outlet obstruction in advanced gastric cancer.
- Principle of the surgery is to bypass gastric contents into a loop of jejunum.

### Operative technique
- The abdominal cavity is opened as above.
- The stomach is assessed and its contents emptied via NG tube if possible.
- Site of anastomosing a loop of jejunum is selected.
- Ideal site is the posterior gastric wall.
- To access this, the greater omentum is taken off the transverse colon and the lesser sac entered.
- Select a convenient part of the posterior gastric wall for the anastomosis.
- Place two stay sutures on the selected area at least 9cm apart
- Bring a loop of jejunum to the stomach without tension and place two stay sutures 6cm apart. A standard stapled anastomosis fashioned using a 90mm linear cutting stapler is ideal.
- For a hand sewn approach (rarely utilised) place a running suture (seromuscular) between the jejunum and the stomach wall.
- Open the stomach wall between the stay sutures using diathermy.
- Place suction tube in the stomach and thoroughly empty the stomach.
- Similarly open the jejunum taking care not to damage the running suture, which will be the most posterior layer of the double layer anastomosis.
- Now place a running suture between posterior walls of the stomach and jejunum. This can be full thickness.
- The running suture is continued to the anterior walls of the anastomosis taking care to bury the corners and fully closing the anastomosis.

- Another running suture is then placed on the anterior wall of the anastomosis to achieve double layered anastomosis.
- Sometimes it is not possible to get access to the lesser sac due to tumour infiltration. It is therefore acceptable to place the anastomosis on the anterior stomach wall, although functionally is not as good as a posteriorly placed anastomosis.
- Roux-en-Y limb formation to divert the bile is an alternative adjunct.
- The abdomen is then closed as before.

# Complications of gastric surgery

Early complications

*Bleeding*
- Intra- or post-operative.
- Post-operative bleeding tends to be torrential and usually requires immediate re-exploration. Often due to the short gastric vessels, splenic/liver tear or bleeding from a loose tie to a vessel, such as the left gastric artery.

*Infection*
- Wound or chest.
- Usually treatable and not life-threatening.
- If pneumonia develops can be fatal in the weak and malnourished.

*Anastomotic leak*
- Most serious complication.
- Usually occurs from day 5 onwards after surgery.
- Management is multifaceted.
- Principle is control sepsis, address nutritional requirements and support organs.
- Patients should be in HDU/ITU setting.
- Surgery is only indicated in the presence of uncontrolled abdominal sepsis.
- Aim is to establish a controlled fistula and treat sepsis with appropriate antimicrobial therapy and percutaneous drainage of any abdominal collections.
- Recovery tends to be long and protracted, and one or two organ failures are common.
- Mortality is high.

General complications
- Cardio-respiratory complications.
- Deep vein thrombosis and pulmonary embolism.
- MRSA and *Clostridium difficile* infection.

Late complications

*Dumping syndrome*
- Symptom complex that occurs after ingestion of a meal.
- Can be early or late.
- **Early dumping** more common and occurs 20–30min after ingestion of a meal and is accompanied by gastro-intestinal cardiovascular symptoms.
- GI symptoms include nausea and vomiting, sense of fullness, belching, abdominal cramps, and explosive diarrhoea.
- Cardiac symptoms include palpitations, tachycardia, sweating, fainting, dizziness, flushing, and visual disturbance.
- It is thought that the sudden passage of high osmolarity food into the small bowel results rapid shift of extracellular fluid into the small bowel lumen. This stretches the lumen and induces an autonomic response.

- This process causes the release of several humeral agents, such as serotonin, bradykinin-like substances, neurotensin, and enteroglucagon, which give rise to the various symptoms associated with early dumping.
- Symptoms usually subside with time, but if prolonged management strategy includes dietary measures in order to reduce carbohydrate intake and to eat small amounts of meals (little and often).
- Those that do not respond to dietary measures may find relief using the somatostatin analogue octreotide acetate.

### Late dumping

- Less common and occurs 2–3h after ingestion of a meal.
- It is due to the rapid delivery of large amount of carbohydrates to the proximal small intestine, which are quickly absorbed. This causes sudden hyperglycaemia, which triggers the release of a large amount of insulin to control the rising blood sugar level.
- Overshooting occurs resulting profound hypoglycaemia, which triggers the release of catecholamines from the adrenal gland, causing tachycardia, sweating, confusion, and dizziness.
- Symptoms similar to hypoglycaemic shock.
- Patients are advised to eat small amounts of meals and to reduce carbohydrate intake.

### Metabolic disturbance

- **Anaemia:** most common metabolic disturbance after gastrectomy. Iron deficiency anaemia is the commonest type, and results from a mixture of decreased iron intake, impaired iron absorption, and chronic subclinical blood loss from the friable mucosa at the anastomosis. Easily corrected by supplemental iron in diet. Megaloblastic anaemia occurs from deficiency of vitamin $B_{12}$ as a result of lack of intrinsic factor secretion from the stomach, which is necessary for absorption. 3-monthly injection of hydroxocobalamin usually corrects the problem. Folate deficiency is usually corrected by diet supplementation
- **Impaired absorption of fat:** due to inadequate mixing of fat with bile salts and pancreatic juices as a result of the Roux-en-Y reconstruction, which bypasses bile and pancreatic fluid, further down in the small bowel. If steatorrhoea is present, pancreatic replacement enzymes given orally is effective.
- **Osteoporosis and osteomalacia:** due to calcium malabsorption and requires calcium supplementation in diet before the onset of bone disease.

### Afferent loop syndrome

- Occurs in Billroth II gastrectomy and gastrojejunostomy bypass procedures.
- Seen when the afferent limb of the small bowel anastomosis is blocked by kinking, adhesions, or herniation.
- Usually requires surgery, such as converting the reconstruction into Roux-en-Y limb.

*Efferent loop syndrome*
- Occurs due to obstruction of the efferent limb of the anastomosis as a result of herniation of the small bowel.
- Requires surgical intervention.

*Alkaline reflux gastritis*
- Usually seen in patients who had Billroth II gastrectomy and gastrojejunostomy bypass surgery.
- Present with persistent epigastric discomfort and indigestion type symptoms.
- Diagnosis is by upper GI endoscopy, which reveals the presence of bile in the stomach and inflamed friable mucosa at the anastomosis.
- If medical therapy fails and complications present, such as intractable iron deficiency anaemia and significant upper GI haemorrhage then surgery is indicated.
- The procedure of choice is converting the Billroth II anastomosis to a Roux-en-Y formation.

# Adjuvant chemoradiotherapy

- Evidence now exists of a clear benefit for post-operative chemoradiation over surgery alone.
- The intergroup trial INT-0116 published 2001 and updated 2004 randomized 603 patients with T3 tumours (with or without nodes) to either surgery alone or surgery plus post-operative combined chemoradiotherapy consisting of 5 monthly cycles of 5-FU and leucovorin with radiation therapy (45Gy). There was a significant increase of median survival (36 vs. 27 months), 3-year recurrence-free survival (48 vs. 31%) and overall survival (50 vs. 41%) with combined modality therapy.

*This is the standard adjuvant therapy for gastric cancer in North America (Table 5.3)*

**Table 5.3** Adjuvant therapy for gastric cancer

| M1 | Palliative therapy |
| --- | --- |
| R0 resection and T1, N0 | Observe |
| R0 and T2 and higher | ECF chemotherapy |
| R1 resection | Radiotherapy plus concurrent 5-FU sensitization followed up by ECF chemotherapy if T2 and higher |
| R2 resection | 5-FU based radiosensitization or ECF chemotherapy or best supportive care if unfit |
| Primary palliative chemotherapy | Reassess and if good response consider surgery |

# Chemotherapy for advanced or metastatic disease

- Designed for palliation of symptomatic patients.
- Combination chemotherapy is used, and most trials show that this approach resulted in better quality of life and overall survival when compared with best supportive care.
- In 1980s the FAM (5-FU, doxorubicin and mitomycin) regimen was the gold standard, especially in North America.
- In a trial by the North Central Cancer Treatment Group FAM was compared with 5-FU alone and 5-FU plus doxorubicin. Results show combination chemotherapy better than single agent.
- Many other combination chemotherapy trialled with no overall clear winner.
- In the UK the chemotherapy combination ECF (epirubicin, cisplatin, and 5-FU) is used for advanced gastric cancer.
- In North America there is no single standard regime, but the combination chemotherapy DCF (docetaxel, cisplatin and 5-FU) is widely used. Alternatives include fluoropyrimidine/folinic acid, cisplatin-, oxaliplatin-, or irinotecan-based regimes.

## Radiotherapy for unresectable disease

- Radiotherapy alone in unresectable disease has minimal value in palliation and does not improve survival. May control chronic bleeding.
- Radiotherapy (moderate-dose external-beam radiation of 45–50Gy) combined with 5-fluorouracil (5-FU) improves survival and is of greater use.

# Palliation

Advanced gastric cancer is not curable, and management strategy involves (Table 5.4) reducing symptoms and maintaining quality of life as long as is feasible.

## Obstruction

- Most troublesome symptom in advanced gastric cancer.
- Occurs when tumour occludes the gastro-oesophageal junction and the pylorus/duodenum.
- Management is initially endoscopic approach. Either balloon dilatation or luminal stenting.
- If endoscopy fails or is not possible, then one can consider surgery in the form of gastric bypass (gastrojejunostomy anastomosis), either open or laparoscopic surgery.

## Bleeding

- Upper gastro-intestinal bleeding is usually due to direct bleeding from the tumour.
- This is best managed endoscopically: diathermy, heat probe, argon laser, adrenaline injection, or clipping.
- Surgical debulking or under-running can be contemplated. Tissue friability and patient performance status usually preclude its use.

## Weight loss/cachexia

- Not always due to poor appetite, but the systemic effects of the advanced cancer.
- High protein diet and supplemental build-up drinks can slow down the progression.
- If possible night-time nasogastric tube feeding may be of use in some patients.
- Laparoscopically-placed feeding jejunostomy is a useful technique, which can maintain nutritional requirements.

**Table 5.4** Management strategies

| | |
|---|---|
| Medically fit, but unresectable tumour | Consider combination chemotherapy as part of a trial. |
| | In the UK ECF is used but numerous trials ongoing using other combinations |
| Medically unfit | Best supportive care: |
| | Obstruction: stent, laser, photodynamic therapy, radiotherapy, surgery |
| | Nutrition: enteral feeding |
| | Pain control: radiotherapy and/or analgesics |
| | Bleeding: radiotherapy, endoscopic therapy or surgery |

# Surveillance

- All patients should be followed up systematically.
- Currently, no national guidelines exist in terms frequency of follow-up and type of investigations that should conducted.
- However, most units treating gastric cancer have guidelines in place that broadly follow the pattern below:
  - first 3 years follow-up should be intensive, since recurrence is most common at this stage;
  - follow-up should be 4–6 months for first 3 years, thereafter annually;
  - history, physical examination, and routine blood profile should be conducted at each follow-up visit;
  - CT scan should be performed yearly, or for first 3 years or sooner if suspicious;
  - yearly gastroscopy on patients who have undergone subtotal gastrectomy.

# Chapter 6

# Liver and biliary cancers

# Clinical presentation and evaluation

### Presentation
- Late and insidious.
- Often asymptomatic in early stages
- Constitutional symptoms weight loss, nausea, loss of appetite, and lethargy.
- Enlargement of the liver and stretching of the liver capsule may result in right upper quadrant pain.
- ***Diaphragmatic irritation:*** referred pain to the right shoulder tip.
- Biliary obstruction, jaundice.
- High risk patients may be participating in a screening programme and, therefore, detected when asymptomatic.
- Incidental finding of hepatic mass.
- ***Rare presentations:*** spontaneous rupture into peritoneal cavity, haemorrhage, bone metastases, ascites.

### Associated paraneoplastic syndromes
Erythrocytosis (erythropoietin), hypercalcaemia (parathyroid-related protein), hypogycaemia (insulin-like growth factor).

### Diagnosis
#### Blood tests
Liver function tests may be non-specifically deranged due to underlying cirrhotic process.

#### Alpha-1 foeto-protein (AFP)
- Glycoprotein produced by embryo then foetus. Low, but detectable level in adult.
- Classically ↑. A level of >500ng/mL and mass on imaging is considered diagnostic with a confidence interval of greater than 95%.
- Sensitivity and specificity are poor.
- Elevated in 60–90% of HCC cases disproportionately more AFP secreting tumours in Asia.
- **AFP L3** percentage rise >10% over AFP more sensitive for small tumours.
- More specific.
- **PIVKA II:** 'Des-gamma carboxy prothrombin protein induced by vitamin K absence', Vitamin K antagonist II, increased in hepatitis and HCC more specific than AFP.
- Latter 2 tests not widely available yet.

#### Hepatis serology
Blood glucose may ↓, calcium and lipids may ↑.

### Imaging
- ***Ultrasound:*** inexpensive, accessible, and non-invasive. Ability to detect HCC depends on operator skill, body habitus of the patient and size, and location of the tumour. Used for screening. Can detect portal vein thrombosis, biliary, and vascular invasion.

- **CT scan:** spiral and contrast. More accurate. Detects vascular and biliary invasion, lymph nodes and extrahepatic spread.
- **Hepatic angiography:** diagnostic accuracy depends on tumour size and vascularity. Due to improvement in other imaging techniques now mainly a therapeutic technique during chemo-embolization.
- **MRI:** best imaging technique for differentiating HCC from other lesions.
- **Diagnostic laparoscopy:** not required for routine work up as standard imaging sufficient. Useful if resectability of tumour in doubt.
- **Liver biopsy:** not required in lesions >2cm or where diagnosis proven on imaging and AFP. Risk of tumour seeding and haemorrhage. False negative rate in lesions<2cm 30–40%.
- **Positive emission tomography (PET):** $^{18}$F-fluorodeoxyglucose taken up by tumour. Sensitivity for detection HCC is low. More useful in cholangiocarcinoma where can detect tumours >1cm. Useful in colorectal liver metastases and occult disease recurrence.
- **Magnetic resonance cholangiopancreatography (MRCP)** and **endoscopic retrograde cholangiopancreatography (ERCP):** allows visualization of biliary system and extent of tumour involvement. Used in pre-operative investigation of cholangiocarcinoma. ERCP invasive, complication rate <9%, but may provide histological diagnosis and allows therapeutic decompression in obstructive jaundice. MRCP less invasive and provides greater detail of anatomy. Does not allow histology or decompression.

## Screening
- High risk groups screened.
- Lack of evidence for cost effectiveness.
- Ultrasound +/or AFP, Alk Phos, Alb used at 3–6-month intervals.
- Rising AFP, but negative imaging: 3 months screening.

### Limitations
- Cost (especially in endemic regions).
- Lack of compliance (especially alcoholic cirrhosis).
- Previously undiagnosed cirrhosis missed.

# Primary liver cancers

Rare. Most common hepatocellular carcinoma (HCC). Others include angiosarcoma, intrahepatic cholangiocarcinoma, epithelioid haemangioendothelioma, lymphoma.

## Hepatocellular carcinoma

- HCC or hepatoma is a primary cancer of hepatocytes. 90% of primary liver cancers.
- Two types: hepatoma most common and fibrolamellar hepatoma rarer, occurs in young people with no primary liver disease.

## Epidemiology

- Geographical variation, ↑ incidence Africa and Asia where it is one of the most frequently diagnosed cancers.
- Rare in the western world.
- Third cause of cancer death worldwide: most common male cancer in China and Korea male:female 7:1.
- Increasing incidence in developed world due to hepatitis C infection
- 5–30% of those infected with hepatitis C develop HCC: latency period 30–50 years.
- 2507 new cases per year in the UK male to female ratio of 3:2.
- Related to high rates of hepatitis B infection, which increases the risk of HCC 100-fold.
- Usually occurs in 60th decade in Western world, 20–50 years in Africa/Asia.

## Aetiology

Most cases in patients with liver cirrhosis. <30% in non-cirrhotic liver. Virally-induced cirrhosis associated with higher rates of HCC than other causes. In cirrhotic patients further risk factors include age, male sex, severity of cirrhosis, obesity and high alcohol intake.

Aflatoxin B1 ingestion. Toxin produced by fungus, *Aspergillus flavus* found in mouldy grain and cereals. Induces mutation in the *p53* tumour suppressor gene. Unclear whether it is a co-carcinogen with HBV.

- Hepatitis virus integration results in altered gene expression. Often inserts into intron 2 of cyclin A resulting in cell cycle deregulation. Also over-expression of transforming growth factor beta. Also modulates P53 function.
- Oncogene activation uncommon. Frequent allelic losses at 1p, 4q, 5q, 11p, 13q, 16p and 16q suggest associated tumour suppressor genes. Loss of heterozygosity (LOH) at chromosome 16 associated with poorly differentiated tumours and advanced disease. DNA hypermethylation found at various loci on chromosome 16, occurs in cirrhosis and chronic hepatitis indicating an early change.

Metabolic liver diseases are also associated with increased incidence; Includes haemochromatosis, porphyria, alpha-1-antitrypsin deficiency, Wilsons disease, cutanea tarda tyrosinaemia.

Benign adenomas of the liver occur in patients using oestrogen con-taining medications, such as the oral contraceptive pill, anabolic steroids, or those with type 1 glycogenolysis. Risk of malignant transformation.

## Pathology

- Cirrhotic livers can contain benign hyperplastic nodules, dysplastic nodules (premalignant) and HCCs.
- HCC 3 subtypes; unifocal expansile (solid mass), infiltrating and multifocal.

## Other rare tumours

### Epithelioid haemangioendothelioma

- Very rare tumour originating from endothelioid cells lining sinusoids.
- Young adults.
- Females > males.
- Diagnosis via scan, MRI most reliable and biopsy.
- Prognosis very variable.
- Surgical resection treatment of choice. Multifocal nature may make transplantation only option. Metastases not contraindication to treatment.
- Radiotherapy, chemotherapy and embolization of no benefit.

### Angiosarcoma

- Rare.
- Arise from endothelial cells.
- Male:female 3:1.
- Age at diagnosis 50–70 years.
- Linked with exposure to vinyl chloride (plastics industry), arsenics, thorium dioxide, anabolic steroids, contraceptive pill, and cirrhosis.
- Rapidly growing, early metastases, and local recurrence. Poor prognosis.
- Surgical resection where possible and chemotherapy.
- Transplant not indicated as high rate of tumour recurrence.

### Primary hepatic lymphoma

- Very rare.
- Associated with AIDS and chronic liver disease.
- Usually B cell lineage.
- Resection if possible and chemotherapy.

# Staging

Staging is vital pre-operatively (Boxes 6.1 and 6.2).
- Number and size of lesions.
- Vascular involvement.
- Regional and distal lymphadenopathy.
- Presence of metastases.
- Ascites, varices, cirrhosis.

## Tumour staging

### Primary tumour (T)
- **TX:** primary tumour cannot be assessed.
- **T0:** no evidence of primary tumour.
- **T1:** solitary tumour without vascular invasion.
- **T2:** solitary tumour with vascular invasion or multiple tumours none more than 5cm.
- **T3:** multiple tumours more than 5cm or tumour involving a major branch of the portal or hepatic vein(s).
- **T4:** tumour(s) with direct invasion of adjacent organs other than the gallbladder or with perforation of the visceral peritoneum.

### Regional lymph nodes (N)
- **NX:** regional lymph nodes cannot be assessed.
- **N0:** no regional lymph node metastasis.
- **N1:** regional lymph node metastasis.

### Distant metastasis (M)
- **MX:** distant metastasis cannot be assessed.
- **M0:** no distant metastasis.
- **M1:** distant metastasis.

- Bone and lung most common site for metastases.
- HCC locally invasive and readily invade blood vessels.
- Biliary invasion rarer.

## Histological grade
- **Gx:** grade cannot be assessed.
- **G1:** well differentiated.
- **G2:** moderately differentiated.
- **G3:** poorly differentiated.
- **G4:** undifferentiated.

Ishak fibrosis score
- **F0:** score 0–4 (none to moderate fibrosis).
- **F1:** score 5–6 (severe fibrosis or cirrhosis).

**Table 6.1** AJCC stage groupings

| Stage | TNM |
| --- | --- |
| I | T1, N0, M0 |
| II | T2, N0, M0 |
| IIIA | T3, N0, M0 |
| IIIB | T4, N0, M0 |
| IIIC | Any, T, N1, M0 |
| IV | Any T, any N, M1 |

For purposes of treatment, patients grouped into 1 of 3 groups:
Localized resectable: stage I and some stage II.
Localized unresectable: stage III.

Other scoring systems
TNM system has limitations and poor prognostic accuracy as survival depends on many patients factors, as well as those related to tumour. Several alternatives have been developed including the Okuda score (Tables 6.2).

**Table 6.2** Okuda score

|  | Negative | Positive |
| --- | --- | --- |
| Tumour size | <50% liver | >50% liver |
| Ascites | Absent | Present |
| Serum albumin (g/L) | >30 | <30 |
| Bilirubin (μ/mol) | <50 | >50 |

Okuda I, no positive factors; Okuda II 1 or 2 positives; Okuda III, 3 or 4 positives.

*Mean survival*
- **Okuda I:** 11.5 months.
- **Okuda II:** 3 months.
- **Okuda III:** 0.5 months.
- In Okuda I group who undergo surgery, survival increases to 25.6 months.
- Overall 5-year survival rates for HCC <10% partially due to co-existing problems, e.g. cirrhosis. 5-Year survival for early resectable HCC is 30–60%.

*Child–Pugh score*

Used as prognostic score for cirrhotic patients undergoing surgery. Not a predictor of mortality from HCC (Table 6.3).

**Table 6.3** Child–Pugh score

| Biochemical parameter | 1 | 2 | 3 |
|---|---|---|---|
| Encephalopathy(grade) | None | Mild | Marked |
| Albumin (g/L) | >35 | 28-35 | <28 |
| Ascites | None | Mild | Marked |
| Prothrombin, time prolonged (s) | 1–4 | 4–6 | >6 |
| Bilirubin (µmol/L) | <34 | 34–50 | >50 |

*Child Pugh scores:*

<7: A (good operative risk), 7–9: B (moderate operative risk), >9: C (poor operative risk).

**Functional liver reserve**

- No consensus about what volume of hepatic remnant is safe for hepatic resection.
- Liver function measured by synthetic activity and hepatic clearance function. Large variety of approaches.
- *MEGX clearance:* lidocaine metabolite clearance, galactose elimination, aminopyrine clearance (depend on hepatic perfusion).
- CT volumetry used to calculate residual liver volume must be correlated with quality of liver. In those with no Hx chronic liver disease percentage remnant liver volume (PRLV) can give indication of functional liver reserve
- Functional volume index: liver methyl $^{11}$C methionine uptake assessment by PET. Popular in Japan.
- $^{99m}$Tc-GSA dynamic SPECT also used for regional hepatic functional reserve estimation.
- *Hepatic venous pressure gradient:* useful measure of potential hepatic decompensation post-resection in cirrhotic patients.

# Management: hepatic resection

- Treatment of choice in non-cirrhotic patient and potentially curative.
- Controversial in cirrhotic patients.

## Stages I and II disease

- Wedge resection, hepatectomy, extended hepatectomy.
- Few patients suitable for surgical resection due to advanced tumour, multiple tumours, or pre-existing severe cirrhosis and poor functional reserve.

## Indications

- Single tumour <5cm with preserved liver function and no metastases.
- Location of tumour must also be considered.

## Contraindications

- Child–Pugh grade C.
- Limited resection only in Child–Pugh grade B.
- Portal hypertension confers high risk of liver decompensation post-operatively.

## Survival

- Dependent on regenerative potential, current interest in optimizing management of liver remnant.
- Peri-operative mortality 6–20%.
- Recurrence rate 50–60% at 5 years.
- Indocyanine green clearance can be used to predict liver function.
- Techniques include selective in-flow occlusion and reduced mobilization.
- Aim to reduce blood flow, which has been shown to increase survival increase survival.

## Portal vein embolization

- For major resection, considered pre-operatively.
- PVE of lobe to be resected results in atrophy of that lobe and concurrent hypertrophy of remaining lobe.
- Good evidence PVE allows larger resections and results in significant reduction in complications and hospital stay.
- Hypertrophy of contralateral lobe may not occur if portal pressure raised, therefore, no benefit.
- Traditionally limited resection preferred, some evidence now advocating removal of tumour and segments, which share portal supply improves survival.
- Complication rate <5%.

## Fibrolamellar variant

- In young, non-cirrhotic patients.
- Resection is treatment of choice even when tumour large as it is slow-growing with low metastatic potential and remainder of liver is functionally normal.

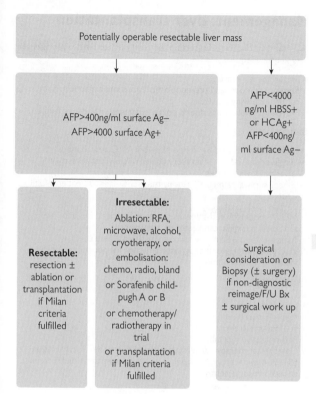

**Fig. 6.1** Management of potentially resectable liver mass.

# Management: liver transplantation

- Treatment of choice if resection technically unfeasible or liver reserve will be inadequate.

- Stage I and II disease.
- Removes tumours and pre-neoplastic lesions and cirrhotic liver, thus, curing underlying disease.
- Prevents complications due to portal hypertension and liver failure.

### Indications

- ***Milan criteria:*** used by United Network for Organ Sharing.
- Single nodule <5cm or up to 3 nodules <3cm without vascular invasion or metastases.
- 5-Year survival rate 60–75% using these criteria. <10% patients fulfil criteria.

- ***MELD:*** model for end-stage liver disease. Priority criteria for liver allocation in eligible candidates for transplant.
- Tumours up to 6.5cm may have similar survival results.
- Vascular invasion worst prognostic indicator for poor outcome following transplantation.

### Problems
- Cost.
- Lack of donors.
- Age >65 may be refused.
- Tumour recurrence.
- Peri-operative mortality.
- Co-adjuvant therapy (such as arterial embolization or local ablation) to limit tumour progression, while awaiting transplantation has been adopted in some centres.

# Local ablative treatment

- Toxic agent applied directly into tumour.
- Stage I and II disease.
- Minimally invasive.
- Well tolerated.
- Has low cost, is repeatable, and preserves normal liver.
- *Indications:* tumour <5cm or 3 nodules <3cm with adequate functional reserve (Child–Pugh A/B) and not suitable for surgery, peripheral lesions.
- *Contraindications:* coagulopathy, ascites, obstructive jaundice, inadequate view on imaging.

## Chemical ablation

- Ethanol or acetic acid becoming superseded by radio-ablation.
- Ethanol results in cell dehydration and necrosis.
- *Complications:* pain, extravasation (can result in portal vein thrombosis), hepatic decompensation, abscess formation, cholangitis, bleeding.
- 5-Year survival. Child A patients HCC <5cm is 47–51%, but tumour recurrence is 65–90% at 5 years.

## Radiofrequency ablation

- Uses heat to cause necrosis of tissue.
- 14 G needle electrode inserted into tumour under image guidance or at laparoscopy/laparotomy alternating current applied.
- Heat generated locally is greater than 100°C.
- More expensive than chemical ablation, but fewer sessions required to induce necrosis.
- Ineffective if tumour adjacent to large vessels.
- *Complications:* perforation of adjacent structures, bleeding, abscess formation.
- *Contraindications:* superficial tumour, biliary-enteric anastomosis. Slightly improved long-term survival over chemical ablation.

## Cryotherapy

- Operative placement of metal probe through which liquid nitrogen or argon gas flows, creating an ice ball in the tumours centre.
- Monitored via ultrasound and is considered adequate when the ice is 1cm beyond the tumours edge.
- Tumours close to vascular structures or bile ducts are not suitable for cryotherapy.

**Table 6.4** Treatment algorithm for inoperable HCC due to poor performance status

| Localized disease inoperable due to poor performance status | Asymptomatic | Ablation<br>Or sorafenib if Child–Pugh A or B<br>Or clinical trial |
|---|---|---|
| | Symptomatic | Ablation: RF, chemo, microwwave<br>Or embolization: chemo, radio, bland<br>Or sorafenib<br>Or supportive care |

### Sorafenib

- Inhibitor of PDGF (platelet-derived growth factor), VEGF receptor 2 and 3 kinases, Raf kinase, and c Kit the receptor for stem cell factor.
- Simultaneous targeting of the Raf/Mek/Erk pathway.
- Licensed for Rx of RCC and advanced HCC. Recent European approval 2007.
- SHARP trial presented, ASCO 2007 efficacy of sorafenib in hepatocellular carcinoma.
- 44% improvement in patients who received sorafenib compared with placebo. Median overall survival and time to progression improved by 3 months.

# Embolic therapies

Arterial embolization or chemo-embolization (see Fig. 6.2).

## Indications

- Multiple diffuse tumours, tumours >5cm, inoperable tumours.
- Palliative to reduce tumour load with adequate hepatic reserve.
- Feeding artery located with fluoroscopy and blocked by gelatine particles.
- Can be combined with chemotherapeutic agents including doxorubicin, cisplatin, epirubicin, mitomycin +/– lipiodol (retained by neoplastic cells).
- May be combined with local ablation. Improves 2-year survival in patients with good liver function and compensated cirrhosis.

## Complications

- *Post embolization syndrome* is common, presents with pain, nausea, and fever. Usually self-limiting, but can result in hepatic decompensation. Contraindicated in Child–Pugh C patients or those with portal vein thrombosis.
- Pancreatitis, pulmonary oedema, gallbladder infarction.
- Complications of arterial puncture and catheterization.
- CT scan at 1 month to assess response.

## Chemotherapy and radiotherapy

Chemotherapy has poor response rate and not used routinely. Recommendations are for entry into clinic trials with novel agents. External beam radiotherapy (EBRT) poor results as tumour radioresistant at low doses and higher doses induce hepatitis. Transarterial, locally delivered chemotherapy has better results. Sometimes used in conjunction with embolization. Results conflicting. No agreed benefit.

## Hormone treatment

Anti-oestrogens and anti-androgens have been trialled with little positive results.

## Future trends

- The proteomics field has provided potential new tumour markers for screening/monitoring treatment, including human hepatocytes growth factor and des-gamma carboxyprothrombin.
- New potential treatments including anti-angiogenesis agents and antibodies to epidermal growth factor are being evaluated.
- Criteria for liver resection and transplantation are continuously being expanded with the development of surgical techniques and sophistication of ITU.
- Microdissection genotyping to assess degree of malignancy of tumour may predict recurrence risk

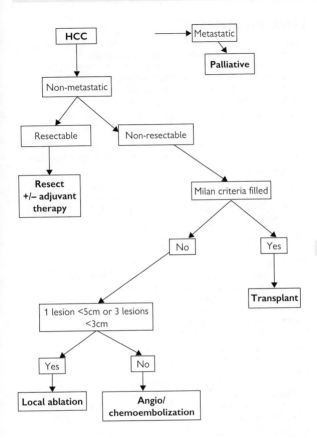

**Fig. 6.2** Algorithm for management of HCC.

# Liver metastases

- Liver is a common site of metastases for a number of tumours, most commonly breast, lung, colon, pancreas, and stomach.
- Isolated liver metastases occur most frequently in colorectal cancer.
- Evidence suggests an improvement in survival rates by resection of isolated hepatic metastases from colorectal, adrenal, renal, and carcinoid tumours.

## Colorectal metastases

### Presentation

Synchronous (15–25% patients with colorectal cancer) or metachronous (20% of patients). Synchronous metastases suggest more aggressive disease.

### Investigation

- To assess degree of liver involvement and extrahepatic disease. US, CT, MRI, PET, intraoperative US (detects deep-seated mets), lapararoscopy.
- *Staging:* biggest influences on survival are grade of primary tumour and degree of liver involvement.

### Resection of colorectal metastases

5-Year survival post-resection 30–40%.

### Indications

- Able to resect hepatic metastases with minimum of 5mm resection margin, whilst leaving adequate hepatic reserve.
- Can resect 70% in non-cirrhotic patient.
- Size of metastases not absolute contraindication, but >3 metastases poorer survival benefit as do tumours >5cm.
- Resectable extrahepatic disease.

### Contraindications

- Need to resect >70% liver (non-cirrhotic).
- Unfit for surgery.
- Unresectable/ablatable extrahepatic disease.
- Multiple small lesions.
- Untreatable primary or unresectable local recurrence.
- Extensive nodal disease.

### Relative contraindications

- Dukes C.
- Portal vein or IVC involvement.
- Suspicious lymph node involvement.

**Table 6.5** Clinical risk score for patients undergoing resection of colorectal liver metastases

| Score | % Survival | | |
|---|---|---|---|
| | 1 year | 3 years | 5 years |
| 0 | 93 | 72 | 60 |
| 1 | 91 | 66 | 44 |
| 2 | 89 | 60 | 40 |
| 3 | 86 | 42 | 20 |
| 4 | 70 | 38 | 25 |
| 5 | 71 | 27 | 14 |

1 point is scored for >1 tumour, size >5cm, node positive primary, disease-free period <12months, CEA >200ng/mL.

- Resectability may be increased by portal vein embolization or a staged procedure.
- Follow-up for 5 years with CT and serial CEA.

*Neoadjuvant chemotherapy*

Oxaliplatin and 5-fluorouracil + folinic acid (FOLFOX) or 5-FU + folinic acid + irinotecan (FOLFIRI). Downsizes metastases allowing resection. North Central Cancer Treatment group treated 44 patients with unresectable metastases with FOLFOX, 40% were able to proceed to resection. NICE guidelines recommend this if metastases initially inoperable but have potential to become operable. Oral analogues of 5-FU (capecitabine or tegafur + uracil) also recommended.

*Adjuvant chemotherapy*

To prevent clinically undetectable lesions growing. Evidence still unclear as to best regime and survival benefit; however, course of systemic chemotherapy recommended to eradicate microscopic disease post-resection. Hepatic artery infusion (HAI) is an option. HAI enables delivery of large doses of chemotherapy to the liver whilst reducing systemic toxicity. Floxuridine (FUDR) often used as 95–99% extracted at first pass in comparison to 19–55% 5-FU resulting in less systemic toxicity. Evidence to demonstrate improved response rate to systemic therapy and increased time to hepatic progression, although not extrahepatic progression. HAI results in higher survival rates than systemic therapy alone Regimes used include 5-FU/leucovorin or floxuridine (FUDR/leucovorin; see Fig. 6.3).

**Non-resectable liver metastases**

- Best supportive care survival is 6 months. Systemic chemotherapy [5-FU +/– folinic acid (leucovorin)] is well tolerated and improves survival to 10–12 months. Delays symptoms. FOLFOX/FOLFIRI improves survival to 20 months. NICE recommends FOLFOX or FOLFIRI as first line treatment. Patients who progress on FOLFOX may benefit from converting to FOLFIRI and vice versa. If oral analogues (capecitabine or tegafur and uracil) used and progression occurs, may benefit from conversion to FOLFOX or FOLFIRI.

- Bevacizumab is a monoclonal IgG1 antibody that inhibits angiogenesis. It may be used in combination with 5-FU/leucovorin chemotherapy. NICE do not recommend it for cost effectiveness reasons. Further trials continue into its use in other regimes.
- Clinical trials are currently investigating the use of cetuximab in combination with FOLFOX/FOLFIRI, but NICE does not recommend this as first line treatment at present for cost effectiveness reasons. Cetuximab is a monoclonal antibody that blocks the epidermal growth factor receptor (EGFR)
- Cryotherapy. Can be used for unresectable disease if no extrahepatic disease and >10 metastases. Also to treat small lesions in contralateral lobe during resection of metastases or in adequate resection margins. Addition of chemotherapy improves survival benefit. No RCTs to demonstrate benefit over standard chemotherapy regimes. Survival benefit unclear.
- Radiofrequency ablation Used to palliate symptoms or in combination with resection. Median survival in unresectable metastases in combination with HAI 24 months. No RCTs to demonstrate benefit over standard chemotherapy. Survival benefit unclear. Ablative techniques are not recommended over resection or in those patients where negative margins can be achieved by resection. If tumour not surgically resectable consider chemotherapy and local ablation vs. chemotherapy (CLOCC) trial. Entry criteria <9 metastases, 4cm diameter, no extrahepatic disease. If not suitable for entry into CLOCC consider ablative therapy.
- Chemo-embolization. Palliation. No evidence to demonstrate improved survival over standard chemotherapy techniques.

**Resection of non-colorectal metastases**

- Not performed often, as non-colorectal metastases tend to be widely infiltrative.
- Exception renal, adrenal, and cortical tumours, no survival benefit in resecting other metastases.
- Palliative effect if bulky metastases causing symptoms.

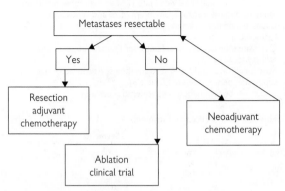

**Fig. 6.3** Summary of management of resectable liver metastases associated with colorectal carcinoma.

# Surgical anatomy

Liver

- Classically anatomically divided into right and left lobe by falciform ligament, and fissures for ligamentum teres and venosum.
- Caudate lobe lies between inferior vena cava (IVC) and fissure for ligamentum venosum.
- Quadrate lobe lies between fissure for ligamentum teres and gallbladder fossa.
- Functionally liver divided in sections then segments according to blood supply and biliary drainage (Table 6.6).
- Caudate lobe (segment I) is considered separately.

**Table 6.6** Liver sections and segments

| Sections | Segments |
|---|---|
| Right anterior | V, VIII |
| Right posterior | VI, VII |
| Left lateral | II, III |
| Quadrate | IV |
| Caudate | I |

*Blood supply*

- Arterial from hepatic artery usually from coeliac trunk. Divides into right and left branches in porta hepatis. Divides into sectional then segmental branches.
- Portal vein divides in right and left branches in porta hepatis. Divides into sectional then segmental branches.
- Venous return is more complex as there is mixing from the two halves. Right, middle, and left hepatic vein drain into IVC directly.
- Lymph drainage is into hepatic nodes in the porta hepatis, along the hepatic artery to pyloric and coeliac nodes. Bare area drains via extraperitoneal lymph nodes to posterior mediastinal nodes.

Gallbladder

- Located in gallbladder fossa on underside of right lobe of liver and next to quadrate lobe.
- Cystic duct is approximately 2–3cm long, drains bile into common hepatic duct. Arterial supply via cystic artery from right hepatic. Crosses Calots triangle, formed by liver, cystic duct, and hepatic duct. Anatomical variations common. May arise from left hepatic artery, hepatic trunk or gastroduodenal artery. May pass in front of or behind cystic or bile duct. Secondary blood supply from liver bed.

*Extrahepatic biliary tree*

Left and right hepatic ducts leave porta hepatic, and join forming common hepatic duct. Common hepatic duct runs in free edge lesser omentum, joined by cystic artery forming bile duct. Bile duct runs from the ampulla in second part of the duodenum. 8cm long and 8mm in diameter, although some increase in diameter occurs with aging. Lower third runs in groove between second part of duodenum and head of pancreas (may be obstructed by pancreatic head tumours) passing in front of right renal vein. Middle third runs behind first part of duodenum. Superior third lies in free edge of omentum in front of portal vein and to right of hepatic artery. Upper third provides easiest surgical access. Blood supply is via branches from cystic, right hepatic, and superior pancreaticoduodenal.

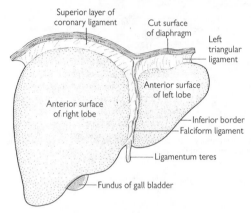

**Fig. 6.4** Liver anatomy anterior view. From Rogers (1992) *Textbook of Anatomy*. With kind permission of Elsevier.

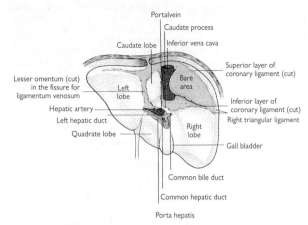

**Fig. 6.5** Liver anatomy posterior view. From Rogers (1992) *Textbook of Anatomy*. With kind permission of Elsevier.

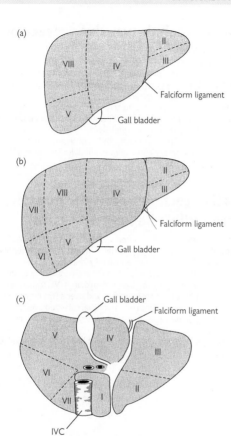

**Fig. 6.6** Liver segments. From Raftery (2000) *Applied Basic Science for Basic Surgical Training*. With kind permission of Elsevier.

# Operative techniques: liver resection

- Cross-match 6 units.
- Ensure correct clotting.
- Undertake outline pre-operative work up as per any major surgery, and assess healthy liver function-bloods, evidence of cirrhosis on US/biopsy, clearance studies, Child–Pugh score.
- Right subcostal incision. Extension across left subcostal margin if needed (inverted V) and further extension by vertical incision from apex of V to xiphisternum (Mercedes Benz).
- Laparotomy to confirm resectability and concurrent disease.
- Portal vein, hepatic artery, and common bile duct identified at hilum, and isolated with sloop.

# Operative techniques: right hepatic lobectomy/left hepatic lobectomy

- Falciform ligament divided on anterior surface to superior IVC. Branches of right hepatic artery, portal vein, and bile duct identified, ligated, and divided. Cystic duct and artery identified, ligated, and divided for right hepatectomy. Liver mobilized posteriorly by dividing peritoneum and retracting the liver forward until IVC visualized. Left, middle, or right hepatic veins identified and over sewn or stapled. Demarcation line between normal and devascularized liver. Liver dissected along demarcation line using ultrasonic scalpel to remove affected lobe.
- Ensure haemostasis is achieved and inspect hilar structures. Saline washout. Consider need for drain.

# Operative techniques: laparoscopic liver resection

- No evidence yet to demonstrate superiority over open techniques. Advocates advise that it reduces operative blood loss and hospital stay (reduced pain and earlier return to activity). Suitable for benign and malignant disease. Laparoscopic US can be used to assess surgical anatomy and tumour.
- A sloop can be placed around porta hepatis (Pringle manoeuvre) to act as a tourniquet in case of haemorrhage. Ultrasonic dissection used to take down triangular ligament. Suprahepatic IVC exposed. For right hepatectomy further dissection required to visualize retrohepatic IVC. Parenchymal resection line marked with surgeons preferred device, e.g. ultrasonic, saline-perfused cautery, diathermy causes pre-coagulation. Small vessels cauterized. Layered application of endovascular stapling devices ligates larger vessels. Fibrin sealents can be applied to cut surface of liver to aid haemostasis. Specimen should be removed in bag to prevent seeding.

# Operative techniques: donor liver retrieval

- Liver mobilized. Hepatic artery and portal vein isolated. Bile duct divided in proximity to duodenum. Superior mesenteric vein cannulated to allow perfusion of cold University of Wisconsin solution (UW). Gallbladder flushed out with cold saline. Cuffs of supra and infrahepatic IVC and coeliac trunk and portal vein allow anastomosis. Liver perfused with UW via hepatic artery and portal vein. Stored on ice during transport. Maximum preservation time 15–18h, although evidence shows shorter preservation time has better outcomes.
- Need to consider anomalous arterial supply in both the donor and recipient liver.

# Operative techniques: orthotopic liver transplant

- Transverse or Mercedes Benz incision. Liver mobilized. Porta hepatis exposed and dissected out to allow ligation and division of hepatic artery and bile duct. Portal vein skeletonized. Vena cava identified and isolated.
- If venous venous bypass required, femoral and axillary vein exposed and cannulated. Venous venous bypass prevent drop in venous return to heart during clamping of IVC. Portal vein and IVC clamped.
- Diseased liver removed. Donor liver implanted, and supra- and infra-hepatic IVC anastomosed. Portal vein anastomosed. Liver reperfused. Haemostasis ensured. Open cholecystectomy performed. Donor hepatic artery anastomosed to common hepatic artery (can use donor infra renal iliac artery as conduit if necessary). End to end bile duct anastomosis +/− T tube or Roux-en-Y hepaticojejunostomy to allow biliary drainage. Direct bile duct anastomosis is more physiological, technically easier and retains sphincter of Oddi function. Stenting of anastomosis with T tube allows monitoring of bile production and consistency in post-operative period and allows cholangiography. Some centres perform side-to-side anastomosis without T tube as T tube can increase risk of biliary leak. However, risk of stricture may be higher without T tube. Prospective randomized trial demonstrated little difference in complication rates for end-to-end and side-to-side anastomosis; therefore, surgeon preference is the deciding factor. Many centres abandoning use of T tube.

# Operative technique: piggy back liver transplant

Avoids venous venous bypass, therefore, quicker and reduced complications. Leaves IVC intact thus maintaining caval blood flow after removal of liver. Vascular clamps applied to all 3 hepatic veins. Liver removed. Donor liver suprahepatic IVC anastomosed to common trunk formed from 3 hepatic veins. Donor infrahepatic IVC ligated. Remainder of operation as above.

## Living donor liver transplant

Initially used for child recipients, now extended to adults. Risk to donor 13% morbidity, although mortality low. Need weight of transplanted liver to be > 1-3 % weight of recipient. Must consider donor's residual liver reserve!

## Liver transplant complications

15% reoperation rate within 5 days. Main reasons bleeding, sepsis, biliary leak, vascular thrombosis. Primary non-function of a successfully transplanted liver can occur. Only treatment is immediate retransplantation. This may be due to damage to donor liver during harvest/preparation process, prolonged warm/cold ischaemic times or reperfusion injury. Surgeon assessment of donor liver texture and fat content important.

## Biliary complications

- Reported rates vary between 7 and 50% (Table 6.7).

**Table 6.7** Biliary complications at different stages

| Early <30 days | Late >30 days |
| --- | --- |
| T tube associated bile leak | Anastomotic stricture |
| T tube obstruction | Non-anastomotic stricture |
| Anastomotic bile leak | Bile leak post-T tube removal |
| Anastomtic stricture | |

- Presentation of biliary complication is non-specific. Consider if abdominal pain, sepsis, worsening LFTs or inflammatory markers, fluctuating ciclosporin levels.
- If suspected, need to visualize biliary tree. Method depends on type of biliary anastomosis. If T tube *in situ* perform T tube cholangiogram. For primary bile duct anastomosis with no T tube, US, CT, ERCP, MRCP or PTC. If Roux-en-Y anastomosis, US, CT +/– PTC.

## Immunosupression

Usually combined approach of Tacrolimus or ciclosporin + prednisolone for several months. Long-term monotherapy with tacrolimus or ciclosporin. Tacrolimus is preferred as number of multicentre, randomized studies have demonstrated lower rejection rate.

## Rejection

- *Acute rejection 30%:* treated by increased immunosuppression.
- *Chronic rejection:* vanishing bile duct syndrome. Major cause of late graft loss. Decreasing incidence with improved immunosuppression.

# Post-operative hepatic ITU care

## HDU/ITU

- Daily bloods. Maintain normal coagulation, haemoglobin, hydration.
- Standard ITU observations and weight, T tube and drain output.
- Antibiotic cover 1st/2nd generation cephalosporin 24–48h.
- Consider parenteral nutrition if gut function doesn't return in few days. Restrict free sodium. Protein restriction if encephalopathic.
- Early ambulation and chest physiotherapy.
- Sepsis. Consider early if deterioration. Send cultures. CT/US to identify collection. Broad spectrum antibiotics. May need drainage of collection/ debridement necrotic liver.
- Ascites. Reaccumulation common. Daily weight and abdominal girth. Colloid and spironolactone to maintain urine output 30–50mL/h.

## Haemorrhage post-resection

- Reduce risk by pre-operative correction of clotting (fresh frozen plasma, vitamin k, and activated factor 7 in conjunction with haematologist advice), meticulous intraprocedure haemostasis (+documentation on operation note). Operative time related to post-operative bleeding risk. Hyperfibrinolytic state occurs post-liver resection, thus higher bleeding risk.
- High index of suspicion in post-operative period. Consider early if deterioration. Resuscitate. Consider CT to confirm if stable.
- Relaparotomy as per any post-operative haemorrhage. Consider Pringle manoeuvre if massive haemorrhage. If site not immediately obvious, consider extrahepatic sites of bleeding, e.g. damage to diaphragm or abdominal wall. If ooze from raw liver bed consider sealants, e.g. fibrin glue, thrombin, Surgicel®. Consider packing and laparostomy for second look.
- **Fibrin glue** (e.g. Tisseal®): fibrinogen and thrombin in two syringes whose tips form common port. Enzymatic action of thrombin on fibrinogen produces fibrin clot in 10–60s depending on thrombin concentration. Bypasses extrinsic and intrinsic pathways, but reproduces final common pathway. Factor XIII is present in fibrinogen component and cross-link's and stabilizes clot. Good for controlling bleeding from multiple pinpoints on large surfaces, e.g. raw liver, and to secure anastomosis. No replacement for good Surgicel® haemostasis or for controlling significant bleeds/larger vessels.
- **Topical thrombin** (Floseal®): thrombin and cross-linked gelatine granules. Acts on fibrinogen. Works on common pathway.
- Surgicel® is oxidized regenerated cellulose. It acts on the intrinsic pathway to cause clot formation. Need functional clotting factors for it to work.
- **Tranexamic acid:** synthetic derivative of amino acid lysine. Prevents plasmin-mediated fibrinolysis.
- Aprotinin (bovine pancreatic trypsin inhibitor) used to reduce bleeding during complex surgery. Acts to slow down fibrinolysis via inhibition of plasmin. Also inhibits kallikrein slowing intrinsic pathway of coagulation. Both TA and aprotinin shown to reduce blood loss and transfusion requirement.

# Bile duct tumours/cholangiocarcinoma

- Rare, <2% cancers.
- Can arise anywhere in biliary epithelium, commonest site is hilar confluence.
- Subdivided into intrahepatic, hilar, distal extrahepatic. Intrahepatic considered as primary liver cancer.

## Presentation

Obstructive jaundice 90%. Jaundice may be absent or late finding in intrahepatic lesions. Pruritus, pain, fever.

## Epidemiology

Rarer than hepatoma. Also more common in Africa and Asia.

## Aetiology

- Often idiopathic. More common in UC and liver flukes. Association with primary sclerosing cholangitis, choledochal cyst, chronic ulcerative colitis. Carcinogens – thorotrast, vinyl chloride, methylene chloride, nitrosamines, aflatoxin.
- Mutations found in tumour suppressor genes (*p53*, *APC*, *p16*, *smad-4*, *bcl-2*) and oncogenes (*K-ras*, *c-myc*, *c-neu*, *c-erbB2*, *c-met*). 25% of tumours display chromosomal aneuploidy. Clinical and prognostic relevance uncertain.

## Pathology

- Adenocarcinoma most common (subtypes non-specific, intestinal, mucinous, clear cell, signet ring, adenosquamous).
- Squamous.
- Small cell (oat cell).
- Undifferentiated.
- Papillary (invasive or non-invasive).
- Carcinoid.
- Mesenchymal tumours rare. Include leiomyosarcoma, embryonal rhabdomyosarcoma, malignant fibrous histiocytoma.
- Outcome varies with type. Papillary has best outcome, adenomucinous worst.

## Spread

Main route lymphatic spread, lymph node metastases present in 50% at presentation. Spread also occurs along ducts. Haematogenous spread rare.

## Diagnosis

- **Bloods:** LFTs obstructive jaundice. CEA, CA 19-9, and CA50 ↑, but non-specific.
- **Imaging:** US first line investigation. Suspect if intra-, but not extrahepatic duct dilatation. May miss small tumours. Can detect level of tumour, liver masses, excludes gallstones. Duplex scan may demonstrate portal vein involvement.
- **CT** more detailed. Detects lymphadenopathy. Doesn't define extent of tumour accurately.

- **MRI** is gold standard. Defines anatomy, extent of duct involvement via MRCP, vascular involvement via MR angiography.
- **Endoscopic ultrasound** (EUS): demonstrates lymphadenopathy. Best for distal and middle third tumours.
- **Cholangiography:** demonstrates anatomy and extent of tumour. Via MRCP, ERCP, or PTC. ERCP and PTC allow decompression if therapeutic relief of jaundice required, and also sampling for cytology. Negative cytology does not exclude cholangiocarcinoma. MRCP non-invasive and may identify blocked duct not seen on ERCP. Often used with MRI for staging.
- **Laparoscopy:** demonstrates peritoneal metastases, but not used for routine staging. Poor at detecting extent of biliary involvement.
- PET and $^{18}$F-2-deoxy-D-glucose. Demonstrates hot spots of uptake by tumour.
- Histological diagnosis is recommended via ERCP, laparoscopy, or laparotomy. Risk of seeding means Surgicel® resectability should be determined first.
- Mini-chromosome maintenance protein 5 (Mcm5) Trials underway to determine whether this can be used as a diagnostic test for biliary tree cancers.

## Recommendations

- US as first line investigation followed by combined MRI and MRCP. Invasive Cholangiography if tissue diagnosis required or therapeutic decompression.
- Following diagnosis metastatic disease should be ruled out by chest X-Ray, CT scan +/– laparoscopy.
- Biliary drainage should be avoided prior to assessing resectability unless cholangitis.

# ERCP

- Endoscope passed through mouth into duodenum and ampulla of vater cannulated.
- Fluoroscopy is the injection of radiocontrast into the bile or pancreatic duct to identify obstruction or stricture.
- Therapeutic procedures include sphincterotomy, stenting, and trawling of stones.
- Major complications in <10%. Pancreatitis, haemorrhage, duodenal perforation, ascending cholangitis. Mortality 1%.
- Stenting allows biliary decompression and relief of jaundice.
- Complications of stents include obstruction, cholangitis, and disease progression.
- Repeated stent exchanges may be necessary impacting on quality of life. Stents are plastic (Teflon, polyurethane, polyethylene) or metal (nickel-titanium alloy, stainless steel). Length range 5–18 cm. Diameter 7–12 Fr.
- Cochrane review of metal vs. plastic stents in patients with malignant obstruction secondary to pancreatic cancer stated that endoscopic placement is preferable option and choice of stent depends on life expectancy of patient.
- Metal stents having longer patency rates, should be used if life expectancy >6 months. Surgical bypass if good expected life expectancy and failure of stenting. Tumour in-growth through mesh of metal stent treated by exchange or insertion of second stent into lumen. Partially covered stents may help alleviate this problem.

# Extrahepatic biliary tumours staging

## Staging

### Primary tumour (T)
- **TX**: primary tumour cannot be assessed.
- **T0**: no evidence of primary tumour.
- **Tis**: carcinoma *in situ*.
- **T1**: tumour confined to the bile duct histologically.
- **T2**: tumour invades beyond the wall of the bile duct.
- **T3**: tumour invades the liver, gallbladder, pancreas, and/or unilateral branches of the portal vein (right or left) or hepatic artery (right or left).
- **T4**: tumour invades any of the following: main portal vein or its branches bilaterally, common hepatic artery, or other adjacent structures, such as the colon, stomach, duodenum, or abdominal wall

### Regional lymph nodes (N)
- **NX**: regional lymph nodes cannot be assessed.
- **N0**: no regional lymph node metastasis.
- **N1**: regional lymph node metastasis.

### Distant metastasis (M)
- **MX**: distant metastasis cannot be assessed.
- **M0**: no distant metastasis.
- **M1**: distant metastasis.

**Table 6.8** AJCC stage groupings

| Stage | Definition | 5-year survival |
|---|---|---|
| 0 | Tis, N0, M0 | 58% |
| IA | T1, N0, M0 | 29% |
| IB | T2, N0, M0 | |
| IIA | T3, N0, M0 | 22% |
| IIB | T1, N1, M0 | |
| | T2, N1, M0 | |
| | T3, N1, M0 | |
| III | T4, any N, M0 | 8% |
| IV | Any T, any N, M1 | 8% |

**Table 6.9** Bismuth stage used for staging hilar tumours

| Stage | Definition |
|---|---|
| I | Up to hilum |
| II | Involves confluence of right and left hepatic duct |
| III | 1st order hepatic duct involved |
| IV | Both hepatic ducts or subsegments |

# Treatment

## Surgery

- **Proximal tumours:** majority unresectable.
- **If resectable:** aim for hilar resection and lymphadenectomy and *en bloc* liver resection +/– caudate resection.
- High peri-operative mortality and low cure rate.
- It is the only potential cure.
- Relieve jaundice via ERCP or percutaneous drainage prior to surgery.
- **Operability** depends on:

  - minimal portal vein involvement;
  - no N2 lymph node involvement;
  - no distant or liver metastases;
  - single focus;
  - no involvement of second order – intrahepatic ducts or major vessels/ducts in both halves of liver;
  - need also to consider patients fitness for surgery and if residual liver remnant is viable;
  - aim >5mm tumour clearance.

- **Perihilar tumour:** least likely to be operable. Resect common and extra-hepatic bile ducts, cystic duct and gallbladder, and lymphadenectomy and Roux-en-Y hepatico-jejunostomy. Bismuth III tumours may require liver resection/hepatectomy. Consider frozen section assesment of bile duct margins.
- **Distal tumour:** distal tumours are those arising from common bile duct. Pancreaticoduodenectomy (Whipples). Survival rates reported as 20–30%.
- **Intrahepatic biliary tumour:** liver resection +/– ablation.
- Liver transplantation contraindicated as associated with rapid disease recurrence within 3 years. Pilot trials of transplant following chemoradiation in selected patients have demonstrated long-term survival in some patients.
- If resection margins negative, generally considered no benefit in adjuvant chemo or radiotherapy. If resection margins positive (R1–2) adjuvant radiotherapy +/– chemotherapy: 5-FU-based or Gemcitabine recommended. F/U imaging every 6 months for 2 years.

## Unresectable tumours

- Relief of jaundice via stenting or Surgicel® bypass. Relieving obstruction improves survival. No evidence to demonstrate Surgicel® bypass superior to stenting.
- No strong evidence to suggest palliative chemotherapy improves survival but current main aim is quality of life benefit. Regimes include gemcitabine+/– cisplatin, 5-FU and leucovorin, irinotecan, and capecitabine.
- Current clinical trials compare single agent gemcitabine vs. gemcitabine + cisplatin (ABC 02) in inoperable tumours, with the use of capecitabine (BILCAP) post-surgery.

- Phase II trials into use of tyrosine kinase inhibitor erlotinib.
  Photodynamic therapy (see 'Carcinoma of the gallbladder', p. 27).
- **_Palliative radiotherapy:_** some benefit, but evidence is not convincing.
- External beam radiotherapy (EBRT) has high complication rate,
  brachytherapy preferred. Iridium-192 used +/− low dose EBRT.
- EBRT requires 5 treatments per week over several weeks.
- Ongoing clinical trials with radiosensitizers and chemotherapeutic
  agents.

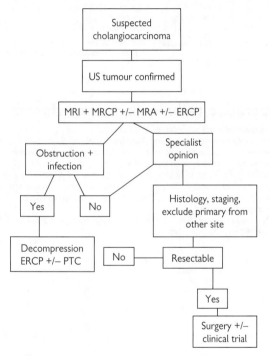

**Fig. 6.7** Management algorithm for suspected cholangiocarcinoma.

**Table 6.10** Extrahepatic biliary carcinoma management

| Resectable | Surgicel® exploration without Bx +− laparoscopic staging | Resect according to protocol above R0 resection: observe or 5-FU/DXT R1-2 resection (margin +ve or Ca in situ at margin or node +ve) 5-FU-based chemo/DXT: external beam or brachy F/U 6 monthly imaging for 2 years |
|---|---|---|
| Unresectable | Biliary drainage if needed Stent/bypass | 5-FU based or gemcitabine chemo Or 5-FU +DXT external beam or brachytherapy Or clinical trial/ supportive |
| Metastatic | Stent if needed | Supportive care +-5-FU based or Gemcitabine or clinical or clinical trial |

# Operative technique: hilar carcinoma

- *Incision:* bilateral subcostal or Mercedes Benz.
- *Divide ligamentum teres and falciform ligament:* divide liver tissue between quadrate and left lateral lobe. Retract quadrate lobe and incise tissue at its base to lower hilar plate. Gallbladder mobilized allowing dissection of hepatic duct. Hepatic duct divided distally and over sewn. Hepatic duct dissected upwards off portal vein and artery to upper limit of resection. Consider frozen specimen to ensure adequate clearance.
- May need to resect liver via right or left hepatectomy or quadrate lobe resection to obtain clearance.

# Operative technique: hepaticojejunostomy

Via Roux-en-Y loop for reconstruction. Upper jejunum identified, 2–3 arterial arcades identified, ligated, and divided. Bowel transected and distal end over sewn. Roux loop brought up posteriorly to transverse colon via mesocolic window. Enterotomy approximately 3cm from distal stump. Single layer interrupted anastomosis 4/0 vicryl. End to side stapled or hand sewn jejunojejunostomy to restore bowel continuity.

# Operative technique: palliative bypass

• Pre-operative work-up as for liver resection.
• Hilar plate lowered to expose left hepatic duct to perform hepaticojejunostomy. If main duct involved will need to expose segment III duct in umbilical fissure. Liver tissue between left lateral segment, and quadrate lobe divided and peritoneum at base of ligamentum teres incised to expose duct. Hepaticojejunostomy carried out as above.

# Carcinoma of the gallbladder

## Epidemiology

- Rare, accounts for 0.2% of all cancers. 500 cases diagnosed in UK per year.
- Poor prognosis, only 25% resectable at presentation.
- Incidence rises with age, most common in 70th decade.
- 1 in 100 found incidentally at laparoscopic cholecystectomy.
- Male to female ratio is 1:3. Geographical variation. High risk in Israelis, native south-western Americans, Mexicans, parts of South America. Familial clustering

## Aetiology

- Thought to be related to gallstone disease and chronic inflammation. Evidence of these processes found in 80% of patients.
- Risk higher in those with large stones.
- Bacterial infection of bile found in 80%.
- Adenomas of the gallbladder occur but it is uncertain whether these confer a risk of malignant change or the time span for this. Malignant polyps are more likely in patients over 50 years of age. They tend to be single and large (<1cm). Polyps should undergo surveillance with ultrasound at 6-monthly to yearly intervals. Polyps >1cm should be removed by laparoscopic cholecystectomy, even when asymptomatic.
- Porcelain gallbladder (calcium-infused wall associated with recurrent inflammation) considered premalignant.
- Other risk factors include smoking, working in metal and rubber industries, choledochal cyst, anomalous pancreatobiliary duct anatomy, obesity, typhoid.
- Rare associations. IBD, polyposis coli.

## Presentation

Usually symptoms of chronic cholecystitis. May present with obstructive jaundice, acute cholecystitis, or empyema. Incidental USS finding.

## Pathology

- Adenocarcinoma 85% of all gallbladder carcinomas. Subdivided into three types. Non-papillary adenocarcinoma (75%), papillary adenocarcinoma (6%), mucinous adenocarcinoma (<2%).
- Remaining 15% squamous cell carcinoma, adenosquamous, small cell carcinoma, sarcoma, neuroendocrine tumour, lymphoma, and melanoma.

# Staging of gallbladder tumours

## Gallbladder tumour stages

### Primary tumour (T)
- **TX:** primary tumour cannot be assessed.
- **T0:** no evidence of primary tumour.
- **Tis:** carcinoma *in situ*.
- **T1:** tumour invades lamina propria or muscle layer.
- **T1a:** tumour invades lamina propria.
- **T1b:** tumour invades the muscle layer.
- **T2:** tumour invades the perimuscular connective tissue; no extension beyond the serosa or into the liver.
- **T3:** tumour perforates the serosa (visceral peritoneum), and/or directly invades the liver, and/or one other adjacent organ or structure, such as the stomach, duodenum, colon, or pancreas, omentum, or extrahepatic bile ducts.
- **T4:** tumour invades main portal vein or hepatic artery, or invades multiple extrahepatic organs or structures.

### Regional lymph nodes (N)
- **NX:** regional lymph nodes cannot be assessed.
- **N0:** no regional lymph node metastasis.
- **N1:** regional lymph node metastasis.

### Distant metastasis (M)
- **MX:** distant metastasis cannot be assessed.
- **M0:** no distant metastasis.
- **M1:** distant metastasis.

**AJCC stage groupings**

*Stage 0*
- *Tis, N0, M0:* 77.5% 5-year survival.

*Stage IA*
- *T1, N0, M0:* 48% 5-year survival.

*Stage IB*
- *T2, N0, M0.*

*Stage IIA*
- *T3, N0, M0:* 27% 5-year survival.

*Stage IIB*
- *T1, N1, M0.*
- *T2, N1, M0.*
- *T3, N1, M0.*

*Stage III*
- *T4, any N, M0:* 9% 5-year survival.

*Stage IV*
- *Any T, any N, M1:* small cell and undifferentiated tumours. 2% 5-year survival.

- *Stage I* or localized disease potentially curable by resection. Few patients diagnosed at this stage, often an incidental finding following routine laparoscopic cholecystectomy. If the tumour confined to the mucosa 5 year survival rate approaches 100%, if invasion into muscular layer this drops to 15%.
- *Stage II-IV* disease is unresectable with the exception of some IIA tumours. Most patients in this category at presentation.

## Surgery for gallbladder tumours

- Porcelain gallbladder indication for prophylactic surgery.
- If tumour suspected during routine surgery send frozen sections to histology, if positive, assess whether curative resection can be performed.
- Exclude peritoneal secondaries.
- Laparoscopic port sites must be resected in all patients as risk of tumour seeding.

### Tumour found incidentally on histology

- TIS/TI no further action required except port site excision.
- T2 should undergo re-exploration.

### If diagnosis known pre-operatively

- TI, simple laparoscopic cholecystectomy +/– lymph node sampling.
- T2–T4, radical cholecystectomy and liver resection (segments 4b +5), and *en bloc* lymph node resection of porta hepatis and superior pancreatic nodes.
- May require right hepatectomy to obtain clear margins if right portal triad involved. Mobilize duodenum to resect retroduodenal nodes.
- If cystic duct involved needs resection and Roux-en-Y reconstruction.
- 5-Year survival in resectable disease 38%. Local invasion predicts outcome.
- Current clinical trial into use of adjuvant capecitabine (BILCAP).

# Adjuvant and palliative treatment for gallbladder tumours

- Unresectable disease, 1 year survival <5%.
- Largely resistant to chemotherapy, may respond to combination chemotherapy resulting in slowing of progression or temporary shrinking of tumour.
- Gemcitabine most commonly used, sometimes in combination with cisplatin, the ABC02 trial is currently underway to determine any difference between the 2 regimes.
- Fluorouracil, doxorubicin, and mitomycin also used.
- External beam radiotherapy may prolong survival. Clinical trials are concentrating on combination chemo and radiotherapy.
- Immunotherapy is currently being investigated with the use of interleukin 2 (IL-2).
- Biliary obstruction should be relieved via percutaneous stenting or Surgicel® bypass.
- Photodynamic therapy (PDT) is used to palliate symptoms. A photo-sensitizing drug (porfimer sodium) is injected intravenously and the area exposed to laser therapy. The patient must stay out of light for 3 days to avoid damage to other cells.
- Phase 3 trials are currently comparing stent alone vs. PDT with stent (PHOTOSTENT) to relieve jaundice.
- Consider enrolment in clinical trials.

# Operative technique: open cholecystectomy

- Per-operative work-up as above. Antibiotic prophylaxis. Cross-match 2 units if extended resection likely.
- Incision. Kochers, right paramedian, or transverse.
- Laparotomy to assess respectability and spread.
- Retract liver upwards + duodenal bulb gently downwards exposing gallbladder.
- Retract gallbladder neck to provide traction. Expose calot's triangle.
- Open peritoneum over neck of gallbladder to allow dissection of space between neck and liver. This should expose cystic artery.
- Once cystic artery identified ligate in continuity and divide.
- Expose cystic duct via blunt and sharp dissection, and identify where it joins bile duct. Double ligate and divide cystic duct.
- Apply traction to gallbladder to assist dissection from the gallbladder fossa via diathermy dissection.
- Ensure haemostasis and no obvious bile leak. Consider need for drain if liver oozing or any concern about bile leak.

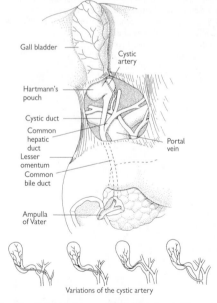

Variations of the cystic artery

**Fig. 6.8** Taken from McLatchie & Leaper (2006). Reproduced with permission of Oxford University Press © 2006.

### Further reading

Rogers AW (ed.) (1992) *Textbook of Anatomy.* Churchill Livingstone.

# Cancers of the pancreas

# Epidemiology, aetiology, and pathology

Incidence

Pancreatic cancer remains a leading cause of cancer death with 230 000 patients registered worldwide every year and 98% of whom die from their disease. It has a grim prognosis and its aggressiveness is demonstrated by the fact that it has a similar annual incidence and mortality rate.

Incidence is increasing in industrialized countries. Its incidence is approximately 10 cases per 100 000 population in both UK and USA with 6220 and 33 370 new cases registered in 2007, respectively. Its peak incidence occurs in the sixth to eighth decades of life (80%). Male:female incidence is approximately 1.2.

- Fourth most common malignancy in the US (4th and 6th commonest cause of cancer-related death in the US and UK, respectively)
- Geographic distribution: highest incidence in affluent western countries such as UK, USA, Canada, Sweden, and Israel. Racial factors also influence the incidence with highest rates in Black Americans, Korean Americans, and female native Hawaiians.

Aetiology

Unknown, but a variety of risk factors has been identified:
- *Smoking:* firmly linked in 25–30% of cases.
- *Chronic pancreatitis:* associated with 5–15-fold increased risk. Debatable as may relate to co-existing ETOH consumption, smoking and selection bias (International Pancreatitis Study).
- *Hereditary pancreatitis\*:* 50–70-fold increased risk. Attributed to a germline mutation on 7q35, which is inherited in an autosomal dominant manner with 80% penetrance.
- *Familial pancreatic cancer\*:* a genetic component present in 5–10% of cases (possibly BRCA2 mutation).
- *Hereditary syndromes:*
  - Peutz–Jeghers – mutation in STK11 tumour suppressor gene;
  - HNPCC – mutation in DNA mismatch repair genes, e.g. MLH1;
  - familial atypical multiple mole melanoma – mutation in p16;
  - FAP – mutation in *APC* gene and typically associated with periampullary cancers;
  - cystic fibrosis – *CFTR* gene mutation.
- *High dietary fat and BMI:* implicated in experimental models.
- *Occupational exposure:* napthylamine and benzidine exposure cause a 5-fold increase in mortality from pancreatic cancer. Also cadmium, radon, and chromium.
- *Diabetes mellitus and hyperglycaemia:* debatable. Probably secondary to pancreatic cancer, rather than causative.
- *Gastrectomy:* 2–5-fold increased risk of pancreatic cancer 20 years post-partial gastrectomy (possibly due to ↓ gastric acidity allowing bacterial overgrowth that elaborate carcinogens.

\*Patients with an inherited predisposition to pancreatic cancer should be referred for genetic counselling and secondary screening.

## Pathology

### Exocrine 98%

- Ductal adenocarcinoma (90%).
- Pancreatic intra-epithelial neoplasia (PanIN, *cis-*).
- Mucinous non-cystic carcinoma.
- Signet ring cell carcinoma.
- Adenosquamous carcinoma.
- Undifferentiated carcinoma (spindle, giant and small cell types).
- Acinar cell carcinoma/cystadenocarcinoma.
- Serous cystadenocarcinoma.
- Mucinous cystadenocarcinoma.
- Pancreaticoblastoma.
- Intraductal papillary mucinous carcinoma with or without invasion (IPMN).
- Solid pseudo-papillary carcinoma.

### Endocrine 1–2%

- These can be sporadic or associated with genetic syndromes, such as MEN-1, von Hippel–Lindau disease, von Recklinghausen's disease, and tuberous sclerosis.
- **Functional:**
  - produce specific hormones;
  - insulinoma (17%), gastrinoma (15%), PPoma (9%), VIPoma (2%), glucagonoma (1%), carcinoid (1%), somatostatinoma (1%), very rare ones such as ACTHoma and GRFoma.
- **Non-functional:** produce non-specific substances, e.g. chromagranin A, HCG, and neurotensin.

### Lymphoma <1%

Has a better prognosis and is more responsive to chemoradiotherapy.

### Metastasis<0.5%

From primaries such as breast, lung, and melanomas.

# Non-invasive pancreatic tumours

Pancreatic cancer is a dismal disease, much emphasis has been placed on identifying and treating its non-invasive precursor lesions, which are thought to be curable. With advances in histopathological and molecular techniques, three important precursors have been identified:
- Mucinous cystic neoplasm (MCN).
- Intraductal papillary mucinous neoplasm (IPMN).
- Pancreatic intra-epithelial neoplasia (PanIN).

## Mucinous cystic neoplasm

MCNs consist of an ovarian type stroma and epithelial lining with varying degree of atypia.
- Hypothesized that ectopic ovarian stroma are incorporated in the pancreas during embryogenesis, and release hormones and growth factors, allowing nearby epithelium to proliferate and form MCNs.
- Pathway from MCN towards invasive carcinoma is distinct from IPMN and PanIN as:
  - MCNs occur almost exclusively in women, and the overwhelming majority located in the body and tail of the pancreas;
  - mean age at diagnosis is younger than that for IPMN (50s vs. 70s);
  - MCNs give rise to invasive mucinous cystic carcinomas and occasionally adenosquamous, osteoclast-like giant cell and choriocarcinomas.

## Intraductal papillary mucinous neoplasm

- IPMNs are grossly visible mucin-producing neoplasms, which arise from the main or branch pancreatic ducts.
- Usually produce a lesion greater than 1 cm in diameter, and are predominantly papillary or rarely flat epithelial neoplasms.
- Morphologically, IPMNs show a variety of cyto-architectural differentiation: gastric, intestinal, pancreaticobiliary, oncocytic.
- Main duct IPMNs are mostly intestinal type and branch duct IPMNs are mostly gastric type.
- Intestinal type IPMNs tend to progress to mucinous non-cystic (colloid) carcinomas, pancreaticobiliary type progress to ductal adenocarcinoma.
- Previously thought that branch duct IPMNs carry lower risk of malignant transformation; therefore, surveillance, rather than resection.
- Recent studies suggest that IPMNs should undergo curative resection as they carry a much better prognosis and much lower risk of cancer recurrence regardless of their type or absence of invasion
- Recurrence rates of non-invasive vs. invasive IPMNs 1.3% and 46%

**Pancreatic intra-epithelial neoplasm**

- PanINs are microscopic papillary or flat epithelial neoplasms arising from pancreatic ducts <5mm in diameter.
- Characterized by columnar or cuboidal cells: varying degrees of cytological atypia and lesser degree of mucin production compared with IPMNs.
- More common in the elderly with a plateau age at 70s.
- PanINs range from 1 to 3 based on factors such as degree of nuclear abnormality, mitoses necrosis, and presence of papillary components.
- Analogous to colorectal adenoma-carcinoma progression, a molecular progression pathway is well recognized for PanIN development into ductal adenocarcinomas.
- Changes occur in a stepwise manner through progressive genetic alterations (Fig. 7.1.).

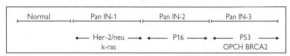

**Fig. 7.1** Molecular progression model of pancreatic cancer.

- Aberrant activation of the Hedgehog and Notch signalling pathways implicated in this progression.
- Both IPMNs and PanINs can develop into ductal adencarcinomas.

• Cumulative oncogenic mutations may occur in a common progenitor that subsequently develop into invasive carcinomas through modification of surrounding environment and various genetic alterations (Fig. 7.2.)

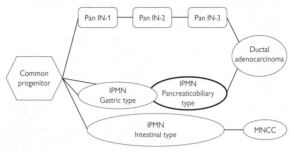

**Fig. 7.2** Precursor progression pathway hypothesis towards invasive carcinoma.

# Adenocarcinoma of the pancreas

Pancreatic adenocarcinoma accounts for 98% of pancreatic malignancies and is associated with a poor prognosis mainly owing to late presentation, thus rendering it irresectable. Overall 5-year survival rate (5YSR) remains <5% (Table 7.1).

- Lymphatic spread is early and common and present in 40–75% of primary tumours <2cm at the time of surgery.
- Perineural infiltration, vascular invasion, and hepatic micrometastases are frequently present at diagnosis.
- Biologically aggressive tumour often clinically quiescent.
- Majority of patients present with either locally advanced (irresectable) or metastatic disease.

**Table 7.1** Staging at presentation and median survival of patients with pancreatic cancer

| Stage | Incidence | Median survival |
|---|---|---|
| Localized (resectable) | 10–20% | 15–19 months |
| Locally advanced | 20–30% | 6–10 months |
| Metastatic | 60% | 3–6 months |

*Pancreatic adenocarcinoma*
Affects:
- **Head of pancreas:** comprises 70–80% of cases and carries a better prognosis as present earlier with obstructive jaundice.
- **Body and tail of pancreas:** 20–30% of cases and worse prognosis.
- **Multifocal:** 5–10% (according to post-mortem and post-resection studies).

# Clinical presentation and evaluation

Main presenting signs and symptoms are:

- *Anorexia and weight loss (80%):* when severe and rapid, suggests irresectability.
- *Pain (75%):* initially upper abdominal and low intensity (visceral in origin and mimicking peptic ulcer disease). With advancing disease, retroperitoneal infiltration of coeliac and superior mesenteric plexus results in a severe persistent back pain, suggesting incurability.
- *Jaundice (70%):* usually an earlier feature of head of pancreas and peri-ampullary tumours accounting for their higher resectability and better cure rates. When present in body and tail tumours, suggestive of hilar or liver metastases, and therefore irresectability.
- *Malnutrition and steatorrhoea (70%):* due to pancreatic duct obstruction.
- *Courvoisier's sign (33%):* in a jaundiced patient, the presence of a palpable gallbladder is unlikely to be secondary to cholelithiasis.
- *Diabetes mellitus (5%):* sudden onset of type 2 DM in non-obese adults with no family history should raise suspicions: 5% of patients with pancreatic cancer develop DM within the previous 2 years.
- *Acute or chronic pancreatitis (5%):* 5% of patients present with an atypical attack, and thus should raise suspicion in the absence of any recognized aetiological risk factors.
- *Ascites, enlarged left supraclavicular nodes (Virchow's) or epigastric mass (5%):* usually indicate irresectability.
- *Gastric outlet obstruction (5%).*
- *Migratory thrombophlebitis:* rarely the first symptom.

# Investigation

- **Establish diagnosis:** radiological +/− tissue diagnosis (see investigation modalities)
- **Stage disease and determine respectability:** assessed radiologically. Defined as absence of metastatic disease and absence of vascular invasion.
- **Assess patients' fitness for surgery:** routine bloods, ECG, and specific cardiorespiratory assessments based on pre-existing disease and symptoms.

## Ultrasound

- Often first line of investigation as it can identify pancreatic tumour, CBD dilation, and importantly presence of possible liver metastases, which would drastically alter further management.
- **Pros:** sensitivity as high as 80–95% in some studies.
- **Cons:** less sensitive in body and tail lesions, large inter-observer variability, bowel gas interference, and provides very limited information regarding resectability and staging.

## CT

- Imaging modality of choice currently, using high quality thin section multidetector 32-slice scanners.
- Accurate in defining the relationship of the primary tumour to the SMV/portal vein confluence, SMA, and coeliac axis. Presence of a fat plane between the tumour and vessels/retroperitoneal soft tissues is critical to predicting resectability and likelihood of achieving R0.
- **Pros:** accuracy of staging and resectability 85–95% with a PPV for non-resectability of 90%.
- **Cons:** suboptimal for small tumours, differentiating cancer from mass-forming pancreatitis or benign enlargement of pancreatic head. Also poor in identifying peritoneal disease, locoregional lymphatic spread and differentiating <1cm hepatic metastases from cysts. NPV for non-resectability is 30%.

## MRI

- Similar accuracy to CT in assessing resectability and staging. MR contrast studies (e.g. gadolinium or manganese-DPDP) can further increase accuracy.
- MRA and MRCP can be constructed to demonstrate ductal and vascular anatomy, and also clarify differential diagnoses such as pancreatitis and identify intraductal tumours.
- **Pros:** can be used in patients with contrast allergies.
- **Cons:** long acquisition time, no advantage over CT and more expensive.

## Endoscopic USS

- Superior to CT in:
  - detection of small tumours and cystic malignant lesions;
  - assessment of vascular involvement and lymphatic staging;
  - assessment of invasion in peri-ampullary lesions.
- Method of choice for obtaining tissue diagnosis whereby confirmation of malignancy is mandatory (locally advanced, metastatic disease, or in patients for neoadjuvant therapy).

## FDG PET functional imaging

$^{18}$F-fluorodeoxyglucose (FDG) is the commonest tracer used in positron emission tomography (PET). It relies on the principle that malignancies demonstrate increased glucose utilization due to an increase in glucose transporter proteins and hexokinase + phosphofructokinase activity.

### Pros

Sensitivity 85–95%, specificity 80–95%. Better in detecting metastases that are sometimes missed on CT and, therefore, change management (Delbeke et al. 1999). Can also be used in assessing treatment response and differentiate local recurrence from post-operative or post-radiation fibrosis. Also helpful in event of rising tumour markers and a negative conventional work-up.

### Cons

Reduced sensitivity (63%) in patients with diabetes or glucose intolerance (competitive inhibition) that is not improved even with correction for serum glucose levels. Poor for <1cm and ampullary carcinomas and T + N staging. False positives in patients with acute or chronic pancreatitis (specificity of 50% in patients with elevated CRP).

## ERCP/MRCP

- Helpful investigation if CT is equivocal and in patients with ampullary tumours as it provides the opportunity for direct visualization, biopsy/ brushing cytology and biliary stenting if obstructed.
- Can be used to differentiate between benign (CBD stone/stricture) and malignant causes of cholestasis.
- Malignancy is suspected if severe stenosis and proximal pancreatic duct dilation. Small early cancers and uncinate tumours easily missed as they only cause duct impingement once large and unresectable.
- MRCP can be also be an adjunct to CT if patient unfit for ERCP and therapeutic intervention is not intended.

## Staging laparoscopy

- Not carried out routinely, but extremely good in identifying sub-radiological metastases, e.g. peritoneal disease or hepatic capsular metastases (4–15% of patients who are deemed resectable with CT).
- Can be used just prior to laparotomy (same sitting) in resectable patients. Laparotomy would thus be avoided if there is evidence of peritoneal disease.
- Enables direct visualization in addition to cytology from peritoneal lavage (M1 disease if positive).

- Indicated in patients with large or body/tail lesions, where confirmation of metastatic disease will preclude surgery and its associated morbidity and mortality.

## Carbohydrate antigen 19-9

- Sialylated Lewis 'a' antigen.
- Not tumour specific.
- Sensitivity (90%), specificity (98%).
- False positive in cholestatsis, cholangiocarcinoma, Mirrizzi's syndrome, chronic pancreatitis, colorectal carcinoma, carcinoma of the stomach, and some liver diseases.
- False negative in patients that do not express the Lewis 'a' antigen (about 5% of the population have fucosyltransferase deficiency required in Lewis 'a' antigen synthesis).
- Good for monitoring treatment response and a good predictor in surveillance for recurrence or metastatic disease.
- Values >200U/mL usually indicate malignancy, whilst most are irresectable when >300U/mL.
- CEA and CA-125 can also be raised in pancreatic cancer.

## Further reading

Delbeke D, Rose DM, Chapman WC, Pinson CW, Wright JK, Beauchamp RD, et al. Optimal interpretation of FDG PET in the diagnosis, staging and management of pancreatic carcinoma. J Nucl Med 1999; **40(11)**:1784–91.

# Management

- Surgical resection offers the only chance of cure for patients with pancreatic cancer.
- Median survival post-resection remain relatively poor (15–19 months) and a 5YSR of ~20%.
- Prognostic indicators for long-term survival are tumour size, DNA content, N0 (no lymphatic metastases), and negative resection margins (R0).
- Patients should be selected for surgery on the basis of curative intent as determined by the probability of achieving R0 resection margins.

It is crucial to achieve R0 status as there is no difference in survival between an R1 resection and non-operative management of these patients with palliative chemotherapy.

Although accurate staging is based on the TNM committee of the International Union Against Cancer and TNM staging is prognostic for overall survival, it is not particularly useful in guiding treatment.

Instead of TNM staging, treatment planning is best served by clinical/radiological staging of the disease together with patient's performance status. This should be carried out in a multidisciplinary setting involving upper gastrointestinal surgeons, radiologists, and oncologists.

The overall consensus reached by the MDT, will group the patients into localized (resectable), locally advanced (unresectable), borderline resectable or metastatic disease, thereby guiding therapeutic planning (Fig.7.3).

### Localized disease

- Primary surgical resection indicated to achieve microscopic clearance (R0) followed by adjuvant therapy (ideally within 4–8 weeks post-operatively) to prevent local and systemic disease recurrence. Achieving R0 status is critical, as numerous studies have shown that patients with residual disease (positive macroscopic or microscopic margins – R1) have survival rates similar to those treated non-operatively.
- Surgery remains the only modality, which offers potential cure. Unfortunately, only 10–20% of patients have resectable (localized) disease at the time of diagnosis with a curative resection rate of 14% and a median survival of 15–19 months.
- 5YSR following resection is 25–30% and 10% for node-negative and positive disease, respectively.
- Recurrence typically occurs in the liver or locally particularly at the retroperitoneal margin due to difficulty in achieving microscopic clearance.

### Locally advanced (unresectable) disease

- Chemotherapy or chemoradiotherapy.
- Palliative interventions.

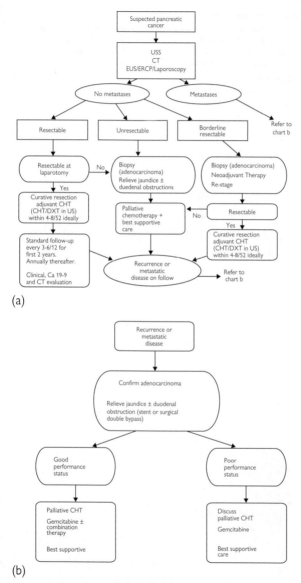

**Fig. 7.3** (a) Primary pancreatic cancer management algorithm.
(b) Algorithm for recurrent or metastatic disease.

*Borderline resectable*
- Consider neoadjuvant chemotherapy to downstage the tumour.
- Re-stage and if resectable, carry out curative surgery followed by adjuvant therapy (ideally within settings of clinical trials).
- If unresectable, then consider chemotherapy or chemoradiotherapy.

*Metastatic disease*
- Chemotherapy (mono or combination).
- Palliative interventions.

# Controversial issues in management

## Pylorus preservation

Pylorus preserving adaptation of the classical proximal pancreatico-duodenectomy (Whipple's procedure) was inaugurated in 1944 by Watson, and popularized by Traverso and Longmire in 1978. This adaptation aimed to reduce the post-gastrectomy complications, such as dumping syndrome, weight loss, marginal ulceration, and biliary reflux encountered with Whipple's procedure.

Multiple studies have tried to evaluate and compare effectiveness of Whipple's vs. pylorus preserving pancreatico-duodenectomy (PPPD). Meta-analysis by Diener (2007) indicated that both operations equally effective, no statistical difference in morbidity, mortality, recurrence and survival but significant reduction in operative time and blood loss with PPPD.

Tran et al. (2004) found no difference in blood loss, operating time or DGE in a prospective randomized multicentre trial.

Operative technique dictated by surgeon's preference and individual cancer centre's protocols and policies.

## Biliary drainage

- Anecdotal historical data is suggestive of increased infective complications and mortality, when jaundiced patients underwent curative pancreatic resection. Pre-operative biliary stenting advocated and widely practiced without prospective randomized trials.
- **Povoski et al. (1999)** *Memorial Sloane-Kettering:* pre-operative biliary drainage, but not pre-operative biliary instrumentation alone, is associated with increased morbidity and mortality rates in patients undergoing pancreatico-duodenectomy (presumably due to instrumentation of cholestasis and dissemination of the infected bile).
- **Sohn et al. (2000)** *(John Hopkins'):* patients with pre-operative stents had a significantly increased incidence of pancreatic fistula and wound infection.
- **Pisters et al. (2001)** *MD Andersen:* increased incidence of wound infection with pre-operative biliary drainage, but no increase in the risk of major complications or mortality.
- **Consensus**: pre-operative biliary stenting (endoscopic or percutaneous) should be avoided and only reserved for:
  - *symptomatic* patients (cholangitis, severe unrelenting pruritis);
  - *jaundiced* patients awaiting neoadjuvant therapy, where there would be a considerable delay prior to surgery;
  - *unresectable/metastatic disease* without gastric outlet obstruction (consider surgical bypass if latter present).

### Pancreatic anastomosis

Pancreatic leaks and anastomotic dehiscence are the most morbid complications of pancreatic resection, and place a major burden on postoperative care and recovery. Countless surgical techniques evaluated, but failed to show superiority. Pancreatic duct internal/external draining stents or fibrin glues have failed to reduce leak rates. Texture of the pancreas (soft) and size of the duct (small) appear to be major risk factors for pancreatic leaks. Meticulous preservation of blood supply essential

**Octreotide** (a somatostatin analogue) has been the subject of several European studies (Buchler 1992, Bassi 1994, Montorsi 1995) show reduced leaks and pancreatic fistulae (although patients with benign disease ere included in studies). Conversely, 2 prospective randomized trials have failed to show a reduced leak rate (Lowy et al. 1997; Yeo et al. 2000). Routine use remains controversial.

### Extended lymphadenenctomy

- Nodal metastases is a significant negative prognostic factor.
- Cause of dismal prognosis post-pancreatectomy in the 1970s and 80s due to residual nodal metastases beyond the field of resection, resulting in early recurrence and disseminated disease.
- Extended lymphadenectomy, instituted in Japan and USA.
- Involves resection of retroperitoneal soft tissue (from lateral border of aorta to right renal hilum + from portal vein to origin of IMA).
- Initial studies from Japanese groups (Ishikawa et al. 1988; Manabe et al. 1989) suggested improved survival but not reproduced by European and North American groups (Geer et al. 1993; Henne-Bruns et al. 2000).
- Two further prospective RCTs have failed to show any survival benefit with extended lymphadenectomy (Pedrazzoli et al. 1998; Yeo et al. 1999, 2002), whilst associated with a higher morbidity rate (pancreatic fistula and delayed gastric emptying) and longer hospital stay.

### Portal vein resection

- Historically, tumour involvement of the SMV/PV or SMA/coeliac axis indicated irresectability.
- **1970s hypothesis:** early recurrence due to inadequate local clearance.
- Vascular resection advocated to achieve more R0 resection margins, hence improving survival.
- Segments of SMV/PV can safely be resected and reconstructed with an autologous or synthetic graft, but it was associated with high morbidity and no improvement in overall survival.
- **Roder et al. (1996):** poor median survival (8 months) in patients with vascular resection and suggested no benefit from this aggressive approach. *Criticism of study:* only 32% of patients with vascular resection actually had R0 resection, which may explain the poor survival observed.
- **Fuhrman et al. (1996) MD Andersen:** no difference in hospital stay, morbidity, mortality, or margin positivity, and concluded it to be a safe procedure.
- **Leach et al. (1998):** similar median survival of 22 vs. 20 months (with and without vascular resection).

- Remains controversial, venous resection advocated by some groups in selected patients. Arterial involvement remains an absolute contraindication to resection.

## Regionalization

- Operative mortality rates have improved dramatically (20% in 1980s vs. <5% currently) attributed to better peri-operative care, operative techniques, and large single-centre experiences.
- Regionalization and institutional volume studied high volume centres report mortality of ~2–3% compared with 7–15% in low volume centres.
- Improved 3YSR when compared with low volume centres (37 vs. 26%), and similar improvements in survival, peri-operative death, length of stay have been observed by European and North American groups.
- Resections should be carried out in large volume centres performing >20 resections per year.

## Further reading

Bassi C, Falconi M, Pederzoli P. Role of somatostatin and somatostatin analogues in the treatment of gastrointestinal diseases: prevention of complications after pancreatic surgery. *Gut* 1994; **35 (3 Suppl)**:S20–2.

Buchler M, Friess H, Klempa I, Hermanek P, Sulkowski U, Becker H, *et al*. Role of octreotide in the prevention of postoperative complications following pancreatic resection. *Am J Surg* 1992; **163(1)**:125–30; discussion 30–1.

Diener MK, Knaebel HP, Heukaufer C, Antes G, Buchler MW, Seiler CM. A systematic review and meta-analysis of pylorus-preserving versus classical pancreaticoduodenectomy for surgical treatment of periampullary and pancreatic carcinoma. *Ann Surg* 2007; **245(2)**:187–200.

Fuhrman GM, Leach SD, Staley CA, Cusack JC, Charnsangavej C, Cleary KR, *et al*. Rationale for en bloc vein resection in the treatment of pancreatic adenocarcinoma adherent to the superior mesenteric-portal vein confluence. Pancreatic Tumor Study Group. *Ann Surg* 1996; **223(2)**: 154–62.

Geer RJ, Brennan MF. Prognostic indicators for survival after resection of pancreatic adenocarcinoma. *Am J Surg* 1993; **165(1)**:68–72; discussion -3.

Henne-Bruns D, Vogel I, Luttges J, Kloppel G, Kremer B. Surgery for ductal adenocarcinoma of the pancreatic head: staging, complications, and survival after regional versus extended lymphadenectomy. *World J Surg* 2000; **24(5)**:595–601; discussion -2.

Ishikawa O, Ohhigashi H, Sasaki Y, Kabuto T, Fukuda I, Furukawa H, *et al*. Practical usefulness of lymphatic and connective tissue clearance for the carcinoma of the pancreas head. *Ann Surg* 1988; **208(2)**:215–20.

Leach SD, Lee JE, Charnsangavej C, Cleary KR, Lowy AM, Fenoglio CJ, *et al*. Survival following pancreaticoduodenectomy with resection of the superior mesenteric-portal vein confluence for adenocarcinoma of the pancreas. *Br J Surg* 1998; **85(5)**:611–7.

Lowy AM, Lee JE, Pisters PW, Davidson BS, Fenoglio CJ, Stanford P, *et al*. Prospective, randomized trial of octreotide to prevent pancreatic fistula after pancreaticoduodenectomy for malignant disease. *Ann Surg* 1997; **226(5)**:632–41.

Manabe T, Ohshio G, Baba N, Miyashita T, Asano N, Tamura K, *et al*. Radical pancreatectomy for ductal cell carcinoma of the head of the pancreas. *Cancer* 1989; **64(5)**:1132–7.

Montorsi M, Zago M, Mosca F, Capussotti L, Zotti E, Ribotta G, *et al*. Efficacy of octreotide in the prevention of pancreatic fistula after elective pancreatic resections: a prospective, controlled, randomized clinical trial. *Surgery* 1995; **117(1)**:26–31.

Pisters PW, Hudec WA, Hess KR, Lee JE, Vauthey JN, Lahoti S, *et al.* Effect of preoperative biliary decompression on pancreaticoduodenectomy-associated morbidity in 300 consecutive patients. *Ann Surg* 2001; **234(1)**:47–55.

Povoski SP, Karpeh MS, Jr., Conlon KC, Blumgart LH, Brennan MF. Preoperative biliary drainage: impact on intraoperative bile cultures and infectious morbidity and mortality after pancreati-coduodenectomy. *J Gastrointest Surg* 1999; **3(5)**:496–505.

Povoski SP, Karpeh MS, Jr., Conlon KC, Blumgart LH, Brennan MF. Association of preoperative biliary drainage with postoperative outcome following pancreaticoduodenectomy. *Ann Surg* 1999; **230(2)**:131–42.

Roder JD, Stein HJ, Siewert JR. Carcinoma of the periampullary region: who benefits from portal vein resection? *Am J Surg* 1996; **171(1)**:170–4; discussion 4–5.

Sohn TA, Yeo CJ, Cameron JL, Pitt HA, Lillemoe KD. Do preoperative biliary stents increase post-pancreaticoduodenectomy complications? *J Gastrointest Surg* 2000; **4(3)**:258–67; discussion 67–8.

Tran KT, Smeenk HG, van Eijck CH, Kazemier G, Hop WC, Greve JW, *et al.* Pylorus preserving pancreaticoduodenectomy versus standard Whipple procedure: a prospective, randomized, multicenter analysis of 170 patients with pancreatic and periampullary tumors. *Ann Surg.* 2004; **240(5)**:738–45.

Yeo CJ. Does prophylactic octreotide benefit patients undergoing elective pancreatic resection? *J Gastrointest Surg* 1999; **3(3)**:223–4.

Yeo CJ, Cameron JL, Lillemoe KD, Sauter PK, Coleman J, Sohn TA, *et al.* Does prophylactic octre-otide decrease the rates of pancreatic fistula and other complications after pancreaticoduodenec-tomy? Results of a prospective randomized placebo-controlled trial. *Ann Surg* 2000; **232(3)**:419–29.

Yeo CJ. Intraductal papillary mucinous neoplasms of the pancreas. *Adv Surg* 2002; **36:**15–38.

# Resectability criteria

Currently, there are no unified international criteria for resection of pancreatic adenocarcinoma. However, particular criteria are favoured by most academic centres when determining potential resectability.

## Most favoured respectability criteria

### Resectable
- No metastases.
- Patent portal vein and SMV.
- No arterial invasion (a clear fat plane between tumour and coeliac + superior mesenteric arteries).

### Borderline resectable
- Incomplete impingement on SMV/PV.
- Encasement of gastroduodenal artery near its origin (hepatic artery).
- SMA abutment.
- Short segment SMV occlusion, with patency proximal and distally*.
- IVC abutment.
- Colonic/mesocolonic invasion.
- Invasion of left kidney, left adrenal, or colon with pancreatic tail cancers.

### Unresectable
- Distant metastases.
- SMA, celiac, or hepatic artery encasement.
- SMV or portal vein occlusion.
- Aorta or IVC encasement or invasion.
- Nodal metastases beyond the field of resection (M1).

*Subject of controversy as some centres carry out venous resection and reconstruction in selected group of patients whereas others consider any venous involvement as unresectable.

# Pre-operative assessment

- FBC, U&Es, LFTs, clotting, group and save, carbohydrate antigen 19-9 (CA 19-9).
- ECG +/– exercise test for assessment of cardiac status +/– echocardiogram if indicated.
- CXR +/– respiratory function tests if indicated.
- Anaesthetic, respiratory or cardiology as indicated.
- MDT meeting discussion pre- and post-operatively.

## Pre-operative preparation

- ***Smoking cessation:*** thromboembolic prophylaxis – anti-thromboembolic stockings, low molecular weight heparin +/– peroperative intermittent pneumatic calf compression.
- ***IV broad-spectrum antibiotics:*** immediately pre-operatively or at induction (cefuroxime/metronidazole or co-amoxiclav).
- ***X-match 4 units blood:*** avoid use if possible due to risks associated with transfusion.
- ***HDU or ITU bed available.***
- ***Epidural placement:*** for post-operative analgesia. Insertion of Foley's urethral catheter.

## Informed consent

***Specific complications:*** inoperability/palliative, incomplete resection, anastomotic leak (pancreatic, biliary, or intestinal), bleeding, intra-abdominal collections and wound infection, damage to loco-regional structures, delayed emptying, pancreatic insufficiency (endocrine/exocrine).

# Staging and prognosis

TNM classification is of limited use in determining resectability in pancreatic cancer as it is applicable only to those who have undergone formal resection (~14% of all cases). It is not suitable for majority of patients who are deemed unresectable, thus precluding histological confirmation of lymphatic involvement.

## TNM classification

### Primary tumour (T)

- **TX:** primary tumour cannot be assessed.
- **T0:** no evidence of primary tumour.
- **Tis:** carcinoma *in situ* (also includes PanIN-III).
- **T1:** tumour limited to the pancreas, ≤2cm in greatest dimension.
- **T2:** tumour limited to the pancreas, >2cm in greatest dimension.
- **T3:** tumour extends beyond the pancreas (into duodenum, bile ducts, or peripancreatic tissues), but *without* involvement of the celiac axis or the SMA.
- **T4:** tumour directly invades into other organs or structures (stomach, spleen, colon) *with* involvement of the celiac axis or the SMA.

### Regional lymph nodes (N)

- **NX:** regional lymph nodes cannot be assessed.
- **N0:** no regional lymph node metastasis.
- **N1:** metastasis in regional lymph nodes.
- **pN1a:** metastasis in a single regional lymph node.
- **pN1b:** metastasis in multiple regional lymph nodes.

### Distant metastasis (M)

- **MX:** distant metastasis cannot be assessed.
- **M0:** no distant metastasis.
- **M1:** distant metastasis.

**Table 7.2** AJCC staging

| Stage 0 | Tis, N0, M0. |
| --- | --- |
| Stage IA | T1, N0, M0. |
| Stage IB | T2, N0, M0. |
| Stage IIA | T3 N0 M0. |
| Stage IIB | T1 N1 M0. |
| | T2 N1 M0. |
| | T3 N1 M0. |
| Stage III | T4 Any N M0. |
| Stage IV | Any T Any N M1. |

Radiological/clinical staging is thus favoured in pancreatic cancer, and useful in predicting prognosis and assessing efficacy of adjuvant, neoadjuvant, and palliative therapies.

**Table 7.3** Clinical staging at presentation and median survival of patients with pancreatic cancer

| Stage | Incidence | Median survival |
|---|---|---|
| Localized(resectable) | 10–20% | 15–19 months |
| Locally advanced | 20–30% | 6–10 months |
| Metastatic | 60% | 3–6 months |

# Surgical anatomy of the pancreas

**Gross anatomy**

- The pancreas lies retroperitoneally in the transpyloric plane (L1), and divided into head, neck, body and tail. It is about 15cm long, and lies obliquely sloping from the head upwards towards the tail and spleen.
- The *head* is moulded into the C-curve of the duodenum. Its posterior surface has a hook-shaped extension, the *uncinate process*, which extends behind the SM vessels in front of the aorta.
- The *neck* lies in front of the SMV/splenic vein confluence (commencement of portal vein) and origin of the SMA. The transverse mesocolon is attached to the lower border of the neck, which lies in the stomach bed. The gastoduodenal artery (GDA) lies posterior to the junction of head and neck.
- The *body* is triangular in cross-section and crosses the aorta at the origin of coeliac trunk. The splenic vein lies closely applied to its posterior surface. It lies behind the lesser sac forming part of stomach bed.
- The *tail* passes forward and upwards, anterior to the left kidney. It is accompanied by splenic vessels and lymphatics within the lienorenal ligament, thus reaching the splenic hilum.

**Embryology**

- The pancreas develops from two separate endodermal buds at the junction of foregut and mid-gut. These buds develop into ducts from which acini and islets originate.
- The smaller ventral bud/segment swings posteriorly to fuse with the larger dorsal bud/segment, trapping the superior mesenteric vessels between them, thereby forming the single adult pancreas.
- The smaller duct takes over the main pancreatic drainage (Wirsung), whilst the duct of the larger segment becomes the accessory duct (Santorini).

**Structure**

- Macroscopically, lobulated organ within a fine capsule. Lobules are made of exocrine acini and group of endocrine cells, which drain their secretions into the principal ducts via ductules. The main pancreatic duct, runs the length of the gland and usually open together with the CBD at the ampulla of Vater. The accessory duct drains the lower part of the head opening independently above it into the duodenum.
- Microscopically, the bulk (98%) of the pancreas is composed of pancreatic *exocrine* cells and their associated ducts. Exocrine pancreas is responsible for secreting digestive enzymes, such as trypsin, chymotrypsin, pancreatic lipase, and pancreatic amylase. Embedded within this exocrine tissue are roughly one million small clusters of cells called the Islets of Langerhans, which are the *endocrine* cells (2%) of the pancreas and secrete insulin, glucagon, somatostatin, and pancreatic polypeptides.

**Relations (from right to left)**

- *Anteriorly:* transverse colon/mesocolon, lesser sac, and stomach.
- *Posteriorly:* CBD, portal and splenic veins, IVC, aorta, origin of SMA, SMV, coeliac plexus, left psoas, adrenal and kidney, hilum of spleen.

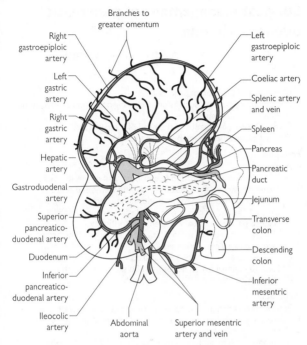

Right gastroepiploic artery
Left gastric artery
Right gastric artery
Hepatic artery
Gastroduodenal artery
Superior pancreatico-duodenal artery
Duodenum
Inferior pancreatico-duodenal artery
Ileocolic artery
Abdominal aorta
Superior mesenteric artery and vein
Branches to greater omentum
Left gastroepiploic artery
Coeliac artery
Splenic artery and vein
Spleen
Pancreas
Pancreatic duct
Jejunum
Transverse colon
Descending colon
Inferior mesenteric artery

**Fig. 7.4** Anatomy of pancreas relations.

## Blood supply
- Most of the blood supply is from the splenic artery, which supplies the neck, body, and tail.
- The head is supplied by the superior and inferior pancreatico-duodenal (PD) arteries.
- Venous drainage is via the splenic and superior PD veins into the portal vein, and via the inferior PD vein into SMV.

## Lymphatic drainage
The lymphatic drainage of the stomach parallels the vasculature:
- *Head:* upper aspect into coeliac group, lower aspect, and uncinate process into superior mesenteric and pre-aortic groups.
- *Neck, body and tail:* into pancreaticosplenic nodes, which accompany the splenic artery.

## Nerve supply
- *Parasympathetic (vagus):* stimulates exocrine secretions and carry pain fibres.
- *Sympathetic (splanchnic nerves):* vasoconstriction and carry pain fibres.

# Surgical management of pancreatic adenocarcinoma

**Operative technique: pancreatico-duodenectomy (Whipple's)**

*Indication*
- Carcinoma of the head of pancreas.
- Peri-ampullary cancers, such as distal cholangiocarcinomas, carcinoma of duodenum, and ampulla.
- Severe chronic pancreatitis of the head of the pancreas.
- Traumatic disruption of the head of pancreas.

*Principles*
- Aim to:
  - resect pancreatic head, duodenum, distal half of the stomach, including pylorus, the gallbladder, and the lower end of CBD together with draining lymph nodes (along hepatic artery, coeliac axis, splenic and pyloric regions) and vascular supply *en bloc*;
  - restore pancreatic, biliary, and enteric continuity.
- Thorough assessment of tumour site, size, presence of metastatic disease, and vascular involvement (SMA and PV) is prudent pre-operatively to avoid unnecessary laparotomies in irresectable disease.
- At least 10 regional lymph nodes must be sampled for optimal histological assessment.

*Preparation*
- Ensure correct patient and notes, and informed concentrate available.
- Correct any coagulopathy by giving 10mg vitamin K pre-operatively ± FFP pre- or peri-induction.
- IV broad-spectrum antibiotics on induction and 2 further doses post-operatively.
- Catheterize.
- General anaesthesia with an epidural for post-operative pain control.

*Procedure*
- Supine position.
- Bilateral subcostal (Chevron), curved transverse or midline laparotomy incision.

### Assessment/trial dissection

- Detailed systematic laparotomy and search for metastatic disease.
- Mobilize the hepatic flexure and right transverse colon in a medial and caudal direction to expose duodenum and pancreas. Kocherize duodenum thus lifting pancreatic head and duodenum forward off the IVC.
- Palpate the head, body, and tail of the pancreas through the lesser omentum to assess localization and extension. Palpate the uncinate process by lifting the transverse mesocolon. Consider total pancreatectomy if extending beyond the head or a multicentric cancer (<10%).
- Palpate for lymphatic spread along the anterior and posterior duodenopancreatic grooves, hepatic, celiac, and superior mesenteric arteries. Some groups advocate extended lymphadenectomy if extension beyond these fields (no survival benefit).
- Ensure primary tumour is mobilizable, i.e. no involvement of pre-aortic fascia posteriorly.
- Ensure there is *no involvement of portal vein* and its tributaries, as this determines resectability in practice. Use the middle coelic vein to guide towards the SMV.
- Use 2 index fingers, one from above along the anterior surface of PV and one finger from below along the SMV to establish a safe plane between the neck of pancreas anteriorly and PV posteriorly. If fingers meet easily then proceed to formal resection. If they don't, do not use force or stray as damage can be caused to several small pancreatic veins, which can bleed profusely. Instead, abandon curative resection and carry out a palliative procedure. Some centres (e.g. MD Anderson group) advocate venous resection and reconstruction with favourable results.

### Formal oncological resection

- Confirmation of resectable disease from trial dissection.
- 2 phases – resection and reconstruction.

#### Resection phase

- **Portal dissection**: dissect the structures within free edge of the lesser omentum. Pass a sloop and retract CBD laterally. Preserve the main hepatic artery. Doubly ligate, and divide right gastric and gastroduodenal arteries.
- Dissect the gallbladder off liver bed and divide the CHD just proximal to its confluence with cystic duct. Apply a bulldog clip on CHD stump.
- Beware of anomalous hepatic arterial tree. An accessory right hepatic artery can arise from the proximal SMA and run posterolateral to PV. Occasionally, the common hepatic artery arises from the SMA or runs posterior to the PV. Care must be taken not to divide this as hepatic necrosis may ensue.
- **Transect the stomach**: use clamps/knife or linear staplers at the junction of body and antrum. A useful landmark is the 3rd or 4th transverse vein on the lesser curve.

- **Division of pancreas:** mobilize the pancreas from the retroperitoneal tissues. Place traction sutures along the superior and inferior borders of the pancreas. Transect the pancreas at the level of PV (knife or diathermy onto a preplaced Kocher dissector behind the pancreas).
- **Division of jejunum:** lift up transverse colon, identify DJ flexure, incise ligament of Treitz, divide upper jejunum (clamps/knife or linear stapler).
- **Removal of specimen:** the whole specimen is only attached by small vessels between duodenum + uncinate and superior mesenteric vessels, most notably the inferior pancreatico-duodenal artery, which lies in the groove between pancreatic head and duodenum. Ligate and divide this vessel followed by very careful dissection of the uncinate off the SMV. The specimen is now completely detached ready for the anastomotic phase.

*Reconstruction phase*

- **Cholodochojejunostomy**: ante or retrocolic tension-free delivery of jejunum followed by an end (biliary) to side (jejunal) anastomosis using a single layer interrupted 4-0 absorbable monofilament suture. Occasionally, a stent is placed *in situ* and some surgeons place a temporary draining T-tube through the anastomosis into the jejunum and remove it on D10 post-operatively following a satisfactory cholangiogram.
- **Pancreaticojejunostomy:** various methods to adapt to different parenchymal consistency and duct size hence reducing risk of leak. Usually carried out 5–10cm distal to the choledochojejunostomy site. Excise a seromuscular disc from the jejunum to match the pancreatic remnant. Incise the jejunal mucosa directly opposite the duct. 2-layer interrupted invaginating end-to-end anastomosis using a 3-0 absorbable monofilament suture. First layer duct to mucosa, second layer pancreatic parenchyma to jejunum. Some groups use a transanastomotic stent (exteriorized through the jejunum and anterior abdomen wall) in patients with cancers with small pancreatic ducts to reduce leaks and strictures. Used less often in chronic pancreatitis or cancers with obstructed dilated pancreatic ducts.
- **Gastrojejunostomy:** Billroth II type end-to-side two-layer anastomosis using a 3-0 absorbable monofilament suture. Should be 25–30cm distal to biliary anastomosis.
- **Closure:** mass closure with 0 PDS, clips to skin.
- **Post-operative care:** 24–48h in HDU/ITU

**Alternative methods**

- Roux-en-Y gastroenteric reconstruction to reduce dumping and biliary gastritis.
- Ligation of pancreatic duct in patients where risk of fistula is high, e.g. soft pancreas (sutures cut through) or small duct. This avoids pancreatic anastamosis, fistulae can still occur, but at lower rate and reduced morbidity. Will need exocrine replacement.
- **Total pancreatectomy:** consider if multicentric cancer or soft friable pancreas/small duct.

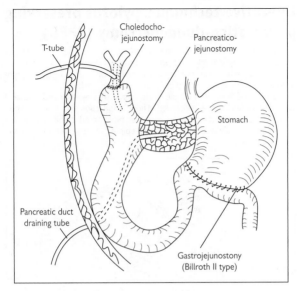

**Fig. 7.5** Whipple's procedure.

## Specific complications (25%)

### Leaks
Usually present on day 3–5, can be biliary, enteric, or pancreatic. Brown/clear fluid with high amylase indicative of pancreatic leaks (15%), which carry a worse prognosis due the corrosive nature of pancreatic juices. Can result in fistulae, sepsis, and haemorrhage. *Management* – CT-guided drainage of collections, antibiotics, NBM, TPN, octreotide. Total pancreatectomy if anastomotic dehiscence.

### Haemorrhage
Bleeding can be gastrointestinal from anastomotic ulceration/erosion or more torrential extra-intestinal from rupture of ligated GDA following a pancreatic leak. *Management* – therapeutic OGD, angiography and embolization of GDA.

### Others
Dumping syndrome, biliary gastritis, afferent loop syndrome, pancreatic insufficiency. Mortality rate <5% in high volume centres.

# Operative technique: pylorus preserving pancreatico-duodenectomy (PPPD)

This pylorus preserving adaptation of Whipple's procedure was inaugurated in 1944 by Watson, and popularized by Traverso and Longmire in 1978 to reduce the post-gastrectomy complications, such as dumping syndrome, weight loss, marginal ulceration, and biliary reflux.

Procedure differs from classic Whipple's in that pylorus and proximal 5cm of duodenum are preserved. Their blood supply is thus retained by careful preservation of right gastro-epiploic arcade. This is achieved by ligation and division of right gastro-epiploic artery and vein on the pancreatic side.

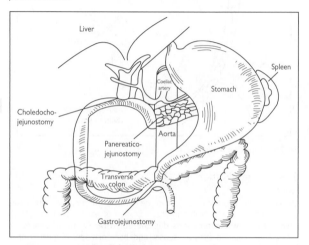

**Fig. 7.6** Pylorus preserving pancreatico-duodenectomy (PPPD).

Dudodenum is then resected 5cm distal to pylorus and the duodenal stump is anastomosed to the jejunum (end-to-side) 25–30cm distal to the biliary anastomosis. This can also be modified through a Roux-en-Y reconstruction.

## Advantages of PPPD
- Reduced post-gastrectomy syndromes.
- Reduced blood loss and operative time.

## Disadvantages of PPPD
- Delayed gastric emptying (DGE).
- Concerns regarding suboptimal clearance of the supra and infrapyloric perigastric nodes, and higher positive margins with negative impact on recurrence and survival.

# Operative technique: distal pancreatectomy

Carried out for cancers or chronic inflammation of the body and tail of the pancreas. For adenocarcinomas and most cases of chronic pancreatitis, a splenectomy is also carried out *en bloc*. Spleen is preserved in endocrine tumours of the body and tail, and less severe cases of chronic pancreatitis.

Prepare patient as per Whipple's procedure.

Assess resectability by excluding metastases and superior mesenteric vessels involvement.

## Procedure

- Mobilize the neck of pancreas from the PV and SMV by incising the peritoneum along the inferior border of the neck of pancreas. Now mobilize the body and tail.
- Mobilize the spleen by dividing its posterior attachments.
- Ligate and divide the short gastric vessels.
- Lift the splenic hilum and pancreatic tail forward, and complete the mobilization of the tail and body towards the midline.
- Identify and doubly ligate the splenic artery followed by the vein (to prevent splenic congestion).
- Splenic vein should be ligated distal to its confluence with IMV to preserve hindgut's venous drainage.
- Transect the pancreas at the level of the neck taking care not to traumatize the underlying PV. Ligate the duct before complete transection. Remove the specimen.
- Under-run the pancreatic stump to further reduce risk of pancreatic leak. Consider a formal drainage procure in the presence of a dilated duct (pancreatico-gastrostomy or jejunostomy with Roux-en-Y reconstruction).
- Place a drain in the splenic bed to monitor haemorrhage and pancreatic fistula.

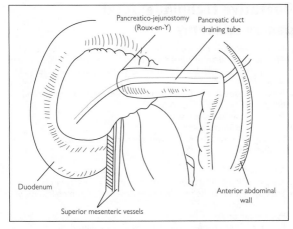

**Fig. 7.7**  Distal pancreatectomy.

## Complications

- Haemorrhage, typically from a tear in the splenic vein.
- Splenic bed haematoma/abscess (fever, left pleural effusion). Manage by CT guided drainage.
- *Pancreatic fistula:* manage by CT-guided drainage and octreotide.
- Pseudocysts.
- Diabetes or exocrine insufficiency.

# Operative technique: total pancreatectomy

Initially advocated routinely for adenocarcinomas in an event of multicentricity and to eliminate any potential pancreatic leak. However, it confers no survival benefit whilst it carries higher morbidity. Thus, reserved for:
- Bulky yet resectable tumours of the head encroaching on neck and body.
- Surgically undetectable insulinomas.
- Total pancreatic necrosis.
- End-stage chronic pancreatitis with endocrine and exocrine insufficiency.

## Procedure

In essence, it is a combination of proximal and distal pancreatectomy.
- Start by mobilizing the neck from the PV followed by mobilization of head and body/tail.
- Pylorus can be preserved.
- Ensure biliary and enteric continuity by either a Billroth I/II or a Roux-en-Y type reconstruction.

## Complications

As for proximal and distal pancreatectomy with the exception of pancreatic leak.

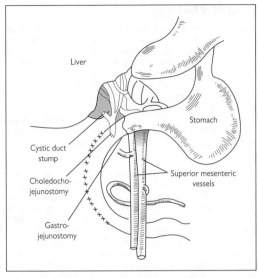

**Fig. 7.8** Total pancreatectomy.

# Adjuvant therapy

Following surgery, prognosis remains fairly poor with a median survival of 15–19 months, and most patients succumb to recurrent or metastatic disease due to unrecognized micrometastatic disease at the time of surgery. Therefore, this is the rationale for adjuvant therapy after curative resection, attempting to increase survival.

Unfortunately, there is no general consensus on standard adjuvant therapy and a great controversy exists across the Atlantic regarding this subject based on the following trials.

Based on current guidelines, Europeans consider chemotherapy (CHT) alone as the optimal adjuvant therapy, whilst North Americans favour chemoradiotherapy (CHT/RT) followed by chemotherapy.

## GITSG Trial

Evidence in favour of the North American combined chemo and radiotherapy protocol was suggested by a small phase 3 trial conducted by the Gastrointestinal Tumor Study Group in 1985 (GITSG). Patients were randomly assigned to either (a) observation only or (b) chemotherapy with 5-FU and concomitant split course radiotherapy (5-FU – 500mg/m$^2$ daily for 3 days together with 20Gy external beam radiotherapy with a 2-week rest interval between courses). This regimen almost doubled median survival compared with the observation only arm (20 months vs. 11 months sand 5YSR of 18 vs. 8%).

This study was, however, criticized due to a number of flaws :
• Lengthy time and poor patient accrual (8 years + 43 patients).
• Delay in treatment (25% of patients did not commence treatment until >10 weeks post-resection).
• Suboptimal RT dose.
• Use of 5-FU without folinic acid (leucovorin).

## EORTC Trial

European Organization for Research and Treatment of Cancer (EORTC) recognized some of the above limitations and carried out a larger trial assigning 114 patients to either (a) observation only or (b) continuous 5-FU infusion and split course radiotherapy (40Gy total). It failed to confirm the benefit of CHT/RT. Results published in 1999, revealed some improvement in survival in the adjuvant therapy group, but such improvements were *not* statistically significant (2-year survival rates of 23% vs. 37%, $p = 0.099$). As a result, European oncologists began to question the effectiveness of radiotherapy.

This study was criticized by North Americans as:
• Underpowered study.
• 20% of patients never received actual treatment in the adjuvant therapy group.
• Suboptimal RT dose.

## ESPAC-1 trial

There was now evidence favouring adjuvant therapy but the best modality remained unanswered. The European Study Group for Pancreatic Cancer (ESPAC) embarked on the largest reported randomized trial to date attempting to answer this question. Commencing in 1994, 541 patients were randomizes in a 2 × 2 factorial design to:

- Observation only.
- **CHT alone:** 6 cycles of 5-FU + folinic acid.
- **CHT/RT:** split course RT (20Gy/fraction) + bolus 5-FU.
- CHT/RT followed by CHT.
  They also analysed the data in a direct head-to-head design:
- CHT/RT vs. no CHT/RT.
- CHT vs. no CHT.
  The results published separately (2001 and 2004), revealed:
- Significant survival benefit for CHT only group, cf. no CHT (2YSR and median survival of 40% and 20.1 months vs. 30% and 15.5 months, respectively).
- **Detrimental effect** of RT (2YSR and median survival – CHT/RT group 29% and 15.9 months vs. 41% and 17.9 months in the no CHT/RT group).
  Criticisms of this trial are:
- **Selection bias:** patient and clinicians could choose which trial to enter, and allow background CHT/RT or CHT if patient was placed in an undesirable arm.
- Inclusion of positive margin patients.
- Not an intention-to-treat analysis.
- Lack of RT quality assurance and unequal dosing for recipients.

As a result of ESPAC-1 trial, European centres abandoned routine use of adjuvant radiotherapy, and opted to investigate and optimize best chemotherapy regimen (ESPAC-3 and CONKO), further deepening the transatlantic divide.

North American groups, however, remain sceptical given ESPAC-1's flaws and have embarked on optimizing the CHT/RT regimen

## RTOG 97-04 trial

Headed by the North American Radiation Therapy Oncology Group, this study intended to evaluate the effectiveness of 5-FU vs. gemcitabine before, and after standard CHT/RT ($50.4Gy + 250mg/m^2$/day 5-FU). It also required prospective quality control of RT, addressing one of the shortcomings of the ESPAC-1 trial.

Results of the 538 patients accrued by this study were published in 2006 and revealed that in patients with carcinoma of the head of pancreas gemcitabine is better than 5-FU when incorporated either side of the CHT/RT regimen (median survival 20.6 months vs. 16.9 months). There was, however *no* difference when cancers of the body and tail were also included.

Gemcitabine also resulted in significantly more haematological side effects, cf. 5-FU, but no difference in non-haematological side effects were observed.

## CONKO trial

European study led by the German CharitéOnkologie, CONKO 001, accrued 368 patients post-resection, who were randomized to gemcitabine vs. observation only. Adjuvant gemcitabine rendered a trend toward overall benefit, improving median disease free survival (13.4 vs. 6.9 months) and median survival (22.1 vs. 20.2). In this study, gemcitabine was generally well tolerated and most patients tolerated the full 6-cycle course.

As a result, gemcitabine has been advocated as first line treatment given its superiority over 5-FU in terms of clinical benefit and improvement in median survival.

## ESPAC-3 trial

This landmark multicentre European trial, whose results are widely anticipated, aims to directly compare 5-FU + folinic acid vs. gemcitabine vs. observation only, since the CONKO trial compared gemcitabine with historical 5-FU results from previous trials. Results are imminent, which should hopefully give further credence to the use of gemcitabine as first line CHT agent in adjuvant therapy of pancreatic adenocarcinoma.

In summary, no definitive protocol has been established in the adjuvant treatment of pancreatic adenocarcinoma and the options are CHT alone (gemcitabine better than 5-FU), or 5-FU based CHT/RT with pre- and post-gemcitabine.

Regardless of the regimen used, individual patient's suitability for adjuvant therapy should be discussed at a multidisciplinary meeting in addition to greatly involving the patient in decision making. Adjuvant therapy should be ideally commenced 4–8 weeks post-resection providing adequate post-operative recovery. Patient should be re-staged (CT and CA19-9) to exclude metastatic disease prior to adjuvant therapy.

## Alternatives in adjuvant therapy

### Interferon-alpha

Based on a small promising phase II trial conducted by Picozzi et al. (2003), combination chemoradiotherapy (Interferon alpha, 5-FU, cisplatin, and EBRT) was shown to improve overall survival (1YSR 95%, 2YSR 64%, 5YSR 55%), which are dramatically superior to standard adjuvant therapy. Unfortunately, 70% of patients developed moderate to severe gastrointestinal side-effects. Furthermore, phase III studies are required to evaluate and optimize this regimen.

### Immunotherapy

- Irradiated allogenic pancreatic adenocarcinoma cells transfected with GM-CSF (granulocyte monocyte colony stimulating factor).
- Phase II trial conducted by Laheru et al. (2007) evaluated this treatment, which was administered 8–10 weeks post-resection, in addition to chemoradiotherapy with 5-FU.
- 1YSR of 88% and 2YSR of 76% with a median survival of 26 months, whilst the vaccine was fairly well tolerated. Again, phase III trials are required to further evaluate this modality.

### Further reading

Picozzi VJ, Kozarek RA, Traverso LW. Interferon-based adjuvant chemoradiation therapy after pancreaticoduodenectomy for pancreatic adenocarcinoma. *Am J Surg* 2003; **185(5)**:476–80.

Laheru D, Jaffee EM. Immunotherapy for pancreatic cancer - science driving clinical progress. *Nat Rev Cancer* 2005; **5(6)**:459–67.

# Neoadjuvant therapy

Rationale for neoadjuvant therapy includes:

- **Downstage tumour:** borderline resectable into resectable and even in resectable disease to increase R0 status.
- **Delayed post-operative recovery** prevents 25% of eligible patients from having adjuvant therapy post-resection.
- **Prevent dissemination and implantation** of tumour cells during surgical manipulation and resection.
- **Prevent unnecessary laparotomy** if patient has progressive or metastatic disease on post-neoadjuvant re-staging.
- Treatment of micrometastases at an earlier stage.

Several studies have investigated the efficacy (no RCTs though) of neoadjuvant therapy in resectable and unresectable disease.

Resectable disease

- Overall survival maximized by the combination of pre-operative chemoradiation and pancreatico-duodenectomy (median survival 21 months, 31% alive without evidence of disease (MD Andersen study).
- Efficacy of neoadjuvant gemcitabine monotherapy against gemcitabine + cisplatin in resectable disease in a phase II trial.
- Combination therapy with cisplatin improved survival (1YSR 61% vs. 46%).
- Following re-staging, 54% of patients had curative surgery, 10% had progressive disease and avoided the burden of unnecessary surgery and 36% of patients had bypass procedures. Unfortunately, ~35% of patients randomized had grade 3/4 haematological toxicity (Palmer 2004).

## Unresectable disease

A few studies have investigated the role of neoadjuvant therapy in converting unresectable to resectable disease. Most encouraging results emanate from the MD Anderson experience (Wolff et al. 2001), which revealed that neoadjuvant therapy with gemcitabine and radiotherapy, improved resectability rate (74%), and median survival (37 months), although 43% of patients required hospitalization (side effects). They thus concluded that gemcitabine is a clinically relevant radiosensitizer in patients with pancreatic adenocarcinoma. However, the toxic effects were significant and appeared to be dose related. A better chance of achieving R0 status was also observed other studies (Pingpank et al. 2001).

The results of prospective trials currently underway, such as ECOG 1200 and the ISGGT should shed further light on the efficacy of neoadjuvant therapy on improving R0 status and survival.

In summary, neoadjuvant therapy is still in investigational and developmental stages, and cannot be endorsed as standard treatment. The current recommendation is that neoadjuvant therapy could be considered for patients with borderline resectable disease and also in context of clinical trials in patients with resectable disease.

### Further reading

Palmer DH, Stocken DD, Hewitt H, Markham CE, Hassan AB, Johnson PJ, et al. A randomized phase 2 trial of neoadjuvant chemotherapy in resectable pancreatic cancer: gemcitabine alone versus gemcitabine combined with cisplatin. *Ann Surg Oncol* 2007; **14(7)**:2088–96.

Pingpank JF, Hoffman JP, Ross EA, Cooper HS, Meropol NJ, Freedman G, et al. Effect of preoperative chemoradiotherapy on surgical margin status of resected adenocarcinoma of the head of the pancreas. *J Gastrointest Surg* 2001; **5(2)**:121–30.

Wolff RA, Evans DB, Gravel DM, Lenzi R, Pisters PW, Lee JE, et al. Phase I trial of gemcitabine combined with radiation for the treatment of locally advanced pancreatic adenocarcinoma. *Clin Cancer Res* 2001; **7(8)**:2246–53.

# Management of locally advanced (unresectable) disease

Prognosis of this large (20–30%) group of patients remains dismal with a median survival of 6–10 months. Attempts have been made to improve their prognosis and quality of life by means of chemoradiotherapy or chemotherapy alone.

## Chemoradiotherapy

This modality has been the mainstay of treatment for locally advanced disease, since the initial reports from the Mayo Clinic followed by outcome from two GITSG trials. Combination of split course external beam radiation (EBRT) and 5-FU chemotherapy, improved median survival by almost 2 folds when compared with radiotherapy alone (10.4 vs. 6.3 months).

The role of other chemotherapy agents have also been evaluated. gemcitabine is a potent radiosensitizer and its use in combination with radiotherapy has been evaluated by two studies (Epelbaum et al. 2002, McGinn et al. 2002). Unfortunately, despite its early promise, neither study demonstrated an improvement in survival with gemcitabine/RT when compared with 5-FU/RT. Furthermore, significant toxicity was observed in the gemcitabine arm.

Superiority of gemcitabine was, however, demonstrated in a small randomized study by Li et al. (2003), where improvements in median survival and time to progression were observed.

Further large phase III randomized trials are thus required to elucidate the best chemotherapy agent to be used in combination with EBRT.

## Chemotherapy alone

Following the European approach and previous findings that radiotherapy can actually be detrimental in an adjuvant setting, the role of chemotherapy alone was evaluated in treatment of locally advanced disease. A French phase III trial carried out by Chauffert et al. (2006), compared chemoradiotherapy (5-FU + cisplatin + 60GyRT) against chemotherapy alone (gemcitabine). Both arms received maintenance gemcitabine alone thereafter. Interestingly, gemcitabine alone inferred a significant survival benefit when compared with combined chemoradiotherapy (median survival 14.3 vs. 8.4 months). Furthermore, increased haematological and non-haematological toxicity were observed in the chemoradiotherapy group and the study was stopped before the planned inclusion date due to poor results observed in this group.

In summary, patients with locally advanced disease and a good performance status, can be given either CHT alone (favoured by Europeans) or combined CHT/RT (favoured by North Americans), albeit with poor overall survival advantage. The efficacy and toxicity need to be thoroughly discussed with the patient before a joint decision is made on treatment. Clearly, novel agents and large phase III RCTs are required to improve prognosis in this group of patients.

## Further reading

Chauffert B, Mornex F, Bonnetain F, Rougier P, Mariette C, Bouche O, et al. Phase III trial comparing intensive induction chemoradiotherapy (60 Gy, infusional 5-FU and intermittent cisplatin) followed by maintenance gemcitabine with gemcitabine alone for locally advanced unresectable pancreatic cancer. Definitive results of the 2000-01 FFCD/SFRO study. *Ann Oncol* 2008; **19(9)**:1592–9.

Epelbaum R, Rosenblatt E, Nasrallah S, Faraggi D, Gaitini D, Mizrahi S, et al. Phase II study of gemcitabine combined with radiation therapy in patients with localized, unresectable pancreatic cancer. *J Surg Oncol* 2002; **81(3)**:138–43.

Li CP, Chao Y, Chi KH, Chan WK, Teng HC, Lee RC, et al. Concurrent chemoradiotherapy treatment of locally advanced pancreatic cancer: gemcitabine versus 5-fluorouracil, a randomized controlled study. *Int J Radiat Oncol Biol Phys* 2003; **57(1)**:98–104.

McGinn CJ, Lawrence TS, Zalupski MM. On the development of gemcitabine-based chemoradiotherapy regimens in pancreatic cancer. *Cancer* 2002; **95(4 Suppl)**:933–40.

# Management of metastatic disease

The majority (60%) of patients with pancreatic cancer have metastatic disease at the time of diagnosis and have a limited survival (3–6 months median survival). Many are frail with poor performance status and often require palliative therapy.

The aim of palliative therapy, whether medical, surgical, or psychological, is to optimize quality of life and prevent suffering. Increased survival is considered a secondary end-point and achievable through palliative chemotherapy.

## Chemotherapy for metastatic disease

### Monotherapy

- 5-FU and mitomycin historically best response rates.
- Replaced by gemcitabine monotherapy as first-line: Burris et al. (1997) gemcitabine vs. 5-FU. gemcitabine significantly improved survival (median 5.6 vs. 4.4 months, 1YSR 18 vs. 2%), quality of life and the clinical response rate (23.8 vs. 4.8%) as measured by disease-related symptoms (pain, maintenance of Karnofsky performance status, and weight gain).
- gemcitabine recently approved by NICE to be considered in patients with a Karnofsky performance score >50.
- gemcitabine is a deoxycytidine analogue and is a prodrug, which needs to be phosphorylated to become an active cytotoxic metabolite.
- Fixed-dose rate (FDR) administration maximizes intracelluar concentrations and hence improve response rates.
- The phase II trial improved survival when administered at $10mg/m^2/min$ when compared with standard 30min infusion, but increased haematological toxicity.
- The phase III trial conducted by the Eastern Cooperative Oncology Group (ECOG 6201) no significant benefit with FDR.

### Combination therapy

Many trials have evaluated whether gemcitabine therapy in combination with other agents would infer an improvement in survival and clinical benefit response. Despite their initial promising improvement in median survival, combination of cisplatin or 5-FU with gemcitabine have failed to demonstrate a statistically significant improvement in overall or progression-free survival (phase III trial; Heinemann et al. 2006).

A promising recent phase III trial (GEM-CAP; Cunningham et al. 2005) has, however, demonstrated a significant improvement in median survival (7.4 vs. 6.0 months) when gemcitabine was used in combination with capecitabine (an oral prodrug, that is enzymatically converted to 5-fluorouracil). Significant myelosupression was, hozwever, observed in the GEM-CAP group.

With advances in understanding of molecular biology of pancreatic cancer, there has been much interest in combination regimen using targeted monoclonal antibodies and gemcitabine.

Several phase II studies have shown good results when gemcitabine was used in combination with cetuximab (EGFR inhibitor) or bevacizumab (monoclonal antibody against vascular endothelial growth factor). However, phase III trials have failed to show any benefit from cetuximab or bevacizumab, but combination therapy with erlotinib (a tyrosine kinase inhibitor) was very promising. This phase III trial carried out by the National Cancer Institute of Canada (Moore et al. 2007), showed statistically significant improvements in overall survival when erlotinib was used in combination with gemcitabine (median – 6.24 vs. 5.9 months and 1YSR – 23% vs. 17%).

### Second-line therapy

A small subset of patients with metastatic disease who have had palliative chemotherapy, will demonstrate disease progression, whilst maintaining a good performance status. These patients could be treated with gemcitabine alone (if not used first time) or a combination of gemcitabine/oxaliplatin or oxaliplatin/capecitabine within the settings of a clinical trial ideally.

In summary, the current recommendation is that patients with metastatic disease with a good performance status should be considered for gemcitabine monotherapy. Combination therapy with capecitabine or erlotinib are also effective, but should be offered to patients within clinical trials. Patients should be closely monitored for toxicity and disease progression, and treatment should be stopped as the optimal goal for management of metastatic disease is to improve quality of life.

## Palliation for metastatic and unresectable disease

This multidisciplinary approach should involve surgeons, oncologist, and anaesthetists, as well as input from occupational therapists and hospices when required not only by patients, but also their families.

### Relief of pancreatic pain

Pancreatic cancer often infiltrates the retroperitoneal coeliac nerve plexus and, as such, pain is a common presenting feature, but when persistent, it is suggestive of irresectable/metastatic disease. Pain is also thought to be secondary to parenchymal pressure (pancreatic duct obstruction) and biliary obstruction.

The following measures can be used to alleviate this disabling symptom:
- Analgesic ladder (WHO) using a combination of simple , non-steroidal and opioid analgesia.
- Coeliac plexus ablation with phenol or ethanol – can be done percutaneous fluoroscopic, or CT-guided, or laparoscopically, and been shown to be effective in 70% of patients.
- Thoracoscopic division of splanchnic nerves.
- EBRT.
- Pancreatic duct stenting.

*Biliary obstruction*

About 70% of patients with pancreatic cancer present with symptomatic biliary obstruction that manifest earlier with cancers of the head of pancreas, and usually secondary to metastatic disease in cancers of the body and tail of pancreas. The options for biliary decompression are:
- ERCP stenting (preferred method).
- PTC.
- Open bypass.

Stent occlusion and ensuing cholangitis is a well recognized complication of stents secondary to disease progression. Plastic stents typically obstruct within 3 months (median patency of 1.8 months), but can be replaced when blocked. In contrast, metal stents are wider and less likely to obstruct with a median patency of 3.6 months, but cannot be replaced.

Patients who have concomitant gastric outlet obstruction would be better served with open double bypass, if they have a good performance status or if metastatic disease is identified at the time of curative resection. Choledocho- or hepaticojejunostomy are preferred to cholecystojejunostomy as they drain more reliably and last longer.

*Gastric outlet obstruction*

This occurs in 10–25% of patients and usually signifies unresectable disease. This can be alleviated by either:
- ***Gastrojejunostomy:*** in patients with good performance status (life expectancy of 3–6 months) or prophylactically in those with unresectable/metastatic disease at the time of curative surgery.
- ***Enteral stent or PEG:*** in those with poor performance status or limited life expectancy.

*Depression*

A common problem in patients with pancreatic cancer, which in its milder form can be addressed in primary and palliative care settings, is that, should risk issues be present, help from psychiatric services may be required. Counselling as a means of adjustment to this life-changing event can often be helpful.

*Nutritional supplements*

Exocrine pancreatic insufficiency is sometimes encountered especially post-resection or due to pancreatic parenchymal or ductal destruction. Replacement with pancreatic supplements (e.g. Creon®) has been shown to improve quality of life and symptom score in patients with advanced disease.

## Surveillance

Following curative resection, patients should be reviewed every 3–6 months for 2 years and annually thereafter. Each consultation would include clinical evaluation in addition to a CT scan and CA 19-9 to exclude recurrence or metastatic disease. Once disease progression is confirmed, further treatment should be discussed at MDT and with the patient, taking into account their wishes and performance status.

## Further reading

Burris HA, 3rd, Moore MJ, Andersen J, Green MR, Rothenberg ML, Modiano MR, et al. Improvements in survival and clinical benefit with gemcitabine as first-line therapy for patients with advanced pancreas cancer: a randomized trial. *J Clin Oncol* 1997; **15(6)**:2403–13.

Heinemann V, Quietzsch D, Gieseler F, Gonnermann M, Schonekas H, Rost A, et al. Randomized phase III trial of gemcitabine plus cisplatin compared with gemcitabine alone in advanced pancreatic cancer. *J Clin Oncol* 2006; **24(24)**:3946–52.

Cunningham D CI, Stocken D, Davies C, Dunn J, Valle J, Smith D, Steward W HP, Neoptolemos JP. Phase III randomised comparison of gemcitabine vs gemcitabine plus capecitabine in patients with advanced pancreatic cancer. *Eur J Can* 2005; **Supplements 3**:4.

Moore MJ, Goldstein D, Hamm J, Figer A, Hecht JR, Gallinger S, et al. Erlotinib plus gemcitabine compared with gemcitabine alone in patients with advanced pancreatic cancer: a phase III trial of the National Cancer Institute of Canada Clinical Trials Group. *J Clin Oncol* 2007; **25(15)**:1960–6.

# Pancreatic endocrine tumours (PET)

- Rare.
- 1–2% of all pancreatic neoplastic lesions.
- Incidence of 0.2–0.4 per 100 000 population per year in UK (0.5–1 per 100 000 in USA), but an increase in incidence has been noted recently, probably due to increased recognition of their clinical features leading to greater awareness and thus diagnosis.
- Autopsy studies indicate a higher incidence of 1.5% (up to 10% in a multi-slice autopsy study although the majority are incidental and asymptomatic findings.
- Typically occur in adults with a peak incidence at 30–60 years.
- They can be *sporadic* or *familial*, in association with a genetic syndrome such as multiple endocrine neoplasia-1 (MEN-1), von Hippel–Lindau disease, von Recklinghause disease, and tuberous sclerosis. 60–80% of patients with MEN-1 have a PET.

## Histology

Originally thought to be arising from embryological neural crest (ectoderm), but recently dismissed and now thought to originate from multipotential endodermal stem cells of the pancreas.

They all demonstrate the ability to uptake amines and produce various hormones or peptides through decarboxylation – hence, the original name of APUDoma (amine precursor uptake and decarboxylation). They have the ability to secrete *multiple* substances, and can arise from anywhere in the gastrointestinal tract, lung, or thyroid gland.

Most are solitary and well demarcated, and range from <1c to >15cm. They can be benign or malignant, and even when malignant, they tend to have an indolent natural history. They carry a better prognosis than adenocarcinomas with a mean survival of 4–5 years.

They typically stain positively for chromogranin, synaptophysin, and neurone-specific enolase.

## Classification

Currently, there is no universally accepted classification for these neoplasms, as they can be classified by their histology, biological behaviour, or their clinical syndrome.

### Clinical classification

Commonest classification used by clinicians, categorizes these tumours into functional or non-functional, based on tumour's excessive secretion of hormones or peptides.

- **Functional (75%):** these tumours typically produce excessive hormones, which are either:
  - entopic (native to pancreas) – insulinoma (17%), PPoma (9%), glucagonoma (1%), somatostatinoma (1%);
  - ectopic (not native to pancreas) – gastrinoma (15%), VIPoma (2%), carcinoid (1%), or very rare ones such as ACTHoma and GRFoma;
  - some PETs produce multiple hormones but cause only one syndrome.

- **Non-functional (25%):** these tumours either secrete excess entopic hormones, insufficient to manifest clinically, or they produce non-specific substances such as chromagranin A, HCG, and neurotensin. Usually diagnosed incidentally on CT or secondary to mass effect of the lesion or metastases.

## WHO classification
This classifies PETs according to their clinicopathological status.
- **Well-differentiated tumours:** benign or low-grade malignancy. Benign – usually<2cm, confined to pancreas, no vascular invasion, no perineural invasion, <2 mitoses per 10 HPF, <2% Ki-67 positive cells. Low grade malignancy – usually ≥2cm, confined to pancreas, vascular or perineural invasion, 2–10 mitoses per 10 HPF, 2–10% Ki-67 positive cells.
- **Well-differentiated carcinomas:** when there is local invasion or metastases.
- **Poorly-differentiated carcinomas:** when >10 mitoses per 10 HPF.
- **Mixed exocrine and endocrine carcinomas:** e.g. adenocarcinoids.
- **Neuroendorine-like lesions.**

## Genetics
- A variety of genetic alterations have been recognized in sporadic and particularly in familial PETs.
- In sporadic PETs, loss of heterogeneity in chromosome 11q and 6q has been observed in some functional and non-functional PETs, respectively.
- In familial PETs, more specific genetic alterations have been observed consistently.
- **MEN-1** (Wermer's syndrome) is an autosomal dominant condition due to mutation in Menin gene (a tumour suppressor gene on 11q13, which regulates JUN-D-mediated RNA transcription). MEN-1 affects ~1 in 30 000 and is characterized by various combinations of parathyroid hyperplasia, pituitary adenomas, pancreatic endocrine tumours, thyroid adenomas and carcinomas, and adrenal adenomas. Patients also tend to have skin lipomas, angiofibromas, and a higher incidence of ovarian lesions and small bowel carcinoids. About 60–80% of patients with MEN-1 develop PETs, most commonly gastrinomas and insulinomas, and rarely, glucagonomas and VIPomas. These lesions tend to be multifocal, may be extra-pancreatic and often the cause of death in patients with MEN-1.
- **vonHippel–Lindau** is an autosomal dominant condition due to a mutation in VHL gene (3p25-26), characterized by development ofphaeochromocytomas, haemangioblastomas of cerebellum, retinal angiomatosis, angiomyolipomas of the kidney and PETs (17%).

**Clinical presentation, natural history and prognosis**

- PETs are slow growing and indolent in nature>
- There is typically a long delay (mean 5–6 years) prior to their diagnosis.
- Initial presentation non-specific with dyspepsia, abdominal pain, diarrhoea, skin rash, weight loss/gain.
- They are often diagnosed as a result of:
  - excess hormone production (see individual sections below);
  - expanding mass effect;
  - incidental finding on CT/MRI;
  - metastatic disease.
- PETs benign or malignant, and with the exception of 90% of insulinomas, all have the potential for malignant transformation and metastases, typically to the liver with hepatic failure the commonest cause of death.
- Emphasis has placed on earlier recognition and intensive management of these lesions including primary resection and even hepatic resection/transplantation in metastatic disease.
- 5YSR of up to 80% have been reported for patients with metastatic disease with aggressive surgical management.

*Prognostic predictors*

The presence of necrosis, >10 mitoses per 10 HPF, vascular invasion, size >2–3cm and presence of liver metastases are associated with worse prognosis. Non-functioning PETs tend to have a worse prognosis as there is a longer delay in diagnosis (no hormonal syndrome) and, thus, usually present with metastases.

**Diagnosis**

Diagnosis is usually initiated by an index of suspicion, which is improving due to greater awareness and understanding. The mainstay of diagnosis is by confirmation of excess hormone/peptide production (if functional) and tumour localization through imaging.

Historically, US, CT, MRI, selective angiography, and portal venous sampling have been the main modalities of diagnosis. However, diagnostic sensitivity has been vastly improved by the advent of EUS and somatostatin receptor scintigraphy (SRS).

- *EUS* is ideal in diagnosis of small PETs and duodenal lesions, and it has the advantage of enabling biopsy for histological valuation.
- *SRS (Octreoscan)* is becoming the gold standard investigation and the most sensitive in localizing 90% of PETs except insulinomas, which usually do not express somatostatin receptors. SRS relies on the intensity of receptor expression (not tumour size). It can be false positive in inflammatory and autoimmune conditions, such as sarcoidosis, TB, SLE, Crohn's, tumours such as melanoma, lymphoma, medullary thyroid carcinoma, and normal structures, such as the gallbladder and breast. SRS is also ideal in diagnosis of metastatic or recurrent disease and predicting and assessing treatment response.

Despite all the advances in imaging modalities, some PETs remain elusive and need surgical exploration for identification. Duodenotomy, pancreatic palpation, selective venous sampling and intraoperative gamma probes can be used to assist localization.

- *Chromgranin A* (or parathyroid secretory protein 1) is a neuroendocrine secretory protein, located in secretory vesicles of neurons and endocrine cells. It is the precursor to several functional peptides including vasostatin and pancreastatin. It is a non-specific marker that is elevated in 60–90% of all PETs except insulinomas, where chromogranin B is a better marker. It is helpful in assessing tumour progression and recurrence and helpful in predicting prognosis.

## Management

- The mainstay of management in PETs involves a combination of medical symptom control through reduction of hormone production, surgery, and non-surgical modalities, such as chemotherapy and radiotherapy.
- Medical symptom control has been revolutionized through introduction of proton pump inhibitors (reduction of debilitating hyperacidity in gastrinomas) and somatostatin analogues (octreotide and long-acting lanreotide) in reducing hormone production in functional PETs, such as gastrinomas, glucagonomas, VIPomas, and some insulinomas.
- Curative surgery offers the only chance of cure in resectable disease, and plays a role through palliative hepatic resection and liver transplantation.
- Other modalities include radiofrequency ablation (RFA) and cryoablation for unresectable liver metastases. Chemotherapy (cisplatin + etoposide- or streptozotocin-based therapy) also play a role in management of advanced and metastatic disease. Radiotherapy can be used for palliation from bony or brain metastases.
- Detailed presentation and management of common PETs are described below.

# Insulinomas

These are beta cell derived insulin secreting tumours and commonest form of PET with an incidence of 0.1–0.4 per 100 000 per year with a slight preponderance in females.

The median age at diagnosis is ~ 50 years, but patients with MEN-1 related insulinomas typically present in their mid-twenties.

Most are slow growing and <2cm. Only 10% are malignant. The majority are solitary, but 10% are multicentric, especially when associated with MEN-1.

## Presentation

Classically, present with episodic *hypoglycaemia* in response to excess insulin production, usually in the early morning or after missing a meal. This usually manifests with CNS dysfunction (blurred vision, confusion, personality change, weakness, convulsion, coma) +/– adrenergic response (sweating, tachcardia, and tremors), which are immediately reversed by glucose administration.

## Diagnosis

### Biochemical diagnosis

Fasting hypoglycaemia (<2.5mmol/L) associated with an elevated insulin level (lack of appropriate suppression) in the absence of exogenous administration of insulin is diagnostic. Failing this, a 72h fasting provocative test could be carried out. Documentation of normoglycaemia during symptomatic episodes excludes the diagnosis of insulinoma.

Measurement of plasma pro-insulin and C-peptide is also helpful if one suspects malingering, as C-peptide will be low in such patients (endogenous pro-insulin divides into c-peptide and insulin in blood, but exogenous insulin does not contain pro-insulin or c-peptide)

### Tumour localization

- CT scanning diagnoses ~70% of cases, and excellent for detection of metastatic disease. EUS and portal venous sampling are complementary should CT fail. EUS is much more sensitive in detection of pancreatic head lesions and suboptimal for body and tail.
- SRS is unhelpful in a majority of cases as 90% do not express somatostatin receptors.

## Differential diagnosis

- Endocrine disorders such as hypopituitarism, Addison's disease, myxoedema, or liver or renal failure may present with hypoglycaemia as a secondary feature.
- Insulinomas are the most common cause of hypoglycaemia resulting from hyperinsulinism, but extrapancreatic insulin-producing tumours should also be considered, as well as self-induced hypoglycaemia, due to the administration of insulin or sulphonylureas.

## Management

### Surgery

- **Small lesions:** enucleation for lesion located away from the duct, pancreatectomy for those near the duct to reduce the risk of fistulae.
- **Large lesions:** Whipple's for head, distal pancreatectomy for body and tail lesions.
- Resection should not be carried out blindly and, if elusive at exploration, intraoperative US and selective portal venous sampling may enable localization.
- Surgery can be curative in 90% of patients with a 10YSR of ~30% post-resection.

### Metastatic disease

- Surgical resection should be considered and is often feasible even when metastases are present. Debulking can also reduce hypoglycaemic episodes.
- **Diazoxide**, a potassium channel activator, can be used to inhibit insulin secretion in patients with metastatic disease or those where lesion is not localizable at exploration. When used with hydrochlorothiazide its hyperglycaemic effect is increased.
- **Octreotide** may also prevent hypoglycaemia in ~50% of patients with an unpredictable response rates.
- **Glucagon** must not be used as it stimulates insulin secretion leading to severe hypoglycaemia.
- **Chemotherapy** with streptozotocin in combination with doxorubicin or 5-FU is used in progressive disease.

# Gastrinomas

- Most common functional PET. Represents the aetiological lesion in Zollinger–Ellison syndrome (triad of gastrinoma, gastric hyperacidity, and atypical recurrent peptic ulcers).
- Present in ~2% of patients with recurrent ulcers despite optimal medical management. 70% of gastrinomas occur sporadically with a mean age of onset 50 years.
- 30% of gastrinomas are associated with MEN-1. Up to 70% of gastrinomas associated with MEN-1 are benign and multicentric,. and affect patients of younger age group compared with the sporadic type.
- Majority of tumours are found in the pancreas and extrapancreatic in up to 40% (duodenum or stomach).

## Presentation

- Increased gastrin production causes acid hypersecretion and ulceration of the gastric mucosa (recurrent symptomatic ulcers, complications such as bleeding and perforation).
- Excessive acid secretion also inactivates small bowel enzymes, resulting in profuse watery diarrhoea and steatorrhoea, and inevitably small bowel ulceration. The mean duration of symptoms prior to diagnosis is ~6 years and thus should be suspected if:
  - recurrent or atypical ulcers;
  - failure to heal despite optimal medical management;
  - personal or family history of MEN-1;
  - peptic ulcers with unexplained diarrhoea.

## Diagnosis

- Raised fasting gastrin concentration (>1000pg/mL) associated with increased basal gastric acid secretion (when not taking H2-blockers or PPI's).
- A secretin test is sometimes used to exclude hypergastrinaemia secondary to G-cell hyperplasia or retained antrum post-gastrectomy.

## Management

- Resection of localized non-metastatic tumours.
- Proton pump inhibitors will almost completely inhibit acid secretion and are highly effective for palliation in metastatic disease.

# Chapter 8

# Small bowel and rare GI cancers

# Epidemiology and presentation

### Epidemiology
Rare. Small bowel malignancies account for 2% of all GI neoplasms. UK incidence 5–9 per 1 million population. US incidence: 7–16 per 1 000 000 population. M>F. 25% have associated cancers in colon, prostate, breast, and other sites.

### Aetiology
Not completely understood. Thought to be due to exposure of mucosa to carcinogens and irritants, causing hyperproliferation and eventually malignant transformation. Low incidence of cancer in small bowel thought to be due to:
- The protective nature of lymphoid tissue and secretory IgA.
- Lower bacterial load, so less conversion of bile into carcinogens.
- Less mucosal irritation of liquid contents of solid stool in colon.
- Rapid intestinal transit, hence, shorter exposure to potential carcinogens.
- Large amounts of benzopyrene hydroxylase in mucosa of small intestine – converts carcinogen benzopyrene into less carcinogenic compound.

For carcinoid, see relevant section.

### Risk factors
Diet (high fat, low fibre), smoking, alcohol.

### Predisposing conditions
Crohns disease, coeliac disease, Peutz–Jeughers, Gardeners' syndrome, FAP, immunodeficiency conditions, autoimmune conditions.

### Presentation
Variable. Abdominal pain (65%), weight loss, and anorexia (50%), bowel obstruction and intussusceptions (25%), palpable mass (25%), perforation (10%), GI bleeding (occult>overt), anaemia. GI symptoms more common in malignant than benign tumours and usually occur late in disease.

### Tumour subtypes
- *Primary:* adenocarcinoma (45%), carcinoid (29%), lymphoma (15%), sarcoma (10%).
- *Secondary:* metastatic melanoma.
- Colon, cervical, and ovarian secondaries via direct spread.
- Breast, lung, and kidney secondaries via haematogenous spread.

# Clinical evaluation

History and examination are non-specific so diagnosis often made late. Need to have index of suspicion and investigate early.

- *Bloods:* FBC, U&E, LFT, haematinics, CEA (raised in most small bowel cancers).
- *Urine:* 24h 5-HIAA if carcinoid suspected.
- *Stool:* FOB test detects occult bleeding.
- *Radiography:* AXR if small bowel obstruction suspected, contrast studies, CT.
- *Endoscopy:* push enteroscopy, double balloon enteroscopy, capsule endoscopy (see 'Enteroscopy', below).
- *Angiography:* rarely used routinely. Can be helpful in diagnosis of carcinoid and leiomyosarcoma – tumour blush demonstrated.
- *Surgical exploration:* exploratory laparotomy/laparoscopy is most sensitive diagnostic modality and should be used when above methods fail to establish diagnosis.

## Investigation

### Contrast studies

- Detects 50–60% small bowel neoplasms.
- *Small bowel follow through (SBFT):* can detect mass lesions, intussusceptions, mucosal defect (e.g. ulcers).
- *Enteroclysis:* double contrast study. Superior to SBFT for detecting neoplasms. A tube is passed into small bowel, and both barium and methycellulose injected. Not very good for picking up flat infiltrating lesions.

### CT scanning

- Good for picking up primary tumour and possible secondaries in liver or mesentery. CT thorax used to help stage disease.
- *MRI:* more sensitive than CT in detection of liver metastases in carcinoid.

### Enteroscopy

- *Wireless capsule endoscopy:* non-invasive method to visualize entire small bowel. Interpretation is time-consuming and operator dependant. Should not be used if small bowel obstruction suspected. *Disadvantage:* no tissue sampling and no possibility for therapeutics unlike enteroscopy.
- *Gastroscopy:* can be used to reach proximal duodenum
- *Push enteroscopy:* a paediatric colonoscope is used orally to intubate the small intestine and then pushed into the jejunum 60cm distal to ligament of Trietz. Goes further than a gastroscope, but not as far as a double balloon enteroscope.
- *Double balloon enteroscopy:* can intubate entire small bowel. Can obtain tissue samples and perform therapeutic interventions. *Disadvantages:* only available in small number of centres, time-consuming, technically challenging, uncomfortable for patient.

# Adenocarcinoma

### Epidemiology

25–50% of small bowel cancers. Age: 50–70. M>F. Highest incidence in duodenum, 65% peri-ampullary. However, in Crohns disease, lower age of onset, highest incidence in ileum.

### Aetiology

Most arise from adenomas, similar adenocarcinoma sequence as color-ectal cancers. *Ki-ras* gene mutations found in 14–53% of small bowel adenocarcinomas, mostly in duodenal disease. APC gene mutations are uncommon (cf. colorectal carcinoma), suggesting different genetic pathway. Adenocarcinomas associated with Crohns and coeliac disease arise de novo.

### Pathology

Well or moderately differentiated in 60%, signet ring, or poorly differenti-ated in 37%.

### Presentation

Non-specific. Symptoms arise at a late stage. Abdominal pain > obstruction > occult GI bleed > anaemia.

### Investigation

Mainstay is imaging. SBFT, double contrast studies, CT abdomen, CT thorax for staging, capsule endoscopy, enteroscopy.

### Staging

TNM classification (see staging section).

### Treatment

*Local disease*

Wide segmental surgical resection, ensuring tumour free margins. Histological confirmation needed. Type of operation is site-specific:

- **First and second part of duodenum:** pancreatico-duodenectomy ensures more radical clearance of tumour bed and regional nodes, cf. segmental resection. Whipples procedure, if difficult to distinguish tumour from pancreatic, distal bile duct or ampulla of Vater carcinoma.
- **Third and Fourth part of duodenum:** segmental resection. Lower mortality than pancreatico-duodenectomy and comparable survival data.
- **Jejunum and Ileum:** wide excision of malignancy and surrounding tissues. Resection of primary and investing mesentery provides staging information and ensures surgical clearance.
- **Distal ileum:** right hemicolectomy.

*Adjuvant therapy*

5-FU and irinotecan-based chemotherapy. Not used routinely, as no clear evidence to define its exact role or benefit. No evidence to suggest survival benefit with use of adjuvant chemotherapy. Combined chemoradiation can be considered for close or positive margins involving retroperitoneum

Neoadjuvant chemoradiotherapy possible use for radiation and concomitant mitomycin and 5-FU.

### Metastatic disease
- **Surgery:** palliative resection of adenocarcinoma to prevent complications of bleeding and obstruction. Resection of isolated hepatic mets should be considered.
- **Chemotherapy:** 5-FU and irinotecan-based regimens
- **Cytoreductive surgery and intraperitoneal chemotherapy** still experimental in cases of peritoneal carcinomatosis.

## Prognosis
- 70–80% small bowel carcinomas are completely resectable at time of diagnosis. 3% have regional nodal metastases, 20–30% have distant metastases.
- Poorer prognosis if mural penetration, nodal involvement, distant metastases, perineural invasion.
- Prognosis worse for jejunal and ileal carcinomas, cf. duodenal carcinomas because of increased frequency of nodal involvement.

### Duodenal carcinoma
5-year survival rates similar to colorectal cancer:
- **Stage I:** 100%.
- **Stage II:** 50%.
- **Stage III:** 45%.
- **Stage IV:** 0%.

### Distal small bowel carcinomas
- **Overall, 5-year survival:** 20–30%.
- **No nodal involvement:** 60–70%.
- **Nodal involvement:** 12–14%.

## Surveillance
Regular follow-up after resection needed. Assessment of recurrence based on:
- History and examination.
- Bloods – FBC, LFT, U&E.
- CXR 6-monthly for first 3 years, then yearly.
- Consider endoscopy for assessment of local recurrence, based on history and investigation findings.

# Staging of small bowel malignancy

Staging system used depends on primary histology. GISTs and carcinoids are not typically staged.

## Adenocarcinoma

TNM classification (Table 8.1).

### AJCC TNM staging for small bowel Adenocarcinoma

- **T0:** no evidence of primary tumour.
- **Tis:** carinoma *in situ*.
- **T1:** tumour invades lamina propria or submucosa.
- **T2:** tumour invades muscularis propria.
- **T3:** tumour invades muscularis propria into subserosa or non-peritonealized perimuscular tissue (mesentery/retroperitoneum) with extension ≤ 2cm.
- **T4:** tumour perforates visceral peritoneum or directly invades other organs or structures (includes other loops of small intestine, mesentery or retroperitoneum>2cm; abdominal wall by way of serosa; invasion of pancreas for duodenal malignancy).
- **N0:** no regional lymph node metastases.
- **N1:** regional lymph node metastases.
- **M0:** no distant metastases.
- **M1:** distant metastases.

**Table 8.1** Stage groupings

| Stage | TNM |
| --- | --- |
| 0 | Tis, N0, M0 |
| I | T1–2, N0, M0 |
| II | T3–4, N0, M0 |
| III | Any T, N1, M0 |
| IV | Any T, any N, M1 |

## Hodgkins and non-Hodgkins lymphoma (Table 8.2)

**Table 8.2** Ann Arbor Staging Classification for Hodgkins and Non-Hodgkins Lymphoma

| Stage | Criteria |
|-------|----------|
| I | Involvement of single lymph node region (I) or single extralymphatic organ or site (IE) |
| II | Involvement of 2 or more lymph node regions on the same side of the diaphragm (II), or an extralymphatic organ and its adjoining lymph node site (IIE) |
| III | Involvement of lymph node sites on both sides of the diaphragm (III) or localized involvement of an extra-lymphatic site (IIIE), spleen (IIIS), or both (IIISE) |
| IV | Diffuse or disseminated involvement of one or more extralymphatic organs, with or without associated lymph node involvement. |

Further subclassified as A or B depending on absence (A) or presence (B) of B symptoms – fever, night sweats, weight loss> 10%.
E refers to extranodal contiguous extension.
Adapted from Carbone et al. 1971; Lister et al. 1989.

### Further reading

Carbone PP, et al. *Cancer Res* 1971; **31**: 1860.

Lister TA, et al. *J Clin Oncol* 1989; **7**: 1630.

# Carcinoid tumours and syndrome

Neuroendocrine tumours of enterochromaffin cells. Part of the APU-Doma (amine precursor uptake and decarboxylation) family.

## Epidemiology
- Most common GI neuroendocrine tumour, however still rare.
- Incidence 3 per 100 000, peak in 6th and 7th decade. F>M.
- Accounts for a third of small bowel neoplasms.

## Aetiology
Cause unknown, genetic link suspected. Multiple endocrine neoplasia type 1 (MEN-1) increases risk for neuroendocrine tumours, including carcinoids. Peptic ulcer disease, pernicious anaemia, atrophic gastritis, Zollinger–Ellison syndrome increase risk for GI carcinoids tumours. Respiratory tract carcinoids are not related to smoking.

## Pathology
- Originate from neuroendocrine enterochromaffin[1] cells: diffuse, but most prevalent in the submucosa of the intestine and main bronchi
- **55% in GI tract:** appendix 38% > jejunum and ileum 25% > rectum 18% > bronchus 10% > colon 6% > duodenum 3%, stomach 3%.
- Less than 1% in the pancreas, gallbladder, liver, ovaries, larynx, and testes, but these have a high incidence of metastases.
- Malignant status based on lymph node invasion and distant metastases, NOT histology.
- Metastatic potential dependent on site and size of primary tumour, not histological features.

## Biochemistry

Carcinoids secrete:

- *Amines:* 5-HT (diarrhoea), 5-HIAA (used for diagnosis), 5-HTP, histamine (pruritis, flushing), dopamine.
- *Peptides*: vasoactive intestinal peptide, insulin.
- *Tachykinins:* neuropeptide K, substance P, kalikrein (bronchospasm).
- *Prostaglandins.*
- *Foregut:* high peptide secretion: ACTH, growth hormone, gastrin. Low tumour 5-HT. High 5-HIAA.
- *Mid-gut:* high tumour 5-HT, high 5-HIAA. Symptomatic levels of 5-HT only if bulky or metastatic.
- Frequently secrete ACTH and growth hormone. Sporadically histamine.
- *Hindgut:* rarely produce 5-HT even if large or metastatic. 5-HIAA normal.

Tryptophan →     5-HT serotonin     →     5-HIAA
                 *Dopa-decarboxylase*         *Monoamine oxidase*

## Classification

Based on origin from embryological divisions of the alimentary tract. Each division demonstrates different histology, behaviour, biochemistry, and malignant potential.

**Table 8.3** Classification of carcinoids

| Embryonic origin | Organs | Histology | Biochemistry | General Features |
|---|---|---|---|---|
| Foregut | Lung, bronchus, stomach, gall bladder, pancreas | Trabecular | High levels of ACTH, GH, gastrin. Low 5-HT. High 5-HIAA | Histamine associated flushing, facial swelling, urticaria. Carcinoid syndrome rare. |
| Mid-gut | Small intestine, appendix, proximal colon | Nodular | High tumour 5-HT and 5-HIAA. Sporadically histamine. Frequently ACTH and GH. | 30% symptomatic – diarrhoea. Most likely to metastasize. 10% develop carcinoid syndrome. 20% occur with synchronous non-carcinoid GI neoplasm |
| Hindgut | Distal colon, rectum, GU tract. | Trabecular | No 5-HT even if large and metastatic. 5-HIAA normal. | Usually asymptomatic. Carcinoid syndrome rare. Good prognosis. |

# Carcinoid: presentation

- Presentation is highly variable, and usually either incidental or late after metastatic progression.
- Many patients with GI carcinoid present with vague abdominal symptoms and are initially diagnosed as IBS.
- Clinical course slow. Takes 10–12 years from onset of tumour growth to carcinoid syndrome.

## Specific signs and symptoms

### Foregut

- **Pulmonary:** recurrent pneumonia, chest pain, cough, Cushings, and acromegaly.
- **Gastric:** epigastric pain chronic atrophic gastritis, pernicous anaemia, Zollinger–Ellison syndrome.

### Mid-gut

Present like other small bowel tumours: vague abdominal colicky pain, anorexia, and weight loss. 15% proceed to obstruction due to intraluminal tumour or mesenteric kinking.

### Hindgut

Largely silent until bleeding or obstructive.

## Carcinoid syndrome

- Caused by release of catecholamines to systemic circulation. 90% due to carcinoid metastases in liver. 10% with primary bronchial and ovarian carcinoids as they drain directly into systemic circulation.
- Characterized by diarrhoea (5-HT), flushing (histamine), bronchospasm (PG, 5-HTP, bradykinin). Less commonly telangectasia (VIP, 5-HT, PG), pulmonary stenosis and right heart failure, hypotension, and glucose tolerance (5-HT).
- 10% of carcinoid tumours (mainly mid-gut) progress to syndrome.

# Carcinoid: investigation

## Investigation

Biochemical tests to confirm secretory tumours or carcinoid. Imaging studies to locate primary tumour and assess for level of invasion, presence of metastases, multifocal carcinoid, and synchronous malignancy. Histology is gold standard to confirm diagnosis.

## Biochemistry

- FBC, U&Es, LFTS.
- 24h urinary 5-HIAA, usually>100mg/day. Not useful in hindgut tumours.
- Chromogranin A (99% of patients with verified carcinoid tumours, sensitivity 80%). Useful for assessing progress and response.
- Substance P (sensitivity: 32%, specificity: 85%). Not routinely used.
- Epinephrine provocation test: sensitivity 100%. Test is positive if infusion of epinephrine causes flushing within 2min and lasts for at least 1min.

## Imaging

*Site specific:* CXR, OGD, colonoscopy, barium follow through, USS abdomen, testis and ovary, CT thorax, abdomen and pelvis, MRI for liver metastases, EUS best for assessing pancreatic disease.

## Nuclear imaging

### Somatostatin receptor scintigraphy (SSRS) testing

Somatostatin receptor subtype 2 (sst-2) are found on 90% of carcinoid tumours. OctreoScan® uses a radiolabelled analogue of somatostatin ($^{111}$In octreotide). Images lesions >0.5cm and allows estimation of receptor density. Predicts response to octreotide treatment.

### Meta-iodobenzylguanidine $^{131}$I (MIBG) scanning

MIBG resembles noradrenaline and serotonin. MIBG is taken up by carcinoid tumour cells and stored in the neurosecretory granules, so can identify tumour. Sensitivity 70%. Used to predict response to MIBG treatment.

# Carcinoid: treatment

### Principles of treatment
- Multidisciplinary approach required.
- Treat the tumour and treat the syndrome.
- Curative treatment possible if local disease.
- Surgical resection is treatment of choice in those fit for surgery.
- If curative treatment not possible, treatment involves retarding progression of disease and controlling symptoms. Specialist palliative nurses should be involved at an early stage. (See algorithm in Fig. 8.1).

### Local disease
- *Extent of resection of carcinoids:* dependent on site, size, and level of invasion.
- *Appendix carcinoids:* distal tumours <1.5cm – appendectomy alone. Proximal tumours – <1.5cm partial caecectomy. >1.5cm, vascular, mesenteric or lymph node invasion or reaction –right hemicolectomy.
- *Small bowel carcinoids:* high incidence of metastases even if <1cm. Wide en bloc resection of small bowel, mesentery, including regional lymph nodes, and omentum. 30% are multicentric, therefore careful assessment of the whole small bowel is mandatory.
- *Gastric carcinoids:* type 1 and 2i <1cm – endoscopic resection and surveillance 6 monthly. >1cm or >5 gastric tumours: antrectomy. Type 3 – partial or total gastrectomy.
- *Colonic carcinoids:* standard resection with regional lymphadenectomy. Clearance of metastatic lymph nodes may contribute to long-term survival.
- *Rectal carcinoids:* <2cm sphincter sparing anterior resection if possible or abdominoperineal resection if low. Tumours >2cm also anterior resection, but some advocate more extensive pelvic exenteration, although the benefits remain unproven.

#### Peri-operative preparation in the presence of carcinoid syndrome
- Need to prevent carcinoid crisis, which occurs secondary to tumour handling, anaesthetic induction, or drugs. Results in prolonged hypo- or hypertension, arrhythmias, flushing, and bronchospasm lasting hours to days.
- Optimize nutrition, hydration, and electrolytes.
- *Octreotide:* 200µg tds SC for at least 1 week pre-operatively or IV infusion 50µg/h for 12h pre-operatively and at least 48h post-operatively. Treatment of carcinoid crisis: Octreotide 300µg IV stat, then IV infusion 50–150µg/h (with caution and cardiac monitoring). Catecholamines are contraindicated.

### Locally invasive or extensive disease
Tumour debulking improves disease-free survival and symptomatic relief in those fit for surgery.

### Metastatic disease
Liver metastases result in carcinoid syndrome so management involves treating this using drugs or interventional techniques.

## Treatment of carcinoid syndrome

### Somatostatin analogues

- Ocreotide reduces secretion of 5-HT, gastrin, cholecystokinin, glucagon, growth hormone, insulin, secretin, pancreatic polypeptide, and vasoactive intestinal peptide. It directly prolongs intestinal transit time and reduces intestinal secretion.
- Useful for diarrhoea and flushing.
- Can also stabilize disease and halt progression.
- Immediate release octreotide. 50µg tds SC, initially, gradually increasing to maximum of 500µg tds. Once stabilized convert to long-acting depot, e.g. IM depot octreotide acetate 20 mg monthly or IM lanreotide fortnightly.
- Rescue injections of octreotide for breakthrough carcinoid syndrome symptoms may be required.
- **Side effects:** fat malabsorption and gallstones. Prophylactic cholecystectomy or ursodeoxycholic acid may be required.

### Interferon therapy

- IFNα used to control symptoms in secreting carcinoids if on maximum dose of somatostatin analogues.
- Reduces hormone production and symptoms of carcinoid syndrome: 50-75% patients in clinical trials.
- Reduced tumour size. Response rates ranged from 0 to 20% in small trials.
- 3–5 megaunits SC or IM 3–5 times a week.
- **Side effects:** flu-like symptoms (fever, fatigue, muscle pain) loss of appetite, weight loss, and anaemia

### MIBG therapy

- Radioactive MIBG is taken up by neurosecretory granules. Most useful in those with a positive MIBG scan.
- Two cycles of therapeutic dose radioactive MIBG may induce long-lasting palliation (8 months) by internal irradiation. Used 3–6 monthly.
- 80% symptom control.
- Non-radioactive MIBG compound effective in palliation, even in patients with a negative scan by tumour acidification and its effect as a false neurotransmitter. Median symptom relief of 4 months.
- **Contraindications:** pregnancy, breast feeding, myelosuppression, renal failure (GFR< 40).

### Chemotherapy

- No clear role for conventional chemotherapy – limited evidence.
- Experimental use of agents such as bevacizumab (angiogenesis inhibitor) and Sunitinib (tyrosine kinase inhibitor). Streptozotocin (STZ): a glucosomine-nitrosourea alkylating agent, modest results: ECOG trial STZ/5-FU vs. STZ/CTZ RR 33/27% OS median 2 years. STZ/5-FU vs. ADR RR 22/21% OS 1 year. Carboplatin, paclitaxel, and topotecan may be of benefit in poorly differentiated carcinoids.

## Treatment of liver metastases

- **Isolated liver metastases:** curative treatment is possible in 10% by resection of liver lesion. Otherwise provides effective symptomatic relief for up to 5 years.

- *Hepatic artery ligation or embolization:* used for patients with non-resectable disease and hormone secreting tumours. The hypervascularity of hepatic neoplasms results in their deriving almost all of their blood supply from the hepatic artery (normal hepatocytes 20%). Occlusion by ligation or embolization causes tumour necrosis, while preserving normal hepatocytes. Decreases symptoms in 60% of cases.
- *Radiofrequency ablation or cryoablation:* percutaneous or laparoscopic. Used for smaller hepatic lesions, but evidence for use lacking.
- *Liver transplant:* use for uncontrollable symptoms in end stage disease, when all other measures have failed. Controversial. Limited organ supply.

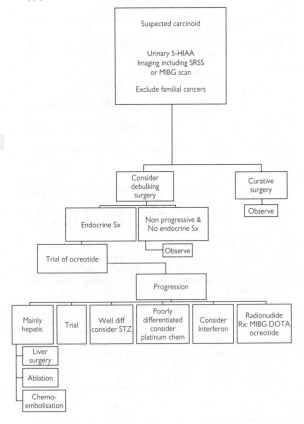

**Fig. 8.1** Algorithm for investigation and treatment of gut carcinoid. Adapted from Gut (2005).

## Symptomatic relief
### Antidiarrhoeal agents
- Antimotility Agents.
- Atropine.
- Diphenoxylate.
- Loperamide.
- Adsorbent agents.
- Kaolin-pectin mixtures and polycarbophil.
- Antisecretory agents.
- Bismuth subsalicylate.
- Bacterial replacement agents.

### Others
- Flushing:
- Phenoxybenzamine and clonidine.
- **Bronchospasm:** salbutamol (albuterol) and low dose aminophylline used to varying success

## Prognosis
- Median survival 5 years with carcinoid syndrome.
- With local disease, prognosis depends on site of origin: mid-gut tumours poor, hindgut tumours good.

## Further reading

Ramage JK, Davies AH, Ardill J, Bax N, Caplin M, Grossman A, et al. Guidelines for the management of gastroenteropancreatic neuroendocrine (including carcinoid) tumours. Gut 2005; **54 Suppl 4**: iv1–16.

# Lymphoma: epidemiology and classification

## Epidemiology
Peak age 60–70 years. M:F 3:2. Predominantly NHL. B cell >> T cell. Tend to be large , 70% larger than 5cm on presentation. Primary GI tract lymphoma rare, 1–4% of small bowel malignancies. Secondary GI involvement common in systemic lymphoma – 10–60%.

## Presentation
Systemic effects: weight loss, anorexia, night sweats. *Direct effects:* colicky abdominal pain, obstruction, bleeding, perforation (25%).

## Classification
WHO classification system of NHL normally used. For GI tract can be thought of as primary vs. secondary, B vs. T cell.

## Primary GI tract lymphoma
More common in Mediterranean and Middle Eastern countries. Defined as:
• Tumour predominantly in GI tract with no liver or spleen involvement.
• Normal white blood count and differential on blood film.
• No peripheral or mediastinal lymphadenopathy
• Divided into B and T cell lymphomas.

## B cell lymphomas
### *Extranodal marginal zone B-cell lymphoma (previously MALToma)*
Most common. Mainly in stomach and distal small bowel. Arise from mucosa associated lymphoid tissue. In stomach, from reactive lymphoid follicles. Usually solitary site, ulcerating, protruding, or infiltrating. Associated with *H. pylori*, autoimmune, and immunodeficiency syndromes.

### *Mantle cell*
Aggressive lymphomas, mainly in colon and small intestine (cf. MALT). Usually present with multiple white fleshy nodular lesions 0.2–2cm, along one or more segments of GI tract. Known as 'lymphomatous polyposis'. Nodal and haematogenous spread early in disease.

### *Burkitts and Burkitts like variants*
Very aggressive and bulky B cell tumours. Mainly ileocaecal region and rectum. Associated with HIV and EBV infection and immunosuppression.

### *T cell lymphoma*
**Enteropathy associated T-cell intestinal lymphoma:** usually associated with coeliac disease, mainly in jejunum. Present as large circumferential ulcers with mesenteric node involvement. Prognosis poor.

## Secondary GI involvement
Common. GI lymph node involvement as part of systemic disease.

Stomach (75%) > small bowel (9%) > ileocaecal region (7%) > rectum (2%)

**Predisposing conditions:**

All are immune type conditions:
- **Immunodeficiency syndromes:** Wiskott–Aldrich syndrome, severe combined immunodeficiency syndrome, X-linked aggamaglobulinaemia.
- **Autoimmune conditions:** rheumatoid arthritis, Sjogrens, SLE, Wegeners; HIV.
- **Iatrogenic immunosuppression:** immunosuppressive therapy, radiation therapy.
- **GI disorders:** Crohns disease (likely to be related to immunosuppression used to treat disease), coeliac disease.

# Lymphoma: clinical evaluation

## Localizing disease

Contrast studies, CT, endoscopy with biopsy, capsule studies. Laparotomy and biopsy for tissue diagnosis if endoscopy fails.

## Staging

Ann Arbor classification system (see staging section). CT is investigation of choice. Bone marrow examination (usually with mantle cell lymphomas).

## Treatment and prognosis

Depends on type. Prognostic factors include stage, grade, extent of tumour penetration.

### Intestinal MALToma

- **Stage IE and IIE:** curative treatment: Eradication therapy for *H. pylori*. *En bloc* resection of involved bowel and contiguous node, usually with post-operative chemoradiotherapy (CHOP).
- **Radiation therapy:** reduces recurrence rates, but does not affect survival – side effects. Radiation enteritis, perforation, and vasculitis.
- Adjuvant combination chemotherapy improves 5-year survival to >50%.
- **Stage IIIE and IV:** combination chemotherapy usually with CHOP. Palliation with radiotherapy in extensive disease, palliative surgery controversial. 5-year survival rates: 50% stage IIIE, 20% stage IV.

### Mantle cell lymphoma

Combination chemotherapy involving rituximab. In younger patients, possible role for aggressive chemotherapy and autologous stem cell transplant. Surgery used for complications e.g. obstruction. Thought to be incurable. Median survival 3–5 years.

### Burkitts lymphoma

*Combination chemotherapy:* various regimens used including CHOP and IVAC. Surgery for palliation of symptoms or to avoid perforation during chemo. Autologous bone marrow transplant in some patients. Median survival from diagnosis ~1 year. However, figures improving with HIV treatment, newer chemotherapy regimens, and immunotherapy with Rituximab.

### T cell lymphoma

Anthracycline-based chemotherapy and maintenance of gluten-free diet. 5-year survival 10%.

# Small bowel sarcoma

Rare malignant tumours arising from mesenchymal tissue.

## Classification

In the GI tract there are 2 types:
- **Gastrointestinal stromal tumours (GIST):** most common, originate from intestinal pacemaker cells (interstitial cells of Cajal).
- **Soft tissue tumours,** which also occur elsewhere in body, e.g. leimoyosarcoma (LMS), fibrosarcoma, liposarcoma, angiosarcoma

## GISTs

- **Incidence:** <1% of GI malignancies. 200–2000 new cases in England and Wales per year.
- **Age :** 40–60 years.
- **Distribution:** stomach (60–70%) > small bowel (25–35%) > colorectal (5%) > oesophagus.
- **Aetiology:** most are sporadic and solitary. 80% GISTs are associated with mutations in tyrosine kinase growth factor receptors (c-KIT), causing constant unregulated cell growth.
- **Pathology:** can be small and asymptomatic, or large with mass and pressure effects, ulceration, and bleeding. GISTs spread to liver, omentum and peritoneum. Nodal spread rare.
- **Presentation:** symptoms rare, but include early satiety, abdominal pain, palpable mass, anaemia. Most are asymptomatic and are picked up incidentally on imaging, or due to complications, e.g. perforation and bleeding.
- **Diagnosis:**
  - *contrast-enhanced CT:* enhance brightly with IV contrast, can be large with necrosis and haemorrhage;
  - *immunocytochemistry:* 80% are positive for CD117 (cell surface marker to c-kit receptor).
- CT abdomen/pelvis. No staging system used.
- **Treatment**
  - *Surgery:* complete resection with intact pseudocapsule is treatment of choice. Meticulous exploration of abdomen to rule out liver and peritoneal spread. No role for extensive mesenteric lymphadenectomy as metastases to mesenteric nodes is rare.
  - *Imatinib:* tyrosine kinase inhibitor, which blocks c-kit receptor. Used for unresectable or metastatic disease. NICE recommends use at 400mg od in 12 week blocks. Response assessed after each block. Treatment continued as long as adequate response achieved.
  - *Palliative:* when no response achieved to imatinib – symptomatic treatment. Palliative surgery indicated for obstruction.
  - *Hepatic arterial chemoembolization:* cisplatin with or without an embolic agent. If isolated liver mets, possible long-term disease control. No long-term data available.
- **Prognosis:** 50% of completely resected GISTs recur within 5 years. Risk of recurrence higher if high grade, higher mitotic rate, larger size. 80% 8-year survival if low grade, less than 18 months if high grade.

**Leimoyosarcoma (LMS)**

- *Incidence:* Rare. LMS >fibrosarcoma,>liposarcoma,>angiosarcoma.
- *Distribution:* jejunum > ileum > duodenum > Meckel's diverticulae.
- *Aetiology:* most arise. LMS are c-kit negative.
- *Pathology:* similar to other sarcomas. Tend to be slow growing and large – 75% are greater than 5cm on presentation (cf. lymphoma). Extramural, rather than intramural extension; hence, bowel obstruction rare. Usually spread haematogenously. LMS spread to lung.
- *Presentation:* usually incidental. Occult bleeding, palpable mass, abdominal pain, perforation. Obstruction rare.
- *Diagnosis:*
  - *contrast enhanced CT:* are usually large with central necrosis and heterogenous enhancement;
  - *upper endoscopy:* can help identify lesions, leiomyomas appear as submucosal masses with smooth margins, endoscopic biopsies rarely helpful as do not yield enough tissue.
  - *EUS:* most accurate method of identifying leiomyomas and differentiating from LMS; allows biopsy of lesions using fine needle forceps. EUS biopsies more useful than endoscopic biopsies.
- *Staging:* TNM classification used for LMS.
- *Treatment:*
  - *Surgery:* usually in tertiary referral centres, for local disease, with minimal invasion, *en bloc* segmental resection with tumour-free margins;
  - specialist oncology involvement.

# Predisposing conditions

Conditions that predispose to cancers of the small bowel.

## Familial adenomatous polyposis (FAP)

- *Definition:* inherited autosomal dominant disorder, predisposes to colorectal and small bowel cancer by causing multiple polyps in bowel.
- *Epidemiology:* 1 in 20 000 live births worldwide, M=F.
- *Pathology:* mutation in adenomatous polyposis coli (APC) gene, located on chromosome 5q21-q22. More than 800 mutations identified, most lead to truncated APC gene product that is not fully functional and leads to oncogenic activity. Some correlation exists between type of mutation and phenotype – mutations in central part of gene predispose to duodenal polyposis, mutations between codons 169 and 1393 associated with profuse colonic polyposis.
- *Extracolonic manifestations:* incomplete penetrance. Duodenal ampullary carcinoma, gastric carcinoma, adenomas, and adenocarcinomas of distal ileum, follicular, or papillary thyroid carcinoma, childhood hepatoblastoma, medulloblastomas.
- *Diagnosis of small bowel malignancies:* endoscopy and biopsy. Gastric fundal polyps can become dysplastic so should be biopsied. Duodenal adenomas have predilection for papilla so possible role for routine biopsy of papilla.
- *Genetic testing* of individual for APC mutation.
- *Treatment:* multidisciplinary approach:
  - *endoscopy:* resection of duodenal and gastric antral adenomas;
  - *surgery:* resection of adenocarcinomas or those with advanced polyposis to prevent progression;
  - *celecoxib:* 400mg bd – trial has shown possible use to reduce extent of duodenal polyposis, though effect on cancer risk unknown.
- *Screening for small bowel cancers:* if involved individual has genetic mutation, can screen other family members at risk. No proven benefit for upper endoscopic screening of individual with colorectal polyposis, but ASGE recommends: upper endoscopy with side and front viewing endoscope in 3rd decade or time of colectomy, and 5 years thereafter.
- *Surveillance:* No clear guidelines. Yearly endoscopy and biopsy for duodenal and papillary adenomas.

## Gardners' syndrome (GS)

- *Definition:* autosomal dominant disorder causing colonic adenomas and extracolonic lesions (both benign and malignant). A variant of FAP where extracolonic lesions > colonic polyposis. Risk of colon cancer same as with FAP.
- *Epidemiology:* 2.3–3 cases per 100 000 persons, M=F.
- *Pathology:* mutation in *APC* gene. 20–30% of cases are due to new mutations.
- *Extracolonic malignancies:* duodenal and peri-ampullary (4%), pancreatic (2%), thyroid (2%), gastric (0.6%), CNS (0.1%), hepatoblastoma. Possibly causes distal small bowel and adrenal adenocarcinomas.
- *Benign extracolonic lesions:* osteomas (20%); dental abnormalities (17%); unerupted teeth, supernumary teeth, dentigerous cysts, and

odontomas; cutaneous lesions – epidermoid and sebaceous cysts, fibromas and lipomas; desmoids tumours; congenital hypertrophy of the retinal pigment epithelium, adrenal adenomas, nasal angiofibromas.

- **Desmoid tumours:** may be the first manifestation of GS, occur mainly intra-abdominally, causing small bowel obstruction and pain. Do not metastasize, but may cause morbidity and mortality when they grow to large size and affect surrounding structures. Growth is stimulated by surgery and impeded by pregnancy. Treatment only indicated if symptomatic or risk to adjacent structures.
- **Treatment:** for cancer, depends on cancer site.
- **Screening and surveillance:** as for FAP.

## Von Recklinghausens (neurofibromatosis Type 1)

- **Incidence:** 1in 2600 to 1in 3000.
- **Aetiology:** autosomal dominant neurocutaneous disorder, caused by mutations of *NF1* gene. 50% familial, 50% sporadic. NF1 codes for neurofibromin, which down regulates a proto-oncogene (p21-ras). Mutation in NF1 therefore results in tumour formation. As neurofibromin is expressed in a variety of tissues, tumours are widespread.
- **Tumour types:**
  - benign and malignant;
  - hamartomous polyps in GI tract;
  - *CNS tumours:* most common, mainly optic pathway gliomas, also astrocytomas;
  - *sarcomas:* nerurofibrosarcoma, rhabdomyosarcoma.

## Peutz–Jeghers

- **Definition:** rare condition characterized by multiple hamartomous polyps in GI tract. Associated with mucocutaneous pigmentation.
- **Genetics:** autosomal dominant, with high degree of penetrance for both polyposis and pigmentation.
- Mutation of *PJ* gene on chromosome 19.

### Presentation

- **Pigmentation:** 95% of patients. Flat, blue-grey/brown spots on lips and peri-oral region, buccal mucosa, hands and feet. Usually present in 1st few years of life and fades after puberty. Buccal lesions remain.
- **GI polyps:** solitary or multiple. 0.1–5cm. Small intestine and colon (64%) > stomach (49%) > rectum (32%). Present in 1st decade, become symptomatic after puberty (cf. pigmentation).
- **Symptoms:** obstruction > abdominal pain > PR bleeding. Intusussception common, present in 50% of patients at some point in life. Can be recurrent requiring multiple operations.
- **Cancers:** 15-fold increased relative risk of cancers cf. general population:
  - *GI cancers:* some thought to arise from hamartomous polyps, others unrelated. Small intestine > stomach > colon > pancreas > biliary and oesophageal.
  - **non-GI:** In females – cervical, uterine, breast, ovarian. In males: sertoli cell testicular tumours.

*Management of small bowel polyps and cancers: endoscopic and surgical, especially for intussusception*
- *Screening:* recommended for 1st degree relatives of affected individuals, using history, examination, looking for pigmentation, genetic testing if mutation present in index case, endoscopy, and contrast studies to look for polyps.
- *Surveillance:* looking for GI and non-GI tumours once diagnosis established.

## Crohns disease
- Associated with increased incidence of adenocarcinoma of the terminal ileum, and lymphoma (relative risk 0.4–2.4%). Lesions arise *de novo*.
- *Risk factors:* duration of Crohns, male sex, fistulating disease.
- No role for screening for small bowel cancer as incidence very low.

## Coeliac disease
Slightly increased risk of gastrointestinal cancers, mainly T cell lymphomas. Also SCC oesophagus, small bowel, and colorectal carcinomas and hepatocellular carcinoma.
- *Incidence:* <5% of individuals with celiac disease have T cell lymphoma.
- *Age:* 6th decade.
- *Symptoms:* suspect if symptoms deteriorate despite compliance with gluten-free diet; late presentation with obstruction, acute GI bleed, perforation.
- *Pathology:* large circumferential ulcer usual in jejunum. Mesenteric node involvement common. Lymphomas usually high grade.
- *Diagnosis:* endoscopy and biopsy of ulcerating lesions. Biopsy of normal appearing mucosa usually reveals villous atrophy.
- *Laparotomy* if endoscopy fails.
- *NB:* in view of association, patients with T cell lymphoma should be tested for coeliac disease.
- *Management:* surgery and chemotherapy. Maintenance on gluten free diet.
- *Prognosis*: poor for T cell lymphoma. 5-year survival 10%.

# Colorectal cancer

# Epidemiology and aetiology

## Epidemiology

The 3rd commonest malignancy in the western world and 2nd commonest cause of cancer death (approximately 10%): UK – 34 000; EU – 217 000. New cases each year: EU – 217 000; USA –150 000. Overall lifetime risk 3–5%.

- Slight male preponderance (age-adjusted odds ratios of 1.44 (male/female ratio) for all colorectal cancers (CRC), 1.34 for colon and 1.73 for rectum).
- Older people more commonly affected, with peak incidence in the sixth decade of life.
- Approximately 394 000 deaths attributable to colorectal cancer worldwide each year.

### Geographic distribution

- Highest incidence North America, Australia, and New Zealand. Incidence in Western Europe is relatively lower than the USA, but higher than Eastern Europe.
- Lowest incidence in Africa, Asia, and South America.
- More common in economically developed regions suggesting a link to specific lifestyle habits associated with these areas and other environmental differences.
- In the USA, Asians, American Indians, and people of Hispanic origin have lower rates of colorectal cancer and lower mortality rates from the disease, while Afro-Caribbeans have a higher incidence of colorectal cancer compared with the general population suggesting racial differences.

### Anatomic site

70% originate in the colon and 30% in the rectum. Of the colonic cancers, 35% are in the sigmoid colon, 20% in the caecum, 15% in ascending colon, 10% in the transverse colon, and 7% in the descending colon with the remainder at either of the two flexures

4–5% synchronous at diagnosis.

Aetiology

- Increased dose-dependent risk in smokers and those with excessive alcohol consumption.
- Obesity, residence in urbanized areas, higher socio-economic status associated with increased incidence of CRC. Increased physical exercise reduces risk of CRC in cohort and case-control studies.
- Relationship between 'western' diet and CRC development proposed after observations in varying rates in different countries and migrant studies.
- Transformation of risk is seen over one generation or 20–30 years following migration from low to high risk country, suggestive of environmental influences, in particular diet-modulated risk. Risk declines when migration is in the opposite direction.
- Fruit and vegetables and integral nutrients possibly protective – evidence inconclusive.
- High intake of fibre in the diet may be protective, although more recent evidence in over 88 000 women suggested no correlation between high-fibre diets and the presence of colorectal adenomas or carcinomas.
- Differences in the benefit of dietary fibre on the development of CRC may be due to variations in types of fibre ingested and the means by which it is assessed.
- Meat intake has been associated with increased risk, although it is unclear if this related to fat, transit time, food preparation, packaging, or storage.

# Colorectal adenocarcinoma biology

## Adenoma-carcinoma sequence

Adenocarcinoma of the rectum and colon is preceded by the adenomatous polyp.

Average time of approximately 10 years from normal colonic mucosa to cancer, including an approximate 5-year period from adenomatous polyp to invasive carcinoma.

The *adenoma-carcinoma* progression hypothesis is supported by the following observations:

- Risk for colonic carcinoma of a population is related to the prevalence of adenomas.
- High grade dysplasia, adenomas, and invasive carcinoma are often co-existent.
- Carcinomas are seen to arise from benign adenomas frequently at histopathology.
- The presence of co-existent, and contiguous adenomas and carcinomas is commonly observed in familial adenomatous polyposis (FAP) and hereditary non-polyposis colorectal cancer (HNPCC).
- Those with FAP develop multiple adenomas in the colon, which, if left, undergo malignant transformation.
- Clinical significance has been demonstrated by the influence of polypectomy on the incidence and mortality of colorectal cancer.

## Adenomas

- Adenomatous polyps are common in developed countries and are age related.
- Commonest lesion in the colon in symptomatic people and in those with a positive screening test.
- At endoscopy, sizes range from a few millimetres to over 100mm and they may be flat, sessile, or pedunculated, single or multiple.
- Disordered non-invasive mucosal cell proliferation leads to adenoma formation and broadly may be tubular, villous or tubulovillous. Monoclonal (originating from a single stem cell) and result from either an inherited or acquired genetic mutation.
- The commonest, *tubular* adenomas have a lobulated external surface corresponding to a fissured mucosal surface microscopically from which branching tubules extend into the normal lamina propria.
- The less common, *villous* adenoma has a disordered appearance due to adenomatous epithelium surrounding thin folia of lamina propria.
- *Tubulovillous* adenomas share characteristics of both tubular and villous types.
- Adenomatous cells are tall and columnar in appearance with basal, oval, or elongated nuclei, which are usually empty of mucin. Mucinous adenoma less common.
- Adenoma cells are similar to mucosa under a state of repair and are dysplastic, appearing somewhat between normal mucosal cells and carcinoma cells.
- Classified according to the grade of dysplastic change

# Inheritance and CRC

- Inheritance of significant importance in the development of colorectal polyposis and carcinoma.
- Combination of environmental factors and genetic susceptibility lead to polyp formation and malignant transformation.
- Inherited predisposition can be seen as one of the well-described syndromes of adenomas and carcinomas or those considered to be 'sporadic'.
- Characterized inherited syndromes may be divided into those with excessive intestinal polyposis and those where only a few polyps may be present, the 'non-polyposis' syndromes.
- Familial adenomatous polyposis (FAP), Gardners' syndrome (GS), and the hamartomatous polyposis conditions of Peutz–Jeghers disease and familial juvenile polyposis make up the inherited polyposis syndromes, which are inherited in an autosomal dominant manner.

## Sporadic CRC
- Remainder of cases (95%) of CRC.
- First-degree relatives affected by colorectal cancer have 2 or 3 times increased risk of developing the disease.
- Proposed that this may be due to partial penetrance of Mendelian genes, although shared environment may also be partially responsible.
- Inherited pre-disposition is the most likely cause as demonstrated by large family studies, particularly where separation has taken place.
- Increased lifetime probability of colorectal cancer from 6% in unaffected families to 18% in affected families.

## Hereditary non-polyposis colorectal cancer (HNPCC)
- 1–5% of colorectal cancer cases.
- Defined by mutation of DNA mismatch repair (MMR) genes.
- Previous FHx criteria now defunct: >3 family members affected or >2 CRC, and 1 endometrial Ca in >2 generations. 1 aged <50 years and 1 a first degree relative of other 2.
- Lifetime CRC risk 80%, gastric Ca 13–20%.
- Encompasses those inherited colorectal cancer syndromes not characterized by a great number of colonic polyps – includes Lynch syndrome I, 'site-specific colorectal cancer' and Lynch syndrome II, 'cancer family syndrome'.
- Both Lynch I and Lynch II are characterized by young age of onset of colorectal cancer, and inheritance is in an autosomal dominant manner with high penetrance.
- In individuals with these syndromes, adenomas are frequent, although polyposis is not extensively present
- HNPCC polyps display more severe pathological features than in the normal population, including larger size and more villous histology.

## Surveillance in HNPCC families

- Colonoscopy every 2 years commencing age 25 or 5 years below earliest familial onset of CRC until age 75 or MMR mutation excluded in individual biochemically.
- OGD every 2 years aged 50–75 years or commencing 5 years before earliest gastric Ca in family.

## Surgery for HNPCC cancers

- **Aim:** cancer control and prophylaxis as risk of metachronous tumours high.
- **Proximal tumours:** colectomy with ileorectal anastomosis recommended.
- **Risk of further rectal Ca:** 3% every 3 years for first 12 years after surgery.
- Surveillance at least yearly.
- Prophylactic surgery for HNPCC family members who are not proven to have mutation is not recommended as overall lifetime familial risk of CRC is 40% in males and 15–30% in females.

# Familial adenomatous polyposis

## Genetics and cancer risk

- Autosomal dominant with very high penetrance.
- >100 colorectal polyps can be 1000s.
- Caused by truncating mutations in the long arm of chromosome in the adenomatous polyposis coli (APC) gene (5q21) mutation identifiable in 60%.
- 25% sporadic non-familial mutations. Some in MYH.
- 90% CRC risk by age 70.
- 7% Gastroduodenal cancer risk.

The polyposis disorders account for <1% of CRC cases, but have advanced the knowledge of the disease gained by studying genetic abnormalities.

## Extra-intestinal manifestations

FAP may present with mesodermal, endodermal, and ectodemal pathology such as:

- *Desmoids:* well circumscribed intra-abdominal benign tumours causing morbidity due to compression. Rx Sulindac, tamoxifen, or resection.
- Osteomas and congenital hypertrophic retinal pigmentation (CHRPE).

## Prophylactic surgery

- Proven FAP offer prophylactic colectomy at age 16–20 years.
- Optimal procedure is restorative proctocolectomy with ileo-anal pouch formation.
- Colectomy with ileorectal anastomosis appropriate in attenuated cases with few polyps.
- Post-IRA yearly surveillance: rectal cancer risk 12–29%.
- If restorative proctocolectomy performed yearly surveillance still necessary for anal cuff.
- 3-Yearly OGD from age 30 for duodenal polyp surveillance, yearly if large number.

## Surveillance for family members

- Polyposis registry should be maintained for family members
- Flexible sigmoidoscopy from age 13–15 to 30 years annually, then 3–5-yearly to age 60.
- *Documented APC mutation or large number of polyps:* prophylactic colectomy and ileorectal anastomosis before age 25, otherwise 6-monthly surveillance if colectomy deferred.

# Other rare polyposis syndromes

Peutz–Jeghers syndrome:
- Rare autosomal dominant, high penetrance.
- Hamartomatous polyps of small bowel, colon, and rectum.
- CRC risk 10–20%. 3-yearly colonoscopy advised.

Juvenile polyposis syndrome
- Rare. 50% associated with *SMAD4* gene.
- Multiple hamartomas of colon (particularly right) and rectum in childhood.
- CRC risk 10–38% gastric Ca 21%.
- Yearly colonoscopy from onset or 15–18 until 35 years of age then 3–5-yearly until age 70 years recommended.
- Prophylactic surgery recommended in those with adenomatous change or large numbers of uncontrollable polyps.

# Inflammation and CRC

Evidence to support the relationship between chronic inflammation and colorectal cancer comes from the study of patients with inflammatory bowel disease. Aspirin and cyclo-oxygenase inhibitors are also appear to be protective against CRC.

## Ulcerative colitis (UC)

- Carcinoma in the presence of ulcerative colitis (UC) is relatively uncommon: 1% of colonic carcinomas.
- Patients with extensive or severe colitis develop cancers at a much higher rate than in the general population particularly after 10 years of the onset of UC.
- Risk of small and large bowel cancer estimated at 4–20 times that of the general population.
- Mean age at onset CRC between 40 and 45 years, although the prognosis of these patients is not worse compared with age-matched controls.
- Extent of disease and length of history and age of onset are important risk factors for the development of colorectal cancer in patients with UC.
- Azathioprine increases risk of lymphoma.

## Crohn's disease

- First case of carcinoma in a patient with Crohn described in 1956.
- In Crohn's, the distribution of cancers is mainly in the colon (70%), with fewer in the small bowel (25%) and some extra-intestinal malignancies (5%).
- Most cancers arise in inflammatory sections of bowel, at stricture sites and chronic fistulae, although cancers in macroscopically un-inflamed bowel are also seen.

# Squamous cell colorectal carcinoma

- Primary squamous cell carcinoma of the colon and rectum is extremely rare, with an incidence of less than 0.25%.
- Commonest site is the rectum and mixed adenosquamous histology may also be expressed.
- Natural history and optimum management have not been defined, clearly although recent reports have proposed the use of primary chemoradiotherarapy, with surgery for refractory or recurrent cases, as with anal squamous cell carcinoma.

# Screening for cancer and premalignant polyps

### Overview

- Colorectal cancer is common – lifetime risk 3–5%.
- Recognized pathway from pre-malignant lesion to cancer (adenoma-carcinoma sequence).
- Adenomas are common, but only few are considered 'high risk', which progress to cancer.
- 'High risk' includes: diameter >1cm; ≥3 adenomas; villous or tubulo-villous; severe dysplasia; >20 hyperplastic polyps above the distal rectum.
- Evidence exists demonstrating that screening for CRC improves overall mortality rates.
- Screening programme ongoing in the USA.
- Currently, not widespread in the UK, but trials ongoing as the NHS Bowel Screening programme.
- Unclear which screening test is best, based on sensitivity, specificity, cost, safety.

### Faecal occult blood (FOB) test

- Uses Guaiac-based products to examine for microscopic blood.
- Easy to use at home by subjects over 3 days by placing stool on a pre-prepared strip.
- Low sensitivity and low specificity.
- Requires dietary modification for reduction in false positive rate.
- Compliance rates not high – subjects are not keen on handling faeces.
- Cost effective when compared with other screening methods and with screening of other malignancies.

### Flexible sigmoidoscopy

- Able to examine up to splenic flexure (60cm) in which about 70% of lesions exist.
- Requires expensive layout – equipment, trained personnel, dedicated facilities.
- Can identify lesions and biopsy/excise lesions.
- Requires patient preparation of lower bowel with enema.
- Does not examine complete colon; therefore, risk of missing proximal lesions.
- Reasonably cost-effective.
- Well tolerated by patients with acceptable compliance.
- Low complication rate.

### Colonoscopy

- Able to identify, biopsy, and excise lesions throughout the colon.
- Considered to be the best method in terms of sensitivity, specificity, diagnosis, and treatment of lesions.
- Too expensive to be used as a general screening tool.
- Associated with risk of complications – bleeding and perforation.

- Investigation of choice for high risk groups – HNPCC and FAP.
- Advised as screening tool in the USA once every 10 years.
- Requires full bowel preparation.

## Double contrast barium enema

- Historical investigation of choice.
- Good sensitivity and specificity for large adenomas and cancers.
- Requires full bowel preparation.
- Not able to biopsy suspicious lesions.
- Demonstrates some intra-observer variability.

## Virtual colonoscopy/CT pneumocolonography

- Relatively new technique using CT.
- High detection rates with high sensitivity and specificity.
- Requires expensive technology, time, and expertise.
- Not able to take biopsies of visualized lesions.
- Risk associated with radiation exposure.
- Better than barium enema for detection of smaller lesions.

## Immunological testing

- Require no dietary modification.
- Common tests include HemeSelect and FlexSure OBT using reverse passive haemagglutination and specific binding of haemaglobin to a specific antibody.
- More sensitive specific than guaiac-based FOB testing:
  - comparable specificity to FOB tests;
  - require special tests to process information (agglutination, immunochromatography, or ELISA), therefore, additional cost implication.

## Gene testing

- Uses gene arrays for detection of CRC mutation associated polymorphisms and microsatellite instability.
- Various mutations may be assessed – APC, p53, K-ras, microsatellite instability and methylation.
- Early reports do not demonstrate adequate sensitivity or specificity for use as a screening test.
- Trials are ongoing and may be of use in the future.

# Colorectal cancer screening recommendations

### Risk stratification

Risk status should be determined well before the earliest potential initiation of screening around age 20: earlier if there is a family history of familial adenomatous polyposis.

**Table 9.1** Patient risk stratification for CRC

| | |
|---|---|
| Low risk | Asymptomatic **and** |
| | Age below 50 **and** |
| | No family history of CRC |
| | **No screening indicated** |
| Average risk | Asymptomatic **and** |
| | Age above 50 **and** |
| | No family history or |
| | Age below 50 and single 1st degree relative diagnosed with CRC at age above 60 |
| Increased risk: | Symptomatic **or** |
| | Previous resection for CRC or colonic adenomas |
| | Known genetic predisposition: FAP/HNPCC **or** |
| | Established IBD **or** |
| | 2 or more 1st degree relatives diagnosed with CRC aged above 60 or 1 below 60 |
| | **All irrespective of patient's age** |

### Average risk

Multiple options recommended in national guidelines:
- FOB test annually. Guaiac test with dietary restriction or immunochemical test without dietary restriction 2 samples from 3 consecutive stools. Examined without rehydration. **Or**
- Offer flexible sigmoidoscopy every 5 years. Or combination of above: FOB test should be done first. **Or**
- Offer colonoscopy every 10 years. **Or**
- Offer double-contrast barium enema (DCBE) every 5 years.
- Positive test on any non-colonoscopy test: perform colonoscopy.

Increased risk

- Colorectal cancer: colonoscopy within 6 months of curative resection if colon not fully assessed pre-operatively. Liver scan within 2 years post-operatively and repeat colonoscopies 5-yearly until 70.
- *Colonic adenomas 1–2 <1cm:* no surveillance or 5-yearly until single colonoscopy is negative.
- *Colonic adenoma 3–4 or any >1cm:* colonoscopy every 3 years until 2 consecutive colonoscopies negative.
- *Colonic adenomas ≥5 or ≥3 with at least 1 >1cm:* annual colonoscopy until risk group changes.
- *Large sessile adenomas:* colonoscopy 3-monthly until no residual material. Surgical resection if any doubt.
- *Colonic adenomas moderate dysplasia:* colonoscopy at 1 year.
- *Colonic adenomas severe dysplasia:* colonoscopy at 3–6onths or treat as for invasive adenocarcinoma polyps (see algorithm).
- *UC and Crohn's colitis:* colonscopy and biopsies every 10cm, 8 years post-onset pan-colitis or 15 years post-left colitis, then 3-yearly in 2nd decade, 2-yearly in 3rd decade, then annually.
- *IBD + PSC ± liver transplant:* colonoscopy at diagnosis of PSC then annually with 10cm biopsies for life.
- *Acromegaly:* colonoscopy  5-yearly above age 40.
- *Urteterosigmoidostomy:* flexible sigmoidoscopy 10 years post-operatively and then annually.
- *FAP* (see ' Familial adenomatous polyposis', p. 446): flexible sigmoidoscopy + OGD and genetic testing at puberty, then annual flexible sigmoidoscopy.
- *Juvenile polyposis and Peutz–Jegers:* colonoscopy + OGD and genetic testing annually from puberty.
- *HNPCC* (see ' hereditary non-polyposis colorectal cancer', p. 444) *or >2FDR CRC:* Colonoscopy ± OGD at 25 or 5 years before earliest CRC. OGD at 50 or 5 years before earliest gastric Ca. Then colonoscopy and OGD every 1–2 years.
- *1 FDR < 60 or 2 FDR>60:* colonoscopy at 40 or presentation if later or 10 years younger than the earliest diagnosis in the family, whichever comes first. Then colonoscopy every 5 years
- *1FDR or 2 second degree > 60:* same as average risk, but starting at age 40 years.

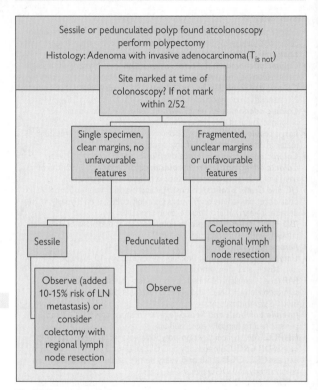

**Fig. 9.1** Management of adenomatous polyp with invasive adenocarcinoma.

**Unfavourable histological features**
- Grade 3 or 4.
- Lymphovascular invasion.
- Unclear margins (no definitive definition 2mm from transaction margin to carcinoma cells within diathermy of transected margin).

# Diagnosis

## Overview
- Accurate diagnosis reduces mortality and morbidity.
- A thorough history and examination and rectal examination is essential.
- Factors that suggest a diagnosis of colorectal cancer are clearly described and atypical presentation is unusual.

## Presentation
- History of rectal bleeding.
- Tenesmus.
- Weight loss.
- Change in bowel habit (towards loose stools most common).
- Previous colorectal cancer or polypectomy.
- Positive family history.
- Palpable abdominal mass.
- Palpable rectal mass (40–80% with rectal Ca).
- Iron-deficient anaemia.
- Emergency bowel obstruction.

### Clinical features less likely to suggest colorectal cancer
- Rectal bleeding with anal symptoms (pain, itching, discharge).
- Change in bowel habit tending towards decreased frequency and harder stools.
- Abdominal pain without evidence of intestinal obstruction.

## Investigations
- Digital rectal examination and rigid sigmoidoscopy.
- FBC/U&Es, LFTs, CEA better for surveillance.
- *Endoscopy, contrast plain X-rays or CT pneumocolon:* determination of which primary investigation should be undertaken is dependent on patient factors [symptoms, family history, co-morbid conditions, e.g. UC, diverticular disease, general patient condition, ability to tolerate bowel preparation, and institutional factors (facilities and expertise available)].

## Endoscopy

- Majority of cancers in patients who present with rectal bleeding +/− change in bowel habit are located <60cm from the anal verge.
- Flexible sigmoidoscopy can detect the majority of these cancers.
- If cancer detected by sigmoidoscopy, a completion colonoscopy is required pre- or post-operatively to investigate for synchronous lesions (4–5%).
- Colonoscopy has a high sensitivity for the detection of colorectal cancer and is advantageous as compared with less invasive means as biopsies may be taken during the procedure, and it does not expose patients to potentially harmful radiation.
- Opportunity for immediate polypectomy, which may be the definitive intervention.
- Narrow band imaging with magnification may allow immediate assessment of dysplastic grade.
- Disadvantages of colonoscopy include incomplete studies in a variable proportion of examinations, the use of respiratory depressant intravenous sedation, often poor colonic localization, and the risk of complications including perforation and bleeding.
- Completion barium enema or CT pneumocolon may still be required.

## Double-contrast barium enema

- Generally well tolerated and widely available.
- Safe, does not require intravenous analgesia or sedation, and has the ability of providing complete colorectal information in most patients, but does require a dose of ionizing radiation.
- DCBE combined with flexible sigmoidoscopy has been shown to have similar diagnostic accuracy as colonoscopy in detection of cancers or polyps ≥9mm in size.
- Small sigmoid polyps may be missed with barium enema, particularly in the presence of diverticular disease.

## CT pneumocolon/CT colonography/virtual colonoscopy

- Requires adequate bowel preparation.
- Does not permit biopsy.
- Better sensitivity for detection of polyps than barium enema.
- Accurate in the identification of colorectal cancer and polyps greater than 10mm in size.
- Useful for staging the tumour and assessment of hepatic involvement, and may be useful in frail and elderly patients.

## Magnetic resonance colonography

Has also been used to assess for colorectal adenomas and cancers with some promising results, but is not in widespread use due to lack of technology and expertise.

# Pre-operative assessment and preparation

## Purpose of pre-operative staging

- Assess local spread and assist in operative planning.
- Assess nodal spread.
- Investigate for distant metastasis.
- Determine need for neoadjuvant therapy.
- Determine curative intent.

## Staging for rectal cancer

- History and clinical examination including rectal examination.
- Local staging by (at least 1.5 Tesla) magnetic resonance imaging (MRI).
- MRI determines circumferential resection margin clearance accurately and some indication of lymph node status.
- MRI was first used in the staging of rectal cancer in 1986. Conventional MRI techniques initially used in staging rectal cancer proved to have limitations due to poor spatial resolution. The introduction of (1) endorectal coils; (2) pelvic phased array coils; (3) thin section high resolution MR imaging, and the ability to combine these electronically, has resulted in greater staging accuracy, and the ability to accurately predict tumour-free surgical resection margins due to improved definition of the mesorectal fascia.
- Involvement of the mesorectal fascia (the surgical plane of dissection) is clearly demonstrated and microscopic clearance of less than 1mm may be predicted.
- Lymph node morphology in conjunction with size (>1cm) may be indicative of tumour deposition.
- New techniques for accurately predicting lymph node status include ultrasmall particle iron oxide (USPIO) contrast-enhanced MRI
- Endo-anal ultrasound is more accurate at predicting early T stages than MRI (T1 and T2)

## Staging for CRC

- IV contrast-enhanced CT abdomen – to assess local spread in colonic neoplasms, and exclude hepatic and distant nodal metastasis.
- IV contrast-enhanced CT chest – to exclude lung metastasis.
- Historical abdominal US and chest radiography have been surpassed for detection of metastatic disease.
- PET scan not routinely indicated.

## Pre-operative assessment

- Blood tests – FBC, U&Es, LFTs, clotting, group and save, carcinoembryonic antigen (CEA).
- ECG +/– exercise test for assessment of cardiac status +/– echocardiogram if indicated.
- CXR +/– respiratory function tests if indicated.
- Respiratory or cardiology review.

- Anaesthetic review – suitability for operation.
- All patients in the elective setting should be discussed at a multidisciplinary team (MDT) meeting pre-operatively and all patients, including those operated on for an emergency, should be discussed post-operatively.

## Pre-operative preparation

- *Psychological preparation:* counsel patients about treatment options. Supply detailed description of peri-operative period prior to obtaining informed consent.
- *Smoking cessation:* thromboembolic prophylaxis – anti-thromboembolic stockings, low molecular weight heparin +/– per-operative intermittent pneumatic calf compression.
- *IV broad-spectrum antibiotics:* immediately pre-operatively or at induction (cefuroxime/metronidazole or co-amoxiclav).
- *X-match 4 units blood:* avoid use if possible due to risks associated with transfusion.
- *HDU or ITU bed available.*
- *Epidural placement:* for post-operative analgesia. Insertion of Foley's urethral catheter.
- *Bowel preparation:* variation in practice – historically bowel preparation given for all colorectal cancer operations if not obstructed one day prior to surgery.
- More recently, bowel preparation reserved for left sided operations.
- Some evidence for no bowel preparation as electrolyte depletion associated with poor return to function.

## Informed consent

- Discuss diagnosis and management options.
- Describe procedure.
- *Explain general complications:* MI, DVT/PE, renal failure, CVA, ITU stay, arrhythmia, pneumonia.
- *Explain specific complications:* anastomotic leak, bleeding, abdominal, pelvic and wound infection, incomplete resection, damage to loco-regional structures – ureter, bladder, prostate, uterus, ovaries and tubes, blood vessels, bowel, nerves (particularly pelvic–uro-genital function), potential need for stoma (temporary/ permanent).

# Staging and prognosis

Risk stratification for prognostic determination to tailor a treatment regimen to an individual patient to maximize survival, and reduce recurrence and progression.

## TNM classification

For rectal adenocarcinoma, lymph nodes considered as loco-regional, include superior, middle, and inferior rectal (haemorrhoidal), inferior mesenteric, internal iliac, mesorectal, lateral sacral, and pre-sacral and sacral promontory nodes.

The TNM pathological classification is determined after histopathological assessment, pT, pN, and pM categories correspond to the clinical T, N and M categories.

## Full clinical TNM classification for colorectal adenocarcinoma

### Primary tumour (T)

- **TX:** primary tumour cannot be assessed.
- **T0:** no evidence of primary tumour.
- **Tis:** carcinoma *in situ* – intraepithelial or invasion of the lamina propria.[1]
- **T1:** tumour invades submucosa.
- **T2:** tumour invades muscularis propria.
- **T3:** tumour invades through muscularis propria into sub-serosa or into non-peritonealized pericolic or perirectal tissues.
- **T4:** tumour directly invades other organs or structures and/or perforates visceral peritoneum.[2,3]

### Regional lymph nodes (N)[4]

- **NX:** regional lymph nodes cannot be assessed.
- **N0:** no regional lymph node metastasis.
- **N1:** metastasis in 1–3 lymph nodes.
- **N2:** metastasis in 4 or more regional lymph nodes.

### Distant metastasis (M)

- **MX:** distant metastasis cannot be assessed.
- **M0:** no distant metastasis.
- **M1:** distant metastasis.

### Histopathological grading (G)

- **GX:** grade of differentiation cannot be assessed.
- **G1:** well differentiated.
- **G2:** moderately differentiated.
- **G3:** poorly differentiated.
- **G4:** undifferentiated.

[1]Tis includes cancer cells confined within the glandular basement membrane (intraepithelial) or lamina propria (intramucosal) with no extension through muscularis mucosae into submucosa.

[2]Direct invasion in T4 includes invasion of other segments of the colorectum through serosa, e.g. invasion of sigmoid colon by local rectal cancer spread.

[3]Tumour adherent to other organs or structures, macroscopically, is classified as T4. However, if no tumour is present in the adhesion, microscopically, the pathological classification should be pT3.

[4]A tumour nodule in the pericolic/perirectal fat without histological evidence of residual lymph node is classified in the pN category as a lymph node metastasis if the nodule has the form and smooth contour of a lymph node. If the nodule has an irregular contour, it should be classified in the T category and also coded as V1 (microscopic venous invasion) or V2, if grossly evident, because there is a strong likelihood that it represents venous invasion

**Table 9.2** Stage groupings

| Stage | 0 Tis | N0 | M0 |
|-------|-------|-----|-----|
| Stage | I T1, T2 | N0 | M0 |
| Stage | IIA T3 | N0 | M0 |
| | IIB T4 | N0 | M0 |
| Stage | IIIA T1, T2 | N1 | M0 |
| | IIIB T3, T4 | N1 | M0 |
| | IIIC Any T | N2 | M0 |
| Stage | IV Any T | Any N | M1 |

Main advantage of the TNM classification is the consideration of the three elements of T, N, and M separately, and recognition that they are independent prognostic indicators.

- Previous criticisms of the TNM system included the confusion in the T4 category between adherence of tumour and actual penetration of another organ, two groups with demonstrably different outcomes.
- Previously described N3 category was criticized as was the M category for being too coarse a prognostic indicator, not able to differentiate between regional metastasis, and widespread or distant disease. In subsequent editions, the confusion regarding the T classification was clarified and the N category was limited to N0, N1, and N2, although the wide net of the M stage persists.
- Numbers of nodes found is of prognostic relevance and clinical significance with various methods employed for improving lymph node detection rates.
- In the UK the mean lymph node harvest is 11.7 nodes with significant variability between centres (range 5.5–21.3 nodes).
- Numbers of nodes examined has been significantly associated with time to relapse and survival among node negative rectal cancer patients.
- In addition, potential clinical significance and methods of detection of *micrometastasis* have also been investigated and are considered to be of importance, particularly as so-called negative nodes have subsequently been found to contain small foci of malignant cells.
- Non-anatomical factors that have a significant effect on prognosis in colorectal cancer include:
  - histological grade;
  - tumour border configuration (infiltrative margin worse);
  - presence of microscopic or macroscopic residual tumour (r1, r2);
  - radial margin involvement;
  - venous invasion (intra-mural, extra-mural);
  - lymphatic invasion;
  - pre-operative carcinoembryonic antigen (CEA).

- Other factors were recognized by the AJCC to have prognostic importance, but were considered to be not sufficiently well established for use in a prognostic system:
  - 18q/deleted in colorectal cancer (DCC);
  - K-ras (codon and specific mutation);
  - microsatellite instability (MSI high or low), p53 mutations;
  - thymidine synthase (TS) expression.
  - Bcl-2/BAX mutations.
  - p27 mutations.
  - microvessel density (MVD).
- Despite improved staging in rectal cancer, patients with similar anatomical extent of tumour spread may have different clinical outcomes.
- This has led to attempts to further refine staging systems for rectal cancer and investigate other factors, which can improve the approach to rectal cancer staging.
- It is becoming increasingly clear that additional factors, whether morphological or molecular, will be needed for future clinical management

## Historical perspective and developments in CRC cancer staging the St Mark's contribution

Prior to more accurate staging methods, clinical examination the only staging process to determine operability and predict probability of a favourable outcome.

In 1927 at St Mark's Hospital JP Lockhart-Mummery developed the first staging system specifically for rectal cancer based on three categories of tumour depth of invasion into the wall of the bowel (A, B, and C). In his series, he found a difference in 5-year survival between the groups.

The St Mark's pathologist Cuthbert Dukes noted the importance of lymph node status in the spread of rectal cancer and in 1932 included lymph node involvement within a new staging system called the Dukes classification of rectal cancer and expanded to include colonic cancer:

- **'A' cases:** carcinoma limited to the wall of the rectum, there being no extension into the extrarectal tissues and no metastases in lymph nodes.
- **'B' cases:** spread by direct continuity to the extrarectal tissues, but no invasion of the regional lymph nodes.
- **'C' cases:** metastases within the regional lymph nodes.

Dukes further modified his staging system in 1935 by sub-classifying the C category as follows:

- **'C1' cases:** regional lymph nodes are involved, or those in which the upward spread has not yet reached the glands at the point of ligature of the blood vessels.
- **'C2' cases:** nodal spread has reached up to the level of the point of ligature of the blood vessels.

This refinement was made in acknowledgement of the sequence of rectal cancer nodal progression from the mesorectal lymph nodes upwards following the arterial supply. It was suggested that cure was more likely if the 'apical' lymph node, the highest lymph node in the resected specimen, was not involved by tumour and this was integral to the new sub-division. In 1967, Turnbull proposed the addition of a 'D' category to reflect the prognostic importance of distant metastasis.

More recently, Jeremy Jass and John Northover added lymphocytic infiltration and tumour border configuration in a staging system for rectal cancer.

# Neoadjuvant therapy: rectal cancer

## Overview

- Neoadjuvant therapy is given prior to surgical procedure.
- No benefit demonstrated in colonic cancer.
- Benefit has been demonstrated in decreasing local recurrence and improving circumferential clearance (R0 resection) in some rectal cancers.
- Rationale is to downstage tumour prior to surgery in those with threatened circumferential margins (mesorectal fascia) as demonstrated on pre-operative MRI.
- Useful in some rectal cancers where local recurrence rates are high.

### Pre-operative radiotherapy and chemoradiotherapy

- May be delivered by conventional fractionation of 45–50Gy in 25 daily fractions over 5 weeks, 4–8 weeks prior to surgery to shrink and potentially down-stage a rectal cancer.
- Conventional long course radiotherapy is more effective when combined with synchronous 5-FU-based chemotherapy given either in weeks 1 and 5, or continuously throughout the radiotherapy course, known as chemoradiotherapy (CRT). Given for patients with advanced local rectal cancers with threatened or involved mesorectal fascia to enable a possible R0 procedure to be undertaken.
- Alternatively, may be given as short course pre-operative radiotherapy (SCPRT) to decrease risk of loco-regional recurrence at a dose of 25Gy in 5 daily fractions over a week followed by surgery after approximately 10 days. Appropriate for rectal patients considered to have clinically and radiologically resectable disease.
- Chemoradiotherapy has been shown clearly to decrease local recurrence, although the evidence for improvement in cancer-specific survival has not been clearly demonstrated.
- Early evidence for SCPRT came from the Swedish Rectal cancer Trial (late 1990s), which demonstrated a reduction in local recurrence from 27 to 11% and a significant improvement in overall 5-year survival from 48 to 58%. This trial has been criticized for the high local recurrence rates in both arms.
- It has been argued that the introduction of total mesenteric excision (TME) surgery with care to remove the rectal cancer with its associated lymph nodes has decreased local recurrence in itself without radiotherapy.
- The Dutch Rectal Cancer Trial demonstrated a significant reduction in local recurrence in the group treated with SCPRT from 8.2 to 2.4%, with both groups undergoing TME surgery. However, significant difference in survival was demonstrated in this trial.
- The UK equivalent ongoing CR07 trial has demonstrated a reduction in local recurrence with the addition of SCPRT from 11.1 to 4.7% at 3 years with a demonstrable and significant benefit on disease-free survival from 74.9 to 79.5%.

- Significant risks of radio and chemoradiotherapy include sphincteric, urogenital neurological dysfunction, enteritis, and toxicity. There are also reports of tissue oedema and increased operative bleeding complicating surgery and higher rates of tissue breakdown, particularly in the perineal wound after abdomino-perineal excision of rectal cancer.
- Post-neoadjuvant downstaging patients should undergo anterior resection. It is uncertain if patients who subsequently have clear margins and have no nodal or metastatic reasons for adjuvant chemotherapy should have chemotherapy. The CHRONICLE: *CH*emothe*R*apy or *N*o chemotherapy in *CLE*ar margins after neoadjuvant chemoradiation in locally advanced rectal cancer is a randomized phase III trial of control vs. capecitabine plus oxaliplatin and is currently recruiting patients

# Management of colonic cancer basic resection algorithm (Fig. 9.2)

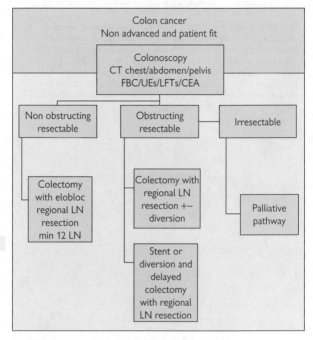

**Fig. 9.2** Management of colonic cancer basic resection algorithm.

Lymphadenenectomy recommendations
- Minimum of 12 nodes needed to establish stage II (T3–4, N0).
- Number of LN correlates with survival in stage III.
- Apex of feeding vessel should be marked to indicate position of apical node.
- Biopsy suspicious nodes outside field of standard *en bloc* resection.

**Table 9.3** Tumour position and resection methods

| Position of tumour | Resection |
| --- | --- |
| Caecum to proximal transverse colon | Right hemicolectomy |
| Distal transverse colon | Extended right hemicolectomy |
| Descending colon | Left hemicolectomy |
| Sigmoid colon | Sigmoid colectomy/high anterior resection |

# Surgical anatomy of the colon and rectum

## Overview

The most distal aspect of the bowel consists of the:
• Caecum and vermiform appendix.
• Ascending colon.
• Transverse colon.
• Descending colon.
• Sigmoid colon.
• Rectum.
• Anal canal and anus.

## Layers of bowel wall

• Mucosal epithelium.
• Muscularis mucosae.
• Submucosa.
• Muscularis propria.
• Subserosa.
• Serosa.

## Caecum

• Blind-ended structure projecting downwards at the first part of the colon below the ileocaecal junction.
• Covered on both sides by peritoneum.
• Three taeniae coli converge on the base of the appendix.
• Covered by peritoneum on the front and two sides.
• Lies on the peritoneal floor of the right iliac fossa.
• *Anterior:* abdominal cavity, small intestinal loops, anterior abdominal wall.
• *Posterior:* iliacus and psoas fasciae.
• *Posteromedial:* right gonadal vessels and ureter.
• *Inferior:* inguinal ligament, pelvic brim.
• *Blood supply:* anterior and posterior caecal vessels, the two terminal branches of the ileocolic artery.
• *Lymphatic drainage:* lymph nodes associated with the ileocolic artery.

## Ascending colon

• About 15cm long extending upwards from the ileocaecal valve to the hepatic (right colic) flexure.
• Superiorly lies on the lateral surface of the inferior pole of the right kidney and in contact with the liver.
• Lies on the iliac fascia and anterior layer of the lumbar fascia – attached by extra-peritoneal fibrous tissue.
• Embryological mesentery originally from the midline to adhere to the posterior abdominal wall peritoneum bringing the ileocolic and right colic vessels.

- Taeniae coli lie in continuation of those in the caecum anteriorly, posterolaterally and posteromedially.
- Appendices epiploicae, bulbous pouches of peritoneum project from parts of the serous coat with supplying blood vessels perforating from the mucosa through the muscle wall.
- Blood supply – ileocolic and right colic arteries derived from the superior mesenteric artery.
- Lymphatic drainage – lymph nodes associated with the arteries.

## Transverse colon

- Usually over 45 cm long.
- Extends from the hepatic flexure to the splenic flexure.
- Hangs down to a variable degree.
- The convexity of the greater curve of the stomach lies in its concavity.
- The stomach and transverse colon are connected by the gastrocolic ligament.
- The greater omentum hangs down from its lower convexity.
- Completely invested in peritoneum – hanging free on the transverse mesocolon, which is attached from the inferior pole of the right kidney across the second (descending) part of the duodenum and pancreas to the inferior pole of the left kidney.
- Splenic flexure is higher than the hepatic flexure.
- Larger and more numerous appendices epiploicae than the ascending colon.
- Blood supply – proximal two-thirds via the middle colic (right and left branches) derived from the superior mesenteric artery; distal third from the ascending branch of the left colic artery derived from the inferior mesenteric artery.
- Anastomotic branches in proximity with the medial margin of the colon form the 'marginal' artery from which short vessels penetrate the bowel wall.
- Veins correspond to arteries, reaching the portal vein via the superior or inferior mesenteric tributaries.

## Descending colon

- Less than 30cm in length.
- Extends from the splenic flexure to the pelvic brim about 5cm above the inguinal ligament.
- As the ascending colon, attached to the posterior abdominal wall by peritoneum.
- Lies on the lumbar and iliac fasciae connected by extra-peritoneal fibrous tissue.
- Three taeniae coli lie in continuity with those of the transverse colon lying one anterior and two posterior.
- Attached are many appendices epiploicae.
- Embryologically contained a midline posterior mesocolon with left colic vessels. Subsequently, colon swung laterally with the mesocolon attached to the posterior abdominal wall.

**Sigmoid colon**

- Previously termed the pelvic colon extending from the descending colon at the pelvic brim to the rectum anterior to S3.
- Usually less than 45cm in length although large variations are common.
- Completely invested in peritoneum hanging free on its mesentery, the sigmoid mesocolon.
- Contains three taeniae coli, which are wider than in proximal colon and merge at its distal end at the top of the rectum.
- Embryologically, the sigmoid mesocolon was attached posteriorly in the midline. Subsequently, hinged laterally and fused with parietal peritoneum on the posterior and left pelvic side wall.
- Blood supply via sigmoid branches derived from the descending left colic artery off the inferior mesenteric artery.
- Veins correspond to arteries. Lymph nodes follow the arteries.

**Rectum**

- Most distal aspect of the gastrointestinal tract except for the anal canal.
- Situated at the termination of the colon.
- A misnomer in humans, the rectum, originally described in monkeys, is derived from the Latin word *rectum*, meaning straight.
- In humans, the rectum is structured with a posterior concavity related to the sacrum and coccyx, and has three lateral curves – upper and lower curves convex to the right and a middle curve convex to the left, with a slight dilation at the distal rectal ampulla.
- Three transverse folds, the rectal valves of Houston, project inwards, caused by the circular muscle of the rectal wall. Approximately 12–15cm long, the rectum is the caudal continuation of the sigmoid colon at the level of the third sacral vertebra (S3), where the bowel peritoneal attachments change from the mesocolon to no mesentery.
- The muscular covering of the rectum is, as with the colon, arranged with an outer longitudinal and inner circular layer.
- The three taeniae coli (longitudinal muscle) of the colon fuse at the level of the rectum to provide a complete outer longitudinal muscle coat, with no appendices epiploicae.
- The rectum passes anteriorly over the coccyx and anococcygeal raphé passing through the pelvic floor into the anal canal, posterior to the perineal body.
- The upper third of the rectum is covered by peritoneum antero-laterally, the middle third only anteriorly and the lower third is below the level of the peritoneum, as it is reflected onto the upper part of the bladder in males or upper vagina in females to give the rectovesicle pouch or recto-uterine pouch (of Douglas), which form the inferior-most aspects of the peritoneal cavity.
- Posteriorly, the rectum is separated from the sacrum and coccyx by the pre-sacral fascia and is related to the piriformis, coccygeus, and levator ani muscles, the sacral plexus, and the sympathetic trunks.

- Anteriorly, in the male, the upper two-thirds of the rectum is related to the sigmoid colon and loops of small bowel, which are located in the rectovesicle pouch. The lower third is in proximity with the posterior surface of the bladder, the termination of the vas deferens, the seminal vesicles on either side, and the prostate, which are all enveloped by the visceral pelvic fascia.
- Anteriorly, in the female, the upper two-thirds of the rectum is in proximity with the sigmoid colon and loops of small bowel which are located uterine pouch (of Douglas). The lower third is related to the posterior aspect of the vagina.
- The lower aspect of the rectum in males and females is attached by Waldeyer's fascia, a layer of connective tissue, to the lower sacrum and retroperitoneal tissue close to the middle rectal vessels known as the lateral ligaments are present on either side which both combine to provide structural integrity together with the levatores ani muscles.
- The blood supply to the rectum is by way of the superior, middle, and inferior rectal arteries. The superior rectal artery, the caudal continuation of the inferior mesenteric artery, enters the pelvis within the sigmoid mesocolon dividing into right and left branches, which are situated behind the rectum and give off branches, which pierce the muscle and supply the mucosa. The right and left branches subsequently anastamose with each other and with the middle and inferior rectal arteries. The middle rectal artery originates from the internal iliac artery and is situated anteromedially to the rectum mainly supplying the muscle. The inferior rectal artery is a branch of the internal prudendal artery and anastomoses with the middle rectal artery at the anorectal junction.
- Venous drainage corresponds to the arterial supply with the superior rectal vein draining into the portal circulation via the inferior mesenteric vein and the middle and inferior rectal veins draining into the internal iliac and internal prudendal veins respectively.
- Lymphatic drainage is to the pararectal or mesorectal lymph nodes. Upper and middle nodes drain into lymphatics which run alongside the superior rectal artery and cranially to nodes accompanying the inferior mesenteric artery. Lower nodes drain into internal iliac nodes via lymphatics, which follow along the middle rectal artery.
- Nerve supply of the rectum is by way of sympathetic nerves derived from the hypogastric plexus and additional nerves from the coeliac plexus which accompany the inferior mesenteric and superior rectal arteries. Parasympathetic nerves arise from S2, 3, and 4 via the splanchnic nerves providing motor function to rectal muscle. Both sympathetic and parasympathetic nerves are accompanied by pain fibres.

# Operative technique: right hemicolectomy

## Indication

Cancers of the caecum, ascending colon, hepatic flexure, and proximal transverse colon.

## Principles

- Aim to resect tumour, lymph nodes and vascular supply *en bloc*.
- Identify tumour and maintain clearance even if required to excise abdominal wall or other locally involved structures.
- Elevate bowel on its embryological mesentery containing its blood vessels, lymphatics, nerves, and associated fat.
- Meticulous dissection between the mesentery and posterior peritoneum is required.

## Procedure

- Ensure correct patient and notes are available.
- Ensure informed consent has been undertaken.
- Ensure CT images are available and have been reviewed in an MDT setting.
- Position patient supine.
- Insert urethral catheter.
- Midline laparotomy incision.
- Open peritoneum.
- Perform exploratory laparotomy including examination of the liver, gallbladder, spleen, stomach, pancreas, small bowel, peritoneum, para-aortic, and mesenteric lymph nodes.
- Palpate greater omentum and remainder of colon to exclude synchronous lesions.
- Examine the pelvic organs.
- Examine the caecum, ascending colon, and transverse colon to identify the tumour.
- Retract the ascending colon medially and divide the peritoneum in the right paracolic gutter. Care is taken to stay anteriorly away from Gerota's fascia.
- Develop the plane between the colon and posterior structures.
- Identify (and protect if possible) the right gonadal vessels.
- Further dissection reveals the right ureter, which should be protected with care.
- Superiorly, dissect between the colon and duodenum (posteriorly). The hepatic flexure is taken down, care is taken here as the small fatty omental perforators have a tendency to bleed. The dissection to the transverse colon. The greater omentum is reflected superiorly and the transverse colon retracted anteriorly. Incision of a single layer of peritoneum open up the same congenital plain that has been entered laterally.

- After the colon is mobilized from its attachments, it should be free on its mesentery which contain the vessels and lymphatics.
- Re-identify the tumour and determine points of subsequent anastomosis – place marking suture.
- Identify the ileo-colic, right colic and right branch of the middle colic vessels.
- Divide the parietal peritoneum overlying the mesentery.
- Clamp, divide, and ligate the ileocolic and right colic vessels close to origin of arteries to ensure maximum lymph node retrieval. The resection can be extended to incorporate the middle colic depending on the position of the tumour.
- Place non-crushing and crushing bowel clamps and divide bowel, or use a GIA stapler
- Approximately 10–20cm proximal to the ileo-caecal valve to the junction between the proximal and middle thirds of the transverse colon should usually be resected.
- Can use linear stapling device or scalpel to divide bowel. Also resect right half of the greater omentum with the specimen.
- Send specimen for histopathological examination.

**Anastomosis** can be hand sewn (usually end-to-end +/– ante-mesenteric slit or oblique transaction for size discrepancy) or stapled, as is preferred by many surgeons.

### Hand sewn
- Place ends in proximity.
- Place stay sutures on mesenteric and anti-mesenteric borders.
- Full thickness or seromuscular bites to anterior layer (various non-absorbable sutures may be used, e.g. vicryl, ethibond, PDS, monocryl.
- Rotate over to place full thickness or seromuscular bites to posterior layer.

### Stapled (usually side-to-side)
- Place ileum and colon side-by-side, and suture anti-mesenteric borders with 3.0 PDS to keep bowel together.
- Make two small holes in each segment of bowel with diathermy.
- Direct linear stapler through each arm heading away from caecum.
- Ensure no bowel or other structures caught in between.
- Engage stapler to anastomose bowel.
- Staple end to close defect.
- Over-sew with 3.0 PDS.

Close mesenteric defect with vicryl, PDS, or prolene suture.

### Closed stapled anastomosis

Alternatively a 2 GIA staple technique can be employed in which the 2 uncut sides of the resection loop are brought side to side at the point of resection. Stay sutures are place and 2 opposing holes are made to introduce a GIA stapler to fashion a side-side anastomosis. A second GIA stapler is placed perpendicular to the anastomosis beyond the defect created and fired. Care is taken to ensure the resulting anastomotic lumen is of good patency. The staple lines should be inspected and over sewn if needed.

- Wash if necessary.
- Mass closure of peritoneum (0 loop PDS or nylon suture).
- Clips or subcutaneous absorbable suture to skin.

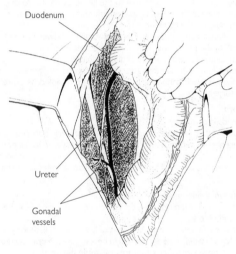

**Fig. 9.3** Right hemicolectomy: posterior relations of right colon. Adapted from McLatchie & Leaper (2006). Reproduced with permission of Oxford University Press © 2006.

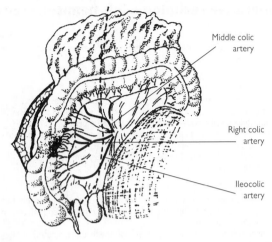

**Fig. 9.4** Extent of resection in right hemicolectomy. Taken from McLatchie & Leaper (2006). Reproduced with permission of Oxford University Press © 2006.

# Operative technique: left hemicolectomy

## Indication

Cancers of the distal transverse colon, splenic flexure, descending colon, sigmoid colon.

## Principles

- Aim to resect tumour, lymph nodes and vascular supply *en bloc*.
- Identify tumour and maintain clearance even if required to excise abdominal wall or other locally involved structures.
- Elevate bowel on its embryological mesentery containing its blood vessels, lymphatics, nerves, and associated fat.
- Meticulous dissection between the mesentery and posterior peritoneum is required.

## Procedure

- Ensure correct patient and notes are available; informed consent has been undertaken; CT images are available and have been reviewed in an MDT setting.
- Position patient in Lloyd–Davies position with approximately 30° hip flexion.
- Insert urethral catheter. Place intermittent calf compressors to decrease risk of deep vein thrombosis.
- Long midline laparotomy incision as will need access to the spleen.
- Open peritoneum.
- Perform exploratory laparotomy including examination of the liver, gallbladder, spleen, stomach, pancreas, small bowel, peritoneum, para-aortic, and mesenteric lymph nodes.
- Palpate greater omentum and remainder of colon to exclude synchronous lesions. Examine the pelvic organs.
- Examine the transverse and descending colon to identify the tumour.
- Remove the small bowel from the abdominal cavity and cover with a pack.
- Retract the descending colon medially and divide the peritoneum along the left abdominal wall (plane of zygosis, white line).
- Develop the plane between the colon and posterior structures. Identify (and protect if possible) the left gonadal vessels.
- Further dissection reveals the left ureter which should be protected with care.
- Superiorly, dissect between the colon and spleen (superiorly) by dividing the phrenocolic ligament. Avoid damage to the spleen or an enforced splenectomy may be required for bleeding.
- Mobilize the sigmoid colon from the side wall. After the colon is mobilized from its attachments, it should be free on its mesentery, which contains the vessels and lymphatics.
- Re-identify the tumour and determine points of subsequent anastomosis – place marking suture.
- Identify the left branch of the middle colic, ascending, and descending branches of the left colic and inferior mesenteric vessels.
- Divide the parietal peritoneum overlying the mesentery.

- Clamp, divide, and ligate vessels close to bowel and close to origin of arteries to ensure maximum lymph node retrieval.
- Place non-crushing and crushing bowel clamps and divide bowel.
- Can use linear stapling device or scalpel to divide bowel. Also resect left half of the greater omentum with the specimen.
- Send specimen for histopathological examination.

### Anastomosis

Usually stapled using a circular stapler introduced via a colostomy or rectally. Alternatively if a hand sewn anastomosis is to be fashioned, then:

- Place ends in proximity.
- Place stay sutures on mesenteric and anti-mesenteric borders.
- Full thickness bites to posterior layer (various non-absorbable sutures may be used, e.g. vicryl, Ethibond, PDS, monocryl.
- Place full thickness or seromuscular bites to anterior layer.
- Close mesenteric defect with vicryl suture. Wash if necessary.
- Mass closure of peritoneum (0 loop PDS or nylon suture).
- Clips or subcutaneous absorbable suture to skin.

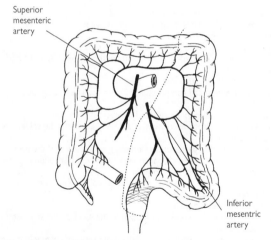

Superior
mesenteric
artery

Inferior
mesentric
artery

**Fig. 9.5** Left hemicolectomy. Taken from McLatchie & Leaper (2006). Reproduced with permission of Oxford University Press © 2006.

# Operative technique: total mesorectal excision (TME) anterior resection

## Indication
Cancers of the distal sigmoid colon and rectum.

## Principles
- Aim to resect tumour, lymph nodes and vascular supply *en bloc* by means of a total mesenteric excision (TME).
- Identify tumour and maintain clearance even if required to excise abdominal wall or other locally involved structures.
- Elevate bowel on its embryological mesentery containing its blood vessels, lymphatics, nerves, and associated fat.
- Meticulous dissection between the mesentery and posterior peritoneum is required.
- A 'high tie' of the inferior mesenteric artery close to its origin at the aorta ensures maximum nodal clearance.

## Procedure
- Ensure correct patient and notes.
- Ensure that CT and MRI scan images are available and have been reviewed at an MDT meeting.
- Ensure informed consent has been undertaken.
- Position patient in Lloyd-Davies position with approximately 30° hip flexion.
- Insert urethral catheter.
- Place intermittent calf compressors to decrease risk of deep vein thrombosis.
- Examine per rectum to assess distal clearance.
- Long midline laparotomy incision as will need access to the spleen.
- Open peritoneum.
- Perform exploratory laparotomy including examination of the liver, gallbladder, spleen, stomach, pancreas, small bowel, peritoneum, para-aortic, and mesenteric lymph nodes.
- Palpate greater omentum and remainder of colon to exclude synchronous lesions.
- Examine the pelvic organs.
- Examine the sigmoid colon and rectum to identify tumour and assess for local invasion.
- Remove the small bowel from the abdominal cavity and cover with a pack.
- Retract the descending colon medially and divide the peritoneum along the left abdominal wall (plane of zygosis, white line).
- Develop the plane between the colon and posterior structures.
- Identify (and protect if possible) the left gonadal vessels.
- Further dissection reveals the left ureter, which should be protected with care.
- Superiorly, dissect between the colon and spleen (superiorly) by dividing the phrenocolic ligament. Avoid damage to the spleen or an enforced splenectomy may be required for bleeding.
- Mobilize the sigmoid colon from the side wall.

- After the colon is mobilized from its attachments, it should be free on its mesentery, which contain the vessels and lymphatics.
- Re-identify the tumour and determine points of subsequent anastomosis – place marking suture.
- Identify the left branch of the middle colic, ascending, and descending branches of the left colic, inferior mesenteric, and sigmoidal vessels.
- Divide the parietal peritoneum overlying the mesentery.
- Clamp, divide, and ligate vessels close to bowel and close to origin of arteries to ensure maximum lymph node retrieval.
- Divide the inferior mesenteric vein either at the same level as the artery or slightly higher level close to the lower border of the pancreas.
- Place non-crushing and crushing bowel clamps, divide proximal bowel, and its mesentery.
- Lift the sigmoid colon vertically to identify the mesorectal fascial plane, the plane of dissection for a total mesorectal excision (TME).
- Identify and preserve the pelvic nerve plexus branches at the level of the sacral promontory.
- Dissect the rectum circumferentially down the mesorectal fascia. Continue the posterior dissection anterior to the presacral fascia preserving the presacral nerves. It is useful to use the St Mark's anterior lipped retractor to help identify and develop the plane with an assistant between the legs.
- Develop the plane laterally and anteriorly taking care not to enter the mesorectal fat.
- Ideal lower clearance is 5cm, although with a low tumour 2cm clearance is acceptable if restorative function is to be achieved in low rectal cancers.
- Can use right-angled stapling device or right-angled clamp, and scalpel to divide bowel.
- Send specimen for histopathological examination fixed in formalin.
- Perform rectal washout usually with povidone-iodine solution.

### Anastomosis
Usually stapled or end-to-end hand-sewn.

*Stapled anastomosis*
- Ensure correct orientation of bowel.
- Determine appropriate size of circular stapler gun (25–31mm) by using a sizing device.
- Place a purse-string non-absorbable (Prolene 0) suture around the proximal bowel tie in the inserted head.
- Insert the circular stapling gun per anal carefully manipulating it towards the end of the rectal stump.
- Open the pin of the stapler to penetrate the rectal stump in the centre and posterior to the staple line.
- Connect the pin to the head of the device ensuring no other tissue is caught up.
- Fire the gun and hold for a few seconds.
- Open the gun and gently rotate it free before carefully removing it and check the completeness of the doughnuts.
- Air test the anastomosis by blowing air per rectum using a rigid sigmoidoscope and look for bubbles in a water filled pelvis.

- Ensure haemostasis, particularly in the pelvis prior to anastomosis, as it is more difficult once the anastomosis has been formed.
- Ensure haemostasis in the region of the left colonic dissection and spleen.
- Examine the anastomosis for adequacy of blood supply and lack of tension. If concerned about the anastomosis consider defunctioning with a loop ileostomy or colostomy.
- Wash and if necessary place a percutaneous drain in the left iliac fossa.
- Mass closure of peritoneum (0 loop PDS or nylon suture) and clips to skin.

*Hand-sewn*

- Place stay sutures on mesenteric and anti-mesenteric borders.
- Full thickness bites to posterior layer (various non-absorbable sutures may be used, e.g. vicryl, Ethibond, PDS, monocryl.
- 'Parachute' the edges so that they lie in apposition.
- Place full thickness bites to anterior layer.
- Aim to invert the anastomosis.

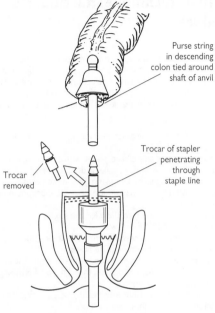

Purse string in descending colon tied around shaft of anvil

Trocar of stapler penetrating through staple line

Trocar removed

**Fig. 9.6** Stapled end-end colorectal anastomosis. Taken from McLatchie & Leaper (2006). Reproduced with permission of Oxford University Press © 2006.

# Operative technique: Hartmann's procedure

## Indication

In the setting of colorectal cancer, this procedure may be considered in cancers of the distal sigmoid colon and rectum, where an anastomosis by way of an anterior resection/sigmoid colectomy is not feasible. This may be in the emergency setting with bowel perforation and faecal contamination, or with largely differing bowel diameters in the case of bowel obstruction.

## Procedure

- The procedure is the same as an anterior resection in terms of left colonic mobilization.
- The rectal stump is usually closed, either with a right-angled stapler or it may be hand-sewn with a single or double layer. If not possible to close, a drain may be placed through it lying in the pelvis.
- The patient should be pre-marked for the most appropriate position for the colostomy.
- Make a circular skin incision to allow for the stoma.
- Dissect down to the abdominal wall.
- Divide the anterior rectus sheath with a cruciate incision.
- Separate the rectus abdominis muscle fibres.
- Divide the peritoneum and insert two fingers to stretch stoma.
- Gently feed descending/sigmoid colon through stoma ensuring no tearing or twisting of mesentery.
- Trim the end of the bowel, ensuring healthy vascular mucosa is present.
- Close abdomen as with anterior resection.
- Suture the stoma with 3.0 undyed vicryl sutures and place a stoma bag over site.

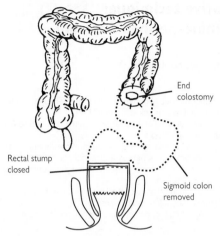

End colostomy

Rectal stump closed

Sigmoid colon removed

**Fig. 9.7** Hartmann's procedure. Taken from McLatchie & Leaper (2006). Reproduced with permission of Oxford University Press © 2006.

# Operative technique: abdomino-perineal excision

## Indication

Low rectal or anal canal cancers.

## Principles

- Aim to resect tumour, lymph nodes, and vascular supply *en bloc* by means of a total mesenteric excision (TME).
- Identify tumour and maintain clearance even if required to excise locally involved structures.
- Elevate proximal bowel on its embryological mesentery containing its blood vessels, lymphatics, nerves, and associated fat.
- Meticulous dissection between the mesentery and posterior peritoneum is required.
- A 'high tie' of the inferior mesenteric artery, close to its origin at the aorta ensures maximum nodal clearance.
- Avoid 'coning' of dissection and entering the mesorectum.

## Procedure

- Ensure correct patient and notes.
- Ensure that CT and MRI scan images are available and have been reviewed at an MDT meeting.
- Ensure informed consent has been undertaken.
- Position patient in Lloyd–Davies position with approximately 30° hip flexion.
- Insert urethral catheter and place intermittent calf compressors to decrease risk of deep vein thrombosis.
- Examine per rectum and in the male, retract the scrotum clear of the anus by way of tape or a silk suture.
- Suture the anus closed with a purse string.
- Long midline laparotomy incision as will need access to the spleen.
- Open peritoneum.
- Perform exploratory laparotomy including examination of the liver, gallbladder, spleen, stomach, pancreas, small bowel, peritoneum, para-aortic, and mesenteric lymph nodes.
- Palpate greater omentum and remainder of colon to exclude synchronous lesions.
- Examine the pelvic organs and the rectum to identify tumour and assess for local invasion.
- Remove the small bowel from the abdominal cavity and cover with a pack.
- Retract the descending colon medially and divide the peritoneum along the left abdominal wall (plane of zygosis, white line).
- Develop the plane between the colon and posterior structures.
- Identify (and protect if possible) the left gonadal vessels.
- Further dissection reveals the left ureter, which should be protected with care.
- Mobilize the sigmoid colon from the side wall.

- After the colon is mobilized from its attachments, it should be free on its mesentery, which contain the vessels and lymphatics.
- Identify the colic, inferior mesenteric, sigmoidal, and superior rectal vessels.
- Divide the parietal peritoneum overlying the mesentery.
- Clamp, divide, and ligate vessels close to bowel, and close to origin of arteries to ensure maximum lymph node retrieval.
- Divide the inferior mesenteric vein either at the same level as the artery or slightly higher level close to the lower border of the pancreas.
- Place non-crushing and crushing bowel clamps, divide the sigmoid colon and its mesentery, either between crushing and non-crushing bowel clamps or with a stapler.
- Lift the sigmoid colon vertically to identify the mesorectal fascial plane, the plane of dissection for a total mesorectal excision (TME).
- Identify and preserve the pelvic nerve plexus branches at the level of the sacral promontory.
- Dissect the rectum circumferentially down the mesorectal fascia. Continue the posterior dissection anterior to the presacral fascia preserving the presacral nerves. It is useful to use the St Mark's anterior lipped retractor to help identify and develop the plane with an assistant between the legs.
- Develop the plane laterally and anteriorly taking care not to enter the mesorectal fat and continue to as far down posteriorly as possible, at least down to the inferior aspect of the coccyx.
- The perineal component of the operation requires an elliptical incision to include the anal canal. The anterior landmark is the midpoint from the anus to the urethral bulb and posteriorly at the coccyx. The shield incision proposed by some may leave an anterior dog-ear.
- The incision is continued through the ischorectal fat and self-retaining retractors are used to expose the plane down to the levatores.
- The anococcygeal raphé is incised anterior to the coccyx.
- Retract the anus anteriorly and incise Waldeyer's fascia transversely.
- Separate the transverse perineal muscles from the external anal sphincter.
- Divide puborectalis and pubococcygeus muscles using a finger between the rectum and anterior structures to aid dissection.
- Care must be taken to avoid entry into the rectum or closely approximated urogenital structures.
- The perineal dissection thus meets the abdominal dissection, and the specimen may be removed, preserved in formalin, and sent for histopathological examination.
- The perineal wound is closed in layers and skin can be closed with either a subcutaneous absorbable suture or, if at risk of breakdown, an interrupted non-absorbable suture may be used.
- It has been shown that the use of neoadjuvant chemoradiotherapy, advocated for low rectal cancers, greatly increases the risk of wound breakdown.
- The use of myocutaneous flaps involving rectus abdominis, gracilis, and gluteus has been proposed with variable results.
- The patient should be premarked for the most appropriate position for the left iliac fossa end colostomy.

- Make a circular skin incision to allow for the stoma.
- Dissect down to the abdominal wall.
- Divide the anterior rectus sheath with a cruciate incision.
- Separate the rectus abdominis muscle fibres.
- Divide the peritoneum and insert two fingers to stretch stoma.
- Gently feed the sigmoid colon through stoma ensuring no tearing or twisting of mesentery.
- Trim the end of the bowel, ensuring healthy vascular mucosa is present.
- Close abdomen as with anterior resection.
- Suture the stoma with 3.0 undyed vicryl sutures and place a stoma bag over.

## Other operative techniques: laparoscopic resection

### Overview

In principle, laparoscopic surgery should be the same procedure, but done with laparoscopic instruments, and should have the same oncological and functional outcome as that achieved by open surgery.

Minimally invasive surgery involves introducing carbon dioxide gas into the abdomen allowing instruments to be introduced to mobilize and resect bowel.

Proponents have been claimed the following in comparing laparoscopic with open surgery:
- Less post-operative pain.
- Faster recovery.
- Better cosmesis.
- Shorter hospital stay.
- Earlier return to work.
- Potential economic benefits.
  Negative points include:
- Steep learning curve.
- Longer operating time, at least at first.
- Technically challenging.
- May be more difficult to control haemorrhage and necessitate conversion to open procedure.
- Less ability to palpate organs for evidence of metastasis.
- Long-term data still not available for recurrence and survival.
- Early reports of port-site recurrence.
- Require large outlay of funds to ensure appropriate operating theatre and equipment is available.

## Pre-operative preparation

- Present laparoscopic option with advantages and disadvantages, and potential need to covert to open procedure as part of obtaining informed consent.
- May be considered as a component of an 'enhanced recovery programme' aiming for early discharge. This requires pre-operative counselling and altering the expectations of the patient.
- Consider the use of mechanical bowel preparation. Differences in opinion exist as to whether this should be used routinely.
- Ensure correct patient with notes and appropriate investigations are available.
- Ensure patient has been discussed appropriately at an MDT meeting.
- Pre-operative deep vein thrombosis prophylaxis should be given, as for open procedure.
- Operating room should be equipped appropriately with table able to rotate while ensuring patient stability and safety.
- Check equipment including camera and gas.
- Nasogastric tube and urinary catheter should be inserted
- Usually, at least two monitors should be available at the eye level of the surgeons.
- Surgeon and camera holder should be on the same side and first assistant should be on other side where the pathology is present.
- As palpation is not possible to identify the tumour, visualization is aided by pre-operative colonoscopic marking.

# Laparoscopic right hemicolectomy

## Principles

- In principle, similar to open procedure with same objectives of resection of right colonic lesions including associated lymphovascular structures.
- In the laparoscopic procedure, the vessels can be divided prior to bowel mobilization.

## Procedure

- Prepare patient as discussed earlier.
- Position monitor for operating surgeon to view on right side of patient.
- Open technique should be used for safe pneumoperitoneum using Hassan technique with dissection through the linea alba in the midline. Alternatively, some surgeons use a Veress needle or Colchester direct insertion technique for gas insufflation to 12mmHg pressure.
- Port-sites depend on surgeon preference, but usually are placed at the umbilicus, supra-pubic, and right and left flanks.
- May use either 0 or 30° laparoscope.
- Can use laparoscopic ultrasound to examine the liver for metastasis.
- The patient is positioned head-down and right side up to facilitate exposure of the caecum, right colon, and terminal ileum.
- The ileocolic, right colic, and right branch of the middle colic vessels are clipped, and ligated or stapled with an endo-stapling device.
- Dissect the caecum and right colon as with the open procedure, retracting the bowel medially, and identifying the right gonadal vessels and ureter.
- In order to visualize the hepatic flexure and transverse colon, the patient is rotated into a head-up position.
- Atraumatic forceps are used to grasp mesentery and bowel, and dissection is less haemorrhagic with the use of the harmonic scalpel. It is preferable not to hold the bowel directly to avoid trauma.
- The bowel is transected, transverse colon followed by terminal ileum using a linear stapler. A grasper is placed on the bowel that is to be exteriorized to aid retrieval.
- Side-to-side anastomosis is usually by way of a linear stapler. This can be performed laparoscopically or extracorporally.
- The specimen is retrieved through a small incision using a wound protector and plastic bag for removal. This is to avoid the previous concern of intra-abdominal, port-site and wound metastasis.
- The mesenteric defect is closed with clips or sutures.
- Mass closure of the RIF, midline or transverse right flank incision is performed. A pneumoperitoneum can then be re-established to check the mass closure suture line.
- Wounds are closed with non-absorbable prolene or absorbable monocryl sutures.
- The nasogastric tube may be removed after the procedure.

# Laparoscopic left hemicolectomy

## Principles

Similar to open procedure with the same indications and principles, with resection of tumour and associated lymphovascular structures.

## Procedure

- Ensure correct patient and notes are available. Ensure informed consent has been undertaken. Ensure CT images are available and have been reviewed in an MDT setting.
- Position patient in Lloyd–Davies position with approximately 30° hip flexion.
- Insert urethral catheter. Place intermittent calf compressors to decrease risk of deep vein thrombosis.
- Surgeon and camera operator stand on patient's right.
- Develop pneumoperitoneum with insufflated carbon dioxide.
- Place ports in a semicircle around umbilical port.
- Rotate patient in a head-down and left side up position to move small bowel away.
- A full peritoneal exploration is performed, small bowel is moved to ensure the aortic bifurcation can be seen.
- For a true oncological radical resection the dissection should proceed from the sacral promontory upwards along the right side of the aorta to the duodenojejunal flexure opening the sigmoid mesocolon at its base, from the medial side dissection should be along Toldt's fascia.
- The sigmoid colon is retracted anteriorly and to the left, and the inferior mesenteric artery (IMA) and inferior mesenteric vein (IMV) are visualized. The artery is then skeletonized and divided at its origin.
- Once the artery is divided a plane of dissection immediately posterior to the artery reveals the left hypogastric nerve that can be swept downwards to preserve bladder and sexual function.
- The inferior mesenteric vein can then be clipped/divided.
- Distal dissection should proceed to the superior rectal branch of the IMA. The colon is then retracted medially to enable lateral dissection along the peritoneal reflection. It is important to apply good retraction so that the space is visualized well enabling dissection off the left paracolic gutter leading to the phrenicocolic ligament and the spleen.
- Superiorly the left branch of the middle colic, ascending and descending branches of the left colic should be identified and clipped or divided with ligature.
- An alternative approach is to formally follow a plain of dissection along the inferior mesenteric vein to its confluence with the splenic vein
- Alternatively, with a mobile specimen the all ligation other than the inferior mesenteric pedicle can take place extracorporally, although this will result in a reduced lymphadenectomy. Identify proximal and distal sites for transection.
- Use a linear stapler to divide the bowel.
- Anastomosis can be performed laparoscopically or externally as for an open resection.

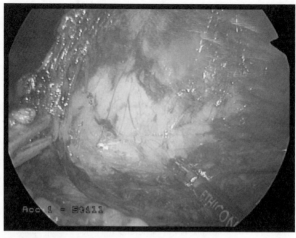

**Fig. 9.8** Dissection along Toldt's fascia.

# Laparoscopic total mesorectal excision (TME): anterior resection

## Principles

The principles of excising the rectum with its lymphovascular supply *en bloc* must be adhered to when performing the procedure laparoscopically.

## Procedure

- The patient must be positioned very carefully, particularly as this potentially long procedure may risk neurovascular damage.
- Trendelenburg position with 15–25° rotation and 5–10° right tilt. Lloyd–Davies to allow access to the perineum facilitating circular stapler insertion per anal.
- Legs to be separated to allow access for assistant and instruments.
- NG tube and urinary catheter to be inserted.
- Heating system in place and intermittent calf compression devices to minimize risk of DVT.
- *Port placement:* supra-umbilicus 12mm, 2 ports in the right mid-clavicular line (1 at the level of the umbilicus and 1 in the right iliac fossa), left mid-clavicular line at the level of the umbilicus, suprapubic, right mid-clavicular line below the sub-costal margin.
- 0–30°scopes may be used.
- After a general laparoscopy, ultrasound assessment of the liver may be performed.
- Pre-operative marking of the tumour is necessary or else intra-operative endoscopy is required to identify the position.
- The patient should be in a sufficiently head down position to enable removal of small bowel loops from the pelvis using an atraumatic grasper, such as a Johan's.
- In females a prolene suture is introduced suprapubically to retract the uterus anteriorly out of the pelvis. This is released at the end of the procedure.
- Incise the parietal peritoneum over the sigmoid mesentery to develop the plane to identify the course of the IMA.
- The IMA is divided close about 1cm from its origin including the left colic artery, after the identification and preservation of the superior hypogastric nerve. Preservation of the left colic artery has been proposed to preserve the blood supply of the anastomosis.
- The IMV is identified to the left of the IMA and divided. Between clips, haemolocks, or ligature.

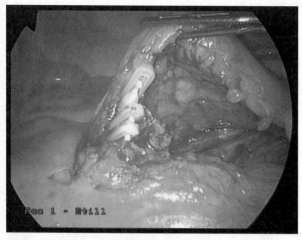

**Fig. 9.9** Anterolateral retraction of the colon exposing the Inferior mesenteric artery with haemostatic clips *in situ*.

- Mobilize the sigmoid colon either medial to lateral or lateral to medial.
- Identify and preserve the left gonadal vessels and left ureter, and avoid damage to the hypogastric plexus.
- The pelvic dissection of the mesorectal fascia is similar in principle to that seen in the open procedure with care to be taken to avoid injury to the prostate, seminal vesicles, and superior hypogastric plexus nerves.
- Start developing the plane posteriorly, anterior to the presacral fascia followed by anterolateral dissection. Care must be taken to ensure coning of the mesorectal specimen does not take place.
- Mobilization of the splenic flexure is often necessary to enable enough length for the anastomosis to be tension-free, and can be performed medial to lateral or vice versa.
- The bowel is divided proximally (may be performed after exteriorization) and distally using a stapler, aiming to ensure at least 2cm distal clearance. A grasper is placed on the bowel to be exteriorized, whilst the pneumoperitoneum is still in place to assist retrieval once an incision is made.
- Place the specimen in a plastic bag for retrieval to prevent tumour dissemination, and remove using a small incision placed either in the left iliac fossa or lower midline. A wound protector may be used.
- The proximal bowel is exteriorized through the same incision to introduce the head of the circular stapling device and a purse-string suture is applied as with the open procedure. A suture can be applied to the end of the spike of the staple gun to assist retrieval laparoscopically once it has pierced the distal stump.

- The gun is then introduced per anal and the ends are joined laparoscopically. Careful anterior retraction of the vaginal vault by an assistant is helpful to ensure its exclusion from the anastomosis.
- Consider the formation of a defunctioning stoma (loop ileostomy or colostomy) for low anatomoses or those in whom neoadjuvant chemoradiotherapy has been given.

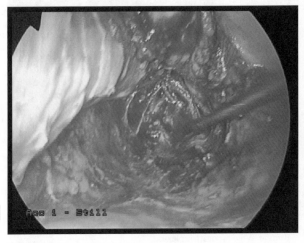

**Fig. 9.10** Pelvic mesorectal dissection to the pelvic floor with the rectum retracted anterolaterally to the left.

# Local excision for rectal cancer

- Curative surgery for rectal cancer aims to provide adequate oncological clearance whilst minimizing the morbidity and mortality associated with the procedure.
- This traditionally involves total mesorectal excision (TME) with anterior resection, and anastomosis or abdominoperineal excision of the rectum with end colostomy formation.
- Local excision has been proposed as an option for patients with early rectal carcinoma in whom radical surgery and its complications may be avoided, as well as for patients in high-risk groups, such as the elderly and those with significant co-morbidity who may not be suitable for administration of general anaesthesia.
- A locally excised specimen is appropriate only if it includes an adequate margin of resected normal tissue, if the tumour grade is not aggressive, and if the disease has not metastasized to loco-regional lymph nodes or distant sites.
- Radiological techniques for staging rectal cancer including endo-anal ultrasound (EUS) and pelvic magnetic resonance imaging (MRI) have been used in determining selection patients for whom local excision is appropriate.
- Commonly used techniques for local excision of low lying rectal cancers include transanal excision and transanal endoscopic microsurgery (TEM).
- In addition to local excision procedures, the use of adjuvant therapy in the form of chemo and radiotherapy has the potential to provide added protection against disease recurrence in those undergoing local excision of early rectal cancers. Despite these improvements in the local curative treatments for early rectal cancer, the main challenge remains the selection of suitable patients.
- Tumour grade, stage, size, and position are all known to be important determinants of success following local resection of early (T1) rectal cancers, but despite close patient selection on the basis of these, recurrence rates have been reported to be as high as 18%.

# Post-operative care and complications

Post-operative care

- Ensure regular review by surgical and anaesthetic teams post-operatively.
- Intensive care or high dependency care may be indicated in some situations.
- Two additional doses of antibiotics are adequate in addition to the dose given at induction. If clean procedure, one dose is sufficient.
- Fluid balance must be carefully monitored.
- Low blood pressure may be a reflection of epidural and not hypovolaemia; therefore, beware of over-filling patient.
- *Monitor urine output:* aim for >0.5mL/kg.
- Respiratory assessment is essential to avoid basal atelectasis and subsequent chest infection.
- *Pain relief:* epidural or patient controlled analgesia assist with pain-free inspiration and prevention of chest sepsis.
- *Nasogastric tube:* monitor output to guide fluid and electrolyte management. May help lessen nausea and vomiting. Some evidence that NG tubes prolong ileus.
- *Nutritional support:* early enteral nutrition is important, and feeding by nasogastric tube or oral intake can be commenced almost immediately post-operatively in most cases.
- Ongoing nutrition support may be required until the patient is eating normally.
- Early mobilization is important to decrease DVTs and chest infections.
- Remove central venous lines early to avoid infection.
- Remove urinary catheters when patient is mobile to avoid sepsis.
- Continue subcutaneous low molecular weight heparin, while patient is hospitalized.
- *Ileus is not uncommon post-abdominal surgery:* correct treatable causes.
- Check post-operative Hb, urea, and electrolytes.
- The enhanced recovery programme includes a reduced volume of normal saline infusion, early removal of NG tubes, good pain control, and early mobilization.

Complications

*Immediate and early*

- *Anaesthetic complications:* drug reaction, cardiac (ischaemia, arrythmia), and respiratory.
- *Renal:* failure.
- Primary, reactionary, and secondary haemorrhage.
- Cardiac failure and pulmonary oedema.
- Injury to autonomic nerves.
- Injury to small or large bowel.
- *Ureteric injury:* requires recognition and repair over pig-tailed stent.
- Damage to pelvic organs.
- *Trauma to vessels:* gonadals, iliacs.

- *Atelectasis:* caused by hypoventilation with pain on inspiration – may develop subsequent pneumonia and respiratory failure i.
- *Thrombo-embolism:* DVT and PE.
- Urinary retention after removal of catheter.
- *Urine infection:* with prolonged catheterization.
- *Intestinal obstruction:* usually ileus, but mechanical obstruction also reported.
- *Stoma:* bleeding, ischaemia.
- *Anastomotic leak:* may result in generalized peritonitis if not localized. After high anterior resection, leak rate is about 5%. Rate increases as anastomosis moves further below the peritoneal reflection (up to 25%). This may be even higher radiologically. Good technique limits this complication, although does not remove it altogether. Aim to ensure tension-free and vascular anastomosis with good suturing technique.
- Anastomotic bleeding has been reported.
- Pelvic collection/abscess.
- *Wound dehiscence:* superficial relatively common; deep rare – usually secondary to intra-abdominal sepsis.
- Ischaemic bowel.
- *C. difficile* infection.

*Late*
- *Sexual dysfunction – males:* erectile problems (damage to nervi erigentes), failure of ejaculation (damage to presacral nerves); females: dyspareunia.
- *Stoma:* herniation, retraction, stenosis.
- *Anastomotic stricture formation:* usually secondary to fibrosis.
- Increased frequency of bowel actions.
- Urgency.
- Incontinence.
- Complications of adjuvant therapy.
- Local +/– distant recurrence.

# Adjuvant therapy

## Overview

- Post-operative chemotherapy, targeted therapy and radiotherapy after surgery with curative intent.
- An important goal in the management of colorectal cancer is the identification of which patients will be cured by surgery alone and which patients may benefit from adjuvant therapies.
- Need to consider risk of local recurrence and risk of distant metastasis.
- Chemotherapeutic agents have been identified, which may be used in conjunction with surgery to decrease recurrence and improve survival.
- New anti-angiogenic compounds have also been introduced with benefit to CRC patients.
- All patients should be discussed at an MDT, at which the attendance of an oncologist is essential.
- Careful consideration must be given and full informed consent should be obtained in all systemic treatments after a full and detailed discussion, more so if therapy is given in the context of a clinical trial after appropriate ethical approval.

## Chemotherapy for colorectal cancer

- Chemotherapy has a definite and effective role in the management of CRC.
- A full discussion is necessary between the clinician and patient regarding risk of recurrence, aims of proposed therapy, alternative treatments, specific risks, and side-effects.
- Commonly used chemotherapeutic agents are cardiotoxic and nephrotoxic, so an assessment of patient co-morbidities is required.
- It is necessary to consider patient preferences in terms of route of administration, necessity for in patient care and transport to and from treatment centre.
- Improved survival has been demonstrated by use of post-operative systemic adjuvant chemotherapy in node positive Dukes' C cancers. Meta-analysis suggests that 6-month treatment with 5-fluorouracil (5-FU) and folinic acid (FA) can increase 5-year disease-free survival from 42 to 58%, and overall survival from 51 to 64% when given after surgery.
- Current guidelines make no differentiation between rectal and colonic disease.
- Oral versions of 5-FU, in particular capecitabine, have been shown to have comparable efficacy and safety profiles to the intravenous drug, and are preferred by patients who do not need intra-venous access.
- The addition of oxaliplatin significantly reduces the relapse rate when compared with 5-FU/FA alone in two randomized trials (MOSAIC and the NSABP C-07 trials) and is approval by the UK National Institute for Health and Clinical Excellence (NICE) for node-positive CRC after potentially curative surgical resection.
- The benefit of chemotherapy for node-negative CRC is not so clear. The IMPACT trial demonstrated no benefit in overall survival although the NSABP trials C-01 and C-04 did show a 5% absolute reduction in 5-year mortality. Also, the UK QUASAR 1 study demonstrated a 4% improvement in survival with 5-FU/FA chemotherapy in patients under 70 years of age. The MOSAIC trial also showed a benefit in Dukes'

B patient with the addition of oxaliplatin, although this is not current standard practice (Table 9.4).
- It is possible to use other poor prognostic factors for recurrence and increased mortality in order to identify 'good Bs' and 'bad Bs' to further sub-stratify patients including T4 or obstructed/perforated cancers, poor differentiation, mucinous tumours, vascular, and peri-neural invasion. Detailed counselling of patients is necessary before providing or withholding treatment or entering them into a controlled trial.
- The COIN study is currently evaluating the use of cetuximab with XELOX in an adjuvant context (see metastatic CRC below).

**Table 9.4** Adjuvant Rx for node negative disease

| Stage | Regime |
|-------|--------|
| (Tis, T1, T2) N0M0 | None |
| T3, N0, M0 low risk | *Consider* capecitabine, 5-FU/FA, **or** FOLFOX, **or** clinical trial, **or** observe |
| T3N0M0 high risk **or** T4N0M0 **or** T3 with localized perforation or unclear margins | FOLFOX **or** capecitabine **or** clinical trial **or** observe |

*High risk features for systemic recurrence*
Grade 3–4/lymphovascular or perineural invasion/bowel obstruction/<12 nodes examined (Table 9.5).

**Table 9.5** Node positive disease

| Stage | Regime |
|-------|--------|
| T1–3, N1–2 M0 T4 N1-2 M0 | FOLFOX **or** capecitabine **or** 5-FU/FA as tolerated |

**Treatment of loco-regional recurrent disease**
- Evidence for the treatment of loco-regional recurrences is not convincing for a particular definitive mode of management.
- In the absence of distant disease, consideration should be given to multi-modality treatment involving radiotherapy (if not given previously), chemotherapy and possible radical salvage surgery.

**Inoperable primary disease**
- Tumours (usually rectal) may be considered inoperable for a variety of reasons. The most common is a large, locally advanced cancer invading or in close proximity to major vascular structures, for example, iliac vessels.
- Patients should be considered for primary combination chemoradiotherapy with repeat imaging to re-assess operability. If still inoperable, palliative chemoradiotherapy may offer palliative symptomatic control.
- These patients should still be considered for a palliative stoma formation or colonic stent if obstruction is likely to intervene and the patient is deemed fit for a procedure.

# Metastatic colorectal disease

Metastases can be:
- Synchronous: metastases known at time of initial diagnosis/resection.
- Metachronous: metastases found after treatment with curative intentresectable with curative intent or irresectable.

## Operable metastatic disease
- Patients with metastatic disease should be discussed in an MDT meeting, preferably in the presence of a hepato-biliary or thoracic surgeon.
- Evidence is clearer for the benefit of hepatic metastatic resection in terms of improved 5-year survival than for pulmonary metastases. 5-year survival 50% post-resection of colorectal liver mets.
- It is not clear whether chemotherapy should be given pre- or post-operatively in the case of metastatic disease.
- Mostly, primary colorectal resection would precede metastatic surgery and usually adjuvant chemotherapy would follow surgical management.
- The ongoing UK-based international phase III trial, EORTC/GITCCG 40983, is currently investigating the relative merits of pre-operative versus post-operative chemotherapy in metastatic disease.
- There is no convincing evidence for the benefit of extra-mesenteric lymphadenectomy.
- Resectability criteria (see Chapter 6 'Liver and biliary cancers' p. 313) criteria evolving, emphasis. Negative surgical margins whilst maintaining liver reserve, rather than number of metastases.

## Irresectable synchronous metastases
Some may be deemed resectable following systemic therapy; therefore, management options are:
- ***Primary systemic chemotherapy:*** FOLFOX, FOLFIRI, XELOX +/– BV if metastases are deemed resectable plan synchronous or staged colectomy and metastasectomy. If not treat according to advanced metastatic protocol.
- Consider colon resection +/– radiofrequency ablation particularly if anaemic or high risk of obstruction.

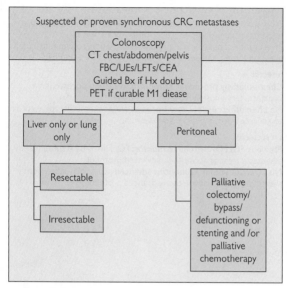

**Fig. 9.11** Management of resectable synchronous metastases.

**Table 9.6** Resectable synchronous liver or lung only mets

| Treatment | Adjuvant |
| --- | --- |
| Colectomy + synchronous **or** subsequent metastectomy or | Advanced chemotherapy regime 6 months **or** |
| Neoadjuvant XELOX, FOLFOX, FOLFIRI +/– BV + synchronous **or** staged colectomy + metastasectomy **or** | Hepatic artery infusion +/– 5-FU IV **or** |
| Colectomy + FOLFOX, FOLFIRI, XELOX +/– BV and staged metastasectomy | Short course chemotherapy and observation particularly if previous neoadjuvant Rx |

Management of metachronous metastases
- Progressive disease detected by serially elevated CEA or definitive evidence of metastases on CT or MRI.
- Investigation should include physical examination, colonoscopy, and CT chest, abdomen, and pelvis if negative arrange PET scan/PET-CT.

*If resectable*
- ***Chemotherapy preceding 12 months:*** resection or resection + hepatic artery infusion Rx (liver mets only).
- ***No chemotherapy >12 months:*** as above or chemotherapy according to advanced protocol prior to resection.

*If irresectable*
- ***Previous FOLFOX within 12 months:*** FOLFIRI +-BV if subsequently resectable treat as above then advanced protocol.
- ***No FOLFOX within 12 months:*** advanced protocol if subsequently resectable treat as above then advanced protocol.

# Chemotherapy and targeted therapy for advanced metastatic disease

- Estimates of metastases at presentation 20–55%.
- 50% of patients apparent complete excision develop metastases.
- 50% of metastatic disease restricted to liver.
- 10% potentially resectable/14% chemotherapy renders liver metastases resectable. Majority therefore proceed to advanced metastatic disease.

*Aim*
- Palliative non-curative.
- Tumour regression, reduced time to tumour progression (TTP), improved overall survival (OS) and quality of life.
- Reduction of metastatic load and metabolic demand.
- If untreated only 50% survive beyond 6 months. Survival beyond 2 years is rare.

*Traditional Rx: 5-fluorouracil + folinic acid*
- 5-FU used for almost 50 years (1958). Tumour regression 20% patients. Median survival 6–12 months. Improved quality of life. Performance status is the best predictor of survival in patients treated with palliative 5-FU chemotherapy.
- The last 5 years have seen the approval of 5 new drugs that have made a massive impact on the efficacy and complexity of treating mCRC patients.

*Cytotoxic drugs*
- **5-FU (IV) folinic acid (FA):** multiple approaches to administration:
  - bolus regimes vs. infusions and combination;
  - Mayo – bolus on 5 consecutive days every 4 weeks;
  - Nordic FU/FA – days 1 + 2 every 2 weeks;
  - De Gramont – modulated infusion FA, bolus FU, and prolonged infusion FU (24–48h); toxicity similar or less than bolus;
  - infusion improves RR, TTP, and OS.
- **Capecitabine (Xeloda®) (po):** oral precursor to 5-FU is equivalent to its intravenous counterpart in terms of efficacy and safety with better tolerance by patients. Metabolized in liver to 5-deoxy-5-fluorocytosine and doxifluridine, which is converted by thymidine phosphorylase, found in high concentrations in tumour tissue, to 5-FU.
- **Irinotecan:** topoisomerase inhibitor derived from Chinese happy tree. First major addition to FU/FA. New era combination Rx 1998. Increases OS 3 months FU/FA resistant pts used as a single 2nd line agent following FU/FA.
- **Oxaliplatin:** platinum-based drug that forms DNA adducts. European approval 1999, USA 2004 (see Table 9.7):
  - 5-FU + FA + oxaliplatin = **FOLFOX.**
  - 5-FU + FA + irinotecan = **FOLFIRI.**

**Table 9.7** FU/FA regimen

|  | Bolus | Infusion | Capecitabine | UFT/FA |
|---|---|---|---|---|
| Oxaliplatin | FLOX$_{Nordic}$ | FOLFOX | XELOC or | TEGAFOX |
|  | FLOX$_{US}$ | FUFOX | CAPOX |  |
|  | bFOL |  |  |  |
| Irinotecan | FLIRI | FOLFIRI | XELIRI or | TE |
|  | IFL |  | CAPIRI |  |

- *OS:* 5-FU/FA max 6–12 months RR 12–23%, FOLFOX max. 20 months RR 34–54%, FOLFIRI max. 21.5 months RR 35–56%, sequential Rx doublet: max 24 months. TTP FU/FA 4–6 months first line doublet 6–12%. Doublet 1st + 2nd line: almost 40% survival at 2 years.
- When compared head to head FOLFOX and FOLFIRI are signifcantly better than 5-FU/FA, but similar to each other in terms of RR, OS and TTP. The choice between them depends on local guidelines and their toxicity profiles.
- *How long should Rx continue?* FU/FA era: continue until disease progression. Initially used for doublets. *Cumulative toxicity high:* drug holidays. Intermittent infusions do not compromise efficacy. Non-progressive mCRC break after 4 months + surveillance + 2nd/3rd line on progression.

## Targeted mAbs
Bevacizumab (Avastin, BV) targets VEGF, inhibiting angiogenesis, reducing tumour growth and increasing drug cytotoxic drug delivery. The inhibition of production of tumour blood vessels that have deranged architecture also increases tumour penetrance of cytotoxic drugs

### Key trials
- *AVF 0780 FU/FA + BV high dose vs. low dose:* low dose better: RR 40 vs. 24% TTP 9 vs. 6 months OS 21 vs. 16 months. FUFA alone in separate study by same group: RR 17%, TTP 5.2 months, OS 13.8 months
- *TREE 1 and TREE2 looked at bFOl, XELOX and FOLFOX without and with BV, respectively:* the addition of BV improved all 3 parameters. In the case of FOLFOX + BV RR53%, TTP 10 months and OS 26 months were found compared with 43%, 8.7 and 19.2 months with FOLFOX alone.
- *The toxicity profile for BV:* includes hypertension, proteinuria, epistaxis, and thrombosis. Thromboembolic events, including myocardial ischaemia, transient ischaemic cerebral attacks and cerebrovascular accidents. Poor wound healing and haemorrhage.
- In the UK NICE have not recommended the use of BV outside clinical trials on a cost effectiveness basis. It is part of the standard protocols of most other countries.

*Cetuximab (Erbitux®, CX) and panitumumab (Vertibix®) targets EGFR*

- *Cetuximab:* chimeric IgG1 monoclonal antibody inhibits epidermal growth factor receptor (EGFR).USA FDA approval 2004: Cetuximab.
- Blocks downstream signalling of EGFR leading to impaired cell growth and proliferation induces antibody dependent cellular cytotoxicity (ADCC). EGFR intracellular signalling cascade stimulates.
- Cell proliferation, protection from apoptosis, loss of differentiation, angiogenesis, cell migration, metastasis formation, all the key processes involved in tumorigenesis. In normal cells: tightly controlled.
- Loss of the regulation of EGFR signalling pathways through over expression and/or gene amplification of EGFR.
- Invasive cancers dependant on EGFR signalling for support of tumour cell motility and survival.

*Key trials*

- *Third line therapy:* BOND 1 and 2 addition of CX to irinotecan improves RR, TTP, and OS. No improvement with addition of BV to CX as third line agent.. EVEREST – escalating CxIri vs. classical CxIri; final data awaited.
- *First line therapy:* ACROBAT FOLFOXCx RR 81%, TTP 12.3 months OS 30.6% excellent results, but not conducted as a head to head study. Final results of FOLFOX/FOLFIRI vs. FOLFOXCx/FOLFIRICx awaited.
- Interestingly, tumour response is not dependent on EGFR positivity, but does correlate with the extent of the acneiform rash that is associated with the use of CX.

**Table 9.8** Overall algorithm: 1. Patients who can tolerate intensive Rx

| 1st Line | 2nd Line | 3rd Line | 4th Line |
|---|---|---|---|
| FOLFOX + BV **or** XELOX + BV | FOLFIRI **or** irinotecan **or** FOLFIRI + CX | Irinotecan + CX | |
| FOLFIRI + BV | FOLFOX **or** XELOX **or** Irinotecan + CX | Irinotecan + CX | |
| | Irinotecan + CX | FOLFOX **or** XELOX | |
| 5-FU/FA + BV | FOLFOX or XELOX **or** | Irinotecan | Irinotecan + CX |
| | Irinotecan **or** FOLFIRI | Irinotecan if tolerated + CX | |

- *For those who cannot tolerate intensive Rx:* Capecitabine +/– BV or 5-FU/FA +/– BV, and reassess functional status and proceed either to protocol above or supportive care.

# Interventional palliative therapies

## Overview

- Treatments for patients deemed incurable should be aimed at improving quality of life.
- Discussion should be undertaken in an MDT setting.
- Patients, relatives and carers should be active participants.
- Aim to provide symptomatic relief and to treat complications of disease – e.g. bleeding, bowel obstruction, bleeding.
- May be considered as a component of palliative care, including psycho-social support, chemoradiotherapy, analgesia, etc., as managed by palliative care physicians and specialist nurses.

## Colonic stents

- Indications include actual or imminent bowel obstruction as a definitive palliative procedure or, as a bridge to formal surgical procedure, either bowel resection or palliative colostomy formation (Fig. 9.12).
- Self expanding metallic stents (SEMS) have a strong structure – either steel or nitinol (nickel and titanium alloy) with a memory, enabling return to a preformed structure 2–5 days after placement.
- Stents are usually placed by an endoscopist and interventional radiologist working together with or without fluoroscopic guidance passing the stent over a guide-wire through the luminal narrowing.
- Re-obstruction rates are quite low with a significant benefit to the vast majority of those undergoing the procedure.
- Complication: perforation, bleeding, migration, re-obstruction, pain.
- Risks and benefits need to be discussed with the patient prior to obtaining informed consent.
- Stenting increases quality of life in the palliative setting.
- It is possible to re-insert stents if migration or re-obstruction occur.
- Stents cannot be used in low rectal tumours, as may obstruct the anal canal causing pain and obstruction.

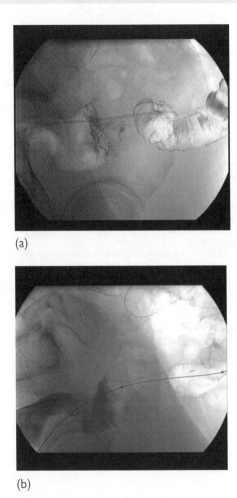

(a)

(b)

**Fig. 9.12** A 22 × 12cm self-expanding nitinol stent has been placed over a tight malignant stricture at the rectosigmoid junction. This will expand over the next 24h.

## Surgery

- Advanced, incurable CRC causes bowel obstruction whether due to locally advanced primary disease or peritoneal disease.
- These are extremely challenging patients as they are often nutritionally compromised and sick.
- Conservative management is preferable, but occasionally surgery is the only way to achieve symptomatic control.
- The most common symptoms requiring control are bowel obstruction and bleeding, and a thoughtful and individually tailored approach is necessary.
- Procedures include bypass, resection, and anastomosis, stoma formation, or a combination using open or laparoscopic techniques.
- In addition, surgical feeding tubes (gastrostomy, jejunostomy) helpful to maintain enteral nutrition.

## Laser therapy

- Light amplification by stimulated emission of radiation treatment has been used in the palliative treatment of non-curable disease.
- Most common indications for laser treatment are bleeding and obstructing disease.
- Most used laser is the neodynium: yttrium-aluminium-garnet (Nd: YAG), usually under sedation with bowel preparation.
- Can be used up to about 30cm from the anal verge.
- More than one session is often required. May be used in combination with other treatment modalities. Complications include bleeding, perforation, and re-stenosis.

## Cryosurgery

- Procedure involves exposing the tumour to extremely low temperature in order to kill surface cancer cells.
- Indications include prohibitive surgical risk, unresectability, and multiple unresectable distant metastases.
- Moderate relief of symptoms of blood loss and/or mucus discharge is achievable. Unsuitable for circumferential tumours. Not used widely.

# Follow-up and surveillance

### Overview

- There is no clearly defined follow-up protocol for patients after receiving treatment for CRC.
- Assessment is aimed to detect evidence of tumour recurrence and providing reassurance for patients.
- A trend has been demonstrated towards an improved survival benefit with high intensity follow-up.
- Questions remain regarding the ideal cost-effect and efficient follow-up regime.
- Intensity of follow-up should be decided by the MDT members.
- Ongoing trials are being undertaken to assess the optimum follow-up for various sub-groups.
- Little evidence that detection of recurrence followed by salvage surgery increases survival.

### Aims of follow-up

- Management of post-operative complications.
- Efficient detection of recurrent disease.
- Detection of metachronous new primary (5–10%).
- To enable discussion of adjuvant therapy.
- To maintain database of research records to allow for improvement of service provision.
- For reassurance of patients and relatives.

### Methods of CRC follow-up

- *Outpatient review:* history and clinical examination to detect symptoms, and signs of new or recurrent disease guiding use of relevant investigations.
- *Serum tumour marker assessment:* carcinoembryonic antigen (CEA), carbohydrate antigen (CA 19-9), tissue polypeptide (TPA), alpha-1-glycoprotein (AGP), alpha-1-antitrypsin (AAT), retinol-binding protein (RBP), haptoglobin, caeruloplasmin, neopterin, protein-bound hexose (PHex). High false positive rates for these protein assays and only a small gain with huge cost implication. CEA has been shown to be the most sensitive and specific for CRC.
- *Colonoscopy:* for detection of recurrence and new primary tumours. Most tumour recurrences are extra-luminal however. American Society of Colon and Rectal Surgeons guidelines are for surveillance colonoscopy 1-year post-operatively and then 3-yearly. Sub-grouping into low, intermediate, and high-risk patients has been proposed as a determinant of regularity of endoscopy.
- *Ultrasound:* for the detection of hepatic metastasis is sensitive, specific, and safe.
- *CT:* proposed for the detection of loco-regional recurrence and hepatic metastasis, but is limited by artefact due to post-operative tissue fibrosis.
- *MRI:* more accurate than CT, but more expensive.

- *Positron emission tomography (PET):* relies on functional uptake of glucose by tumour cells – requires lesions to be at least 1cm. False positive results due to inflammation.
- Ongoing UK Follow up After Colorectal Surgery (FACS) trial assessing 4 groups:
  - symptomatic follow-up in primary care;
  - tumour marker measurement in primary care;
  - intensive hospital follow-up with CT;
  - combination of groups 2 and 3.

# Colorectal cancer and the future

## Overview

- Interesting developments are being seen currently in all areas of colorectal cancer detection, diagnosis, and management.
- In the future, the use of gene testing may allow for prediction of 'at risk' individuals and give an individual genotypic profile for each tumour.
- Screening may be introduced that would result in a stage shift towards early, more curable disease.
- Imaging is continuing to improve, allowing the accurate prediction of nodal stage in addition to tumour and metastatic disease. This would enable widespread use of local excision procedures in known node-negative patients.
- Endoscopic excision technologies are continuing to evolve to allow for intraluminal surgery.
- Laparoscopic surgical techniques are evolving resulting in shorter hospital stay and earlier return to normal functioning.
- Improvements in sphincter-saving procedures are permitting lower anastomoses for rectal cancer surgery.
- Analysis of pathological specimens is allowing for increased quality control and greater knowledge about various prognostic indicators.
- Knowledge of tumour growth and spread, in particular, angiogenesis-mediated growth, is resulting in targeted therapy for CRC.

## Gene testing

- The increase in knowledge of specific genetic mutations, both inherited and sporadic has led to the introduction of DNA microarrays for the identification of subjects at risk of developments of premalignant polyps and colorectal cancers.
- It may be possible from a blood test using PCR to determine subjects at higher risk to enable a targeted, rather than a blanket, screening programme.

## Future of imaging

- Accurate detection of lymph node metastases is important for the determination of prognosis and for optimal management of patients with rectal carcinoma. Few papers have assessed diagnostic accuracy of nodal involvement using MRI with endorectal coil. Comparison of nodal involvement for CT, ES, MRI, and MRI with endorectal coil has demonstrated sensitivity of 52, 71, 65, and 82%; specificity 78, 76, 80, and 83%; and accuracy 66, 74, 74, and 82%, respectively.
- Pre-operative staging of the primary tumour has advanced significantly in recent years, lymph node assessment has remained poor. Currently, mesorectal nodal enlargement (5, 6, 10mm) is the only consistently used imaging criterion on which the diagnosis of metastasis is made. However, there is no definitive, validated size criterion for the assessment of malignancy in mesorectal lymph nodes. Nodal enlargement has major limitations in that metastases in small lymph

nodes or lack of metastases in larger lymph nodes are wrongly described. A significant number (up to 45%) of malignant nodes are smaller than 5mm and not correctly defined presently. Lymph nodes smaller than 5mm may be prognostic indicators of local recurrence.

- Ultrasmall superparamagnetic iron oxide (USPIO) particles are novel magnetic resonance (MR) contrast agents, which were developed with the specific intention for use in MR lymphography.
- Clinical tolerance is excellent. Mild, self-limiting side-effects include lumbar discomfort, rash and transient hypotension with an overall incidence of less than 4%.
- Iron oxide contrast-enhanced MR lymphography has emerged as an effective method of assessing lymph node involvement by tumour. The technique relies on macrophages that phagocytose the small particles of iron oxide as part of their normal scavenging role within the reticuloendothelial system, and deposit the contrast in lymph nodes. Uptake of contrast results in a change in the MR signal, a phenomenon seen in normal lymph nodes, but largely absent in lymph nodes involved by tumour.
- Early studies have been promising for the accurate pre-operative detection of lymph node metastasis. If high diagnostic accuracy is proven, local excision procedures could become far more targeted towards patients with known node negative early rectal cancer.

## Endoscopic excision

- Polypoid lesions on stalks can usually be excised using standard endoscopic techniques.
- Newer techniques, including endoscopic mucosal resection (EMR), have been successfully used to remove early flat or sessile cancers.
- High frequency endoluminal ultrasound has also been used to assess depth of penetration of lesions.
- Argon plasma coagulation (APC) has also been introduced and shown to treat resection margins after piecemeal EMR to remove any residual neoplasia.
- Further developments include the multi-channel operating endoscope with the ability to improve therapeutic options.

## Angiogenesis

- Angiogenesis is the process of the formation of new blood vessels from pre-existing ones. An important consideration in tumour development, growth and metastasis is the vasculature supplying tumour cells.
- New vessels form as a result of budding or sprouting from pre-existing ones, as well as developing from circulating endothelial cells from walls of vessels or after bone marrow mobilization.
- It has been observed that vessels dilate, in part at least, due to the action of nitric oxide (NO) and increase in vascular permeability due to various angiogenic factors through their action on intercellular adhesion molecules.
- Plasma protein extravasation promotes the migration of activated endothelial cells by acting as an early endothelial supporting structure. Further endothelial cellular growth is mediated by factors, such as angiopoietin 2, which are aided by breakdown of the extracellular

matrix by proteinases, including the diverse family of matrix metalloproteinases (MMPs). As the surrounding tissue is broken down, it is possible for endothelial cells to grow into the created space, directed by various angiogenic factors towards the tumour. Subsequently, the cells form into solid structures, which eventually develop lumens and form as disorganized blood vessels that mature to allow functional metabolite and oxygen delivery, albeit in a non-uniform manner.

- As growth and metastases in other tumours were found to be angiogenesis-dependent, colorectal cancer growth, spread, and prognosis has also been correlated with the formation of new blood vessels.
- Increased microvessel density (MVD) in premalignant and malignant colorectal lesions has been demonstrated as compared with surrounding normal tissue and polyps have been found to be less vascularized than invasive cancers.
- Increased angiogenesis has been correlated with transmural tumour extension, high primary colorectal cancer MVD is associated with an increased incidence of haematogenous metastases and increased MVD has been correlated with an increased risk of tumour recurrence.
- Vascular endothelial growth factor (VEGF) is a 34–42kDa protein, which promotes vascular permeability and acts as an endothelial cell mitotic promoter resulting in angiogenesis and lymphangiogenesis. In addition to stimulation of endothelial cell mitotic activity and promotion of vascular permeability, VEGF also acts to decrease apoptosis and hence contributes to endothelial cell stabilization and continuing growth. In addition to VEGF secretion by cancers, it has also been demonstrated that it is produced by tumour associated macrophages, which are recruited by cancers to potentiate growth.
- A positive relationship has been demonstrated between VEGF staining and microvessel density, lymphovascular and perineural invasion, and metastasis in colorectal cancer and VEGF over-expression has been correlated with tumour progression and poor outcome.
- The recombinant monoclonal VEGF antibody bevacizumab (Avastin®) was developed by Genetech Inc, San Francisco, USA and approved for intravenous use. Subsequently, increased response rate, disease-free survival, and overall survival were demonstrated with the use of bevacizumab in metastatic colorectal cancer with limited toxicity.
- The addition of bevacizumab to standard chemotherapy resulted in improved response rates, longer median time to disease progression and longer median survival from 14 to over 20 months.
- A randomized controlled study of oxaliplatin plus 5-FU (FOLFOX) with and without bevacizumab and demonstrated an increased survival time and improvement in time to progression and response rates in the bevacizumab group. Hence, data suggests that anti-VEGF therapy is most effectively used in combination with standard chemotherapeutic agents rather than alone.

- Bevacizumab may stabilize tumour vascular structure to allow chemotherapeutic agents to reach the tumour, rather than acting as a directly tumoricidal agent.
- Treatment with bevacizumab in patients with rectal cancer reduces vessel counts and interstitial pressure, although the decrease in pressure may cause decreased resistance to allow for greater delivery of standard drugs to the site of the tumour.
- Another approach involves targeted blockade of VEGF receptors. Vatalinib, developed by Schering AG and Novartis inhibits the intracellular tyrosine kinase of the VEGF-R2, specifically blocking the most ubiquitous of the VEGF family, VEGF-A.
- Early work described vatalinib to cause minimal toxicity and to disrupt tumour vasculature as demonstrated by dynamic magnetic resonance imaging. This study was the antecedent to the colorectal oral novel therapy for the inhibition of angiogenesis and retarding metastases (CONFIRM) -1 and CONFIRM-2 trials, investigating oxaliplatin and 5-FU with vatalinib and without it.
- The first of these trials was conducted in patients who did not receive chemotherapy and the second included patients who had received first-line irinotecan and 5-FU. However, early data from CONFIRM-1 showed no benefit on disease-free survival, although sub-group analysis (patients with raised lactate dehydrogenase) revealed some effect. Formal publication of data from the CONFIRM-1 and CONFIRM-2 trials are awaited.
- Further work is being undertaken on monoclonal antibodies for epidermal growth factor (EGFR), including cetuximab and pantumomab as EGFR is over-expressed in up to 80% of colorectal cancers.
- *ADCC agents – catumaxumab:* trifunctional antibody targeting EpCam and CD3 forming tri-cell antibody complex promoting antibody dependent cell cytotoxicity. Phase III trials currently underway to assess response in patients with malignant ascites and fluid borne metastases.

# Anal cancer

# Epidemiology and presentation

### Incidence
Rare. 4% of large bowel malignancies. Increases with age. Slight female pre-dominance. 300 new cases per year in the UK. Incidence is higher in men who practice anal-receptive sexual intercourse.

### Pathology
- Squamous cell cancer (90%). Three types of squamous cell anal cancer: large cell keratinizing, large cell non-keratinizing (also called transitional), basaloid.
- Adenocarcinoma (5%).
- Melanoma (1%).
- Lymphoma.
- Sarcoma.

### Pattern of spread
Locally (cephalad direction) anal sphincters, rectovaginal septum, peri-neal body, vagina, scrotum. Lymph node metastases to perirectal, inguinal, haemorrhoidal and lateral pelvic nodes. Haematogenous spread to liver, lung, and bones is late, and is associated with locally advanced disease.

### Presentation
- Rectal bleeding.
- Pain or pressure in the area around the anus.
- Itching or discharge from the anus.
- A lump near the anus.
- A change in bowel habit.
- Faecal incontinence.
- Vaginal discharge with posterior vaginal wall invasion.
- Asymptomatic (20%).

# Squamous cell anal cancer

## Aetiology

Cause unknown, but several risk factors have been identified:

- Age (over 50).
- Sexually transmitted infection with human papillomavirus (HPV).
- Multiple sexual partners.
- Having receptive anal intercourse.
- Chronic immunosuppressed states as in human immunodeficiency virus (HIV) and recipients of a solid organ transplant.
- Cigarette smoking.

HPV is the most common sexually transmitted disease that has been linked to the development of anal cancer (HPV subtype 16 and 18 commonest), as well as cervical, vaginal, penile, and vulvar carcinoma. 80% patients with squamous cell carcinoma (SCC) of the anus are infected with HPV.

The rate of anal cancer is twice as high in HIV +ve men vs. HIV −ve men.

## Investigation

### Examination

Careful note of size, position, extent of tumour, and mobility. Presence of perirectal, inguinal, and femoral lymph nodes. Gynaecological examination assessing vaginal-mucosal involvement. Proctoscopy and sigmoidoscopy with biopsy. Patients unable to tolerate pelvic examination and biopsy should be done under anaesthesia. Palpable inguinal nodes can be assessed by biopsy or fine-needle aspiration (FNA) cytology.

### Loco-regional staging

Transrectal ultrasonography is useful to determine the extent of invasion and involvement of adjacent organs. MRI of the pelvis.

### Systemic staging

- CXR, CT chest/abdomen detects visceral metastatic disease. PET used to investigate indeterminate lesions, or assessment of suspected residual or recurrent disease.
- Consider HIV test in patients at risk of contracting HIV infection.

## Staging

### TNM definitions of anal cancer
- **TX:** primary tumour cannot be assessed.
- **T0:** no evidence of primary tumour,
- **Tis:** carcinoma *in situ*.
- **T1:** tumour 2cm or less.
- **T2:** tumour larger than 2 but less than 5cm.
- **T3:** tumour larger than 5cm.
- **T4:** tumour of any size that invades nearby organ(s), such as the vagina, urethra or bladder.
- **NX:** regional lymph nodes cannot be assessed.
- **N0:** no regional lymph node spread.
- **N1:** metastasis in perirectal lymph node(s).
- **N2:** metastasis in unilateral internal iliac or inguinal lymph node(s).
- **N3:** metastasis in perirectal and inguinal lymph nodes, bilateral internal iliac, or inguinal lymph nodes.
- **MX:** presence of distant metastasis cannot be assessed M0: No distant metastasis M1: Distant metastasis to internal organs or lymph nodes of the abdomen.

### Stage grouping by TNM involvement
- **Stage 0 (carcinoma in situ):** Tis, N0, M0.
- **Stage I:** T1, N0, M0.
- **Stage II:** T2 or 3, N0, M0.
- **Stage IIIA:** T1–3, N1, M0 or T4, N0, M0.
- **Stage IIIB:** T4, N1, M0, or Any T, N2–3, M0.
- **Stage IV:** any T, any N, M1.

Staging of anal cancer uses a system created by the American Joint Committee on Cancer (AJCC).

# Treatment

## Radiotherapy

Anal squamous cell carcinoma is a radiosensitive tumour. External beam radiation and brachytherapy have been used successfully for local control and cure in 70–90% of selected patients. 75% Sphincter preservation. Nodal involvement or tumours > 5cm decreases cure rates to 50%.

*Complications:* incontinence, anal stenosis, ulceration, and necrosis.

## Combined-modality treatment

- **The 'Nigro' regime:** introduced in 1974 involved combination of radiotherapy, 30Gy, 5-FU (1000mg/m$^2$ × 4 q 28 days × 2) and mitomycin C (15mg/m$^2$ day 1). Modifications of this regime have lead to complete regression in 59–95% and 5-year survival of 70–100% of patients.
- **Two randomized trials:** European Organization for Research and Treatment of Cancer (EORTC) and the UK Coordinating Committee on Cancer Research (UKCCCR) compared radiotherapy alone with combined chemoradiotherapy (ACT I trial).
- **Findings:** no difference in overall survival, but chemoradiotherapy improved local control (benefit is greater on larger tumours). Radiation Therapy Oncology Group (RTOG) and Eastern Cooperative Oncology Group (ECOG) had shown that a combination of 5-FU and mitomycin-C with radiation was more effective than 5-FU and radiation. Combined-modality therapy is now the standard for the primary treatment of anal SCC.
- **The ACT II trial** aims to assess whether CDDP or MMC – produces a higher CR rate post-treatment, produces a higher grade 4 acute toxicity and whether maintenance chemotherapy will improve recurrence-free survival. Split course radiotherapy is changed to a continuous course. Patients have been randomized to maintenance chemotherapy.
- **Cisplatin chosen in combination with 5-FU:** active in advanced disease, producing high CR rates in combination with radiotherapy and has activity in other squamous cell carcinomas. Additional chemotherapy will be given after treatment. Neo-adjuvant chemotherapy has not been shown to improve survival when given in combination with radiotherapy in other tumour sites. Currently recruiting a target of 950 patients.

## Surgery

- **Historically:** treatment was abdominoperineal resection (APR) of the rectum and anal canal, with permanent end-colostomy.
- Overall 5-year survival ranged between 30 and 71%.
- Surgery is now reserved for patients needing temporary stoma formation prior to radiotherapy and chemotherapy if they are thought to cope poorly with side effects of pelvic radiotherapy, at risk of rectovaginal fistula, or have lost sphincter function.
- APR is reserved for patients who have residual disease or recurrence after chemoradiation.
- Local excision with curative intent has been performed for small, superficial tumours (<2cm) with 5-year survival ranging from 60 to 70%.

### Residual/ recurrent local disease

Abdominoperineal resection for selected patients offers 50% 5-year survival, similar results have been obtained with salvage chemoradiation. Surgery is associated with high morbidity, particularly delayed perineal wound healing and wound infection. Primary reconstruction of the perineum with rectus abdominis myocutaneous flap can prevent wound complications.

### Metastatic disease

Palliative intent. Salvage chemotherapy has some efficacy, and resection of liver and lung mets is possible if the primary disease is under control.

### Treatment of patients with HIV infection

Advances in highly active antiretroviral therapy have extended the life expectancy of patients with HIV. There is an increasing incidence of anal SCC in the HIV infected population. Treatment is with chemotherapy and radiotherapy. Patients with CD4 counts <200 and those who have had an AIDS defining illness have a higher incidence of treatment related complications and may require dose adjustments.

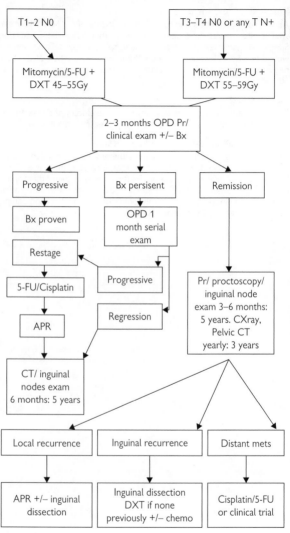

**Fig. 10.1** Management of anal cancer.

**Table 10.1** Key trials assessing optimal multi-modal treatment for anal carcinoma

| Trial | n | Question | RT | RT gap | Chemo | Result |
|---|---|---|---|---|---|---|
| UKCCR ACT I | 585 | CRT vs. RT | 45Gy 20–25 fractions | 6 weeks 15Gy | 5-FU 1g/m² days 1–4 and 29–32 MMC 12mg/ m² day 1 | Risk of local Rx failure sig decreased in CRT group |
| EORTC | 110 | CRT vs. RT | 45Gy 25 fractions | 6 weeks 15–20 | 5-FU 750mg/m² days 1–5 and 29–33 MMC 15mg/ m² day 1 | Local control significantly improved in CRT group |
| RTOG ECOG | 291 | Role of MMC | 45–50.4Gy 25–28 fractions | None | 5-FU 1g/m² days 1–4 and 29–32 MMC 10mg/m² day 1 and 29 one group only | Local control significantly improved with MMC |
| ACT II | 950 | Cisplatin vs. MMC | 50.4Gy in 28 fractions | None | 5-FU 1000mg/m² days 1–4 and 29–32 by 24h continuous infusion and mitomycin 12mg/m² day 1 only, IV bolus or Cisplatin 60mg/m² days 1 and 29 by IV infusion  Maintenance chemo: 2 courses 5-FU and cisplatin 4 weeks after end of primary chemoradiation repeated after 3 weeks 5-FU 1000mg/m² days 1–4 and cisplatin 60mg/m² day 1 by IV | Recruiting at present |

### Surveillance

The objective is to diagnose local recurrence at an early stage. If there are no useful tumour markers, regular follow-up (every 3 months for 2 years then biannually for 3 years) with digital rectal examination and proctoscopy. CT or MRI yearly is recommended for patients with T3/4 N2 disease. EUA +/– biopsy and MRI are used to assess recurrent/ residual disease. HPV pap smears also used.

### Anal intra-epithelial neoplasia (AIN)

Analgous to cervical cancer, the development of invasive squamous cell carcinoma may occur following transition of low grade squamous intraepithelial lesion (LSIL) to high grade squamous intra-epithelial lesion (HSIL). Incidence of AIN is rising in high-risk groups, particularly those infected with HIV. The aetiology of AIN is intricately linked with human papilloma viruses. Like cervical cancer, anal carcinoma may be preventable through identification and treatment of its precursors. Given the known high-risk groups for anal cancer, studies have addressed screening in these populations. Anal swabs for cytology are a possible screening method for AIN and anal cancer. Sensitivity of anal cytology 50–80%.

### Anal adenocarcinoma

Extremely rare. Originating from anal canal glands. Behaves like rectal carcinoma and treatment is surgical resection with APR in localized disease with adjuvant radiotherapy +/– chemotherapy. 5-year survival 60%, recurrence rates 30–50%.

### Anorectal melanoma

Extremely rare. No proven role for chemotherapy/radiotherapy. Radical resection with APR poor 5-year survival (17–25%). Wide local excision (WLE) with sphincter preservation has been used. No series has demonstrated a survival advantage for APR over WLE.

# Renal cancer

# Haematuria protocols

All haematuria requires urgent investigation of urinary tract.

- *History:* pain, duration, associated lower urinary tract symptoms, weight loss, known prostate enlargement or cancer, anticoagulation or antiplatelet agents, steroids, family history of prostate/renal/bladder cancer, smoking history, occupational history.
- *Examination:* full examination including digital rectal examination.
- *Urine*: dipstick analysis (blood, leucocytes, nitrites, protein); urine cytology; sexually-transmitted diseases screen in young or if suspicion on history.
- *Bloods:* full blood count, renal function, PSA in men >45 years. In those on anticoagulation or with macroscopic haematuria, prothrombin time and APTT.
- *Imaging:* ultrasound and abdominal plain film radiograph is sufficient for microscopic haematuria in which cystoscopy and urine cytology are clear. Intravenous urography or CT-IVU in macroscopic haematuria.

## Flexible cystoscopy

- *Consent.* lidocaine 1% gel instilled into urethra. In young men use twice the amount (20mL) of gel and leave for a full 2–3min before inserting scope.
- Insert scope following lumen throughout. Once into bladder, observe for two ureteric orifices and then check bladder neck, lateral walls and, posterior and anterior walls systematically. Carry out J-manoeuvre to look back on bladder neck.
- On way out of bladder, observe urethra carefully.

## Bilateral retrograde studies

At time of cystoscopy under general anaesthesia to screen upper urinary tracts (ureters and renal pelvis) may be indicated if imaging was equivocal.

# Renal cell carcinoma

### Incidence

Comprises 2–3% of all cancers, with 10 per 100 000. 7000 cases per year are diagnosed with increasing incidence probably due to increased use of imaging with incidental detection. There are 3600 deaths per year.

### Aetiology and risk factors

Male:female 3:2. Age group >40 years (peak 50–70 years). *Risk factors:* obesity, smoking, acquired cystic disease, end-stage renal disease, hypertension, urinary tract infections, kidney stones, kidney infection, radiation treatment for other cancers, phenacetin (analgesic now banned), occupation (blast-furnace, iron/steel industry), carcinogens (asbestos, cadmium, petroleum, dry-cleaning solvents).

### Presentation

Incidental on imaging (50%). Presents with flank pain, macroscopic haematuria, and palpable abdominal mass (6–10%); paraneoplastic syndromes (30%, e.g. hypertension, cachexia, weight loss, pyrexia, neuromyopathy, amyloidosis, elevated erythrocyte sedimentation rate, anaemia, abnormal liver function, hypercalcaemia, polycythaemia); symptoms associated with metastatic disease (cough, bone pain; 25–30%).

### Histology

Renal parenchymal cancers (renal cell carcinoma) comprise 5 sub-groups:
• Conventional clear cell (75–80%).
• Papillary (chromophilic; 10–15%).
• Chromophobe (4–5%).
• Collecting duct carcinoma.
• Unclassified.
Transition cell carcinoma can occur in the renal pelvis from transition urothelium, but has same aetiology as bladder transition cell carcinoma.

# Investigation of renal cell carcinoma

### Blood tests
Haemoglobin, erythrocyte sedimentation rate, renal function, alkaline phosphatase, and serum-corrected calcium.

### USS renal tract
Usually discovered incidentally for other medical condition. Mass on USS requires full evaluation with CT.

### Contrast CT
*Chest/abdomen/pelvis:* diagnosis of malignancy (increased enhancement of solid lesion by 15–20 Hounsfield units; necrotic areas may be present; cystic lesions have thickened enhancing walls), extrarenal extension, renal vein extension, contralateral kidney, condition of adrenals and liver, lymph node status, metastatic disease to lungs (more accurate than plain chest radiograph).

### MRI
Indicated for contrast allergy, renal impairment, formal evaluation of renal vein, or inferior vena caval tumour thrombus extension.

### Bone-scan
If metastatic disease is indicated from size of tumour, lymph node status, symptoms, and increased serum calcium/alkaline phosphatase.

### Core-biopsy
Core biopsy is not sufficiently accurate to warrant routine use in equivocal small masses.

# Localized renal cell carcinoma: staging

Prognostic factors classified into anatomical, histological, clinical, and molecular.

## Anatomical

Tumour size, venous invasion, renal capsule invasion, adrenal involvement, and lymph node and distant metastasis (summarized according to 2002 TNM staging).

### Primary tumour

- **TX:** primary tumour cannot be assessed.
- **T0:** no evidence of primary tumour.
- **T1:** tumour <7cm in greatest dimension, limited to the kidney.
- **T1a:** tumour <4cm in greatest dimension, limited to the kidney.
- **T1b:** tumour >4cm, but <7cm in greatest dimension, but not more than 7cm.
- **T2:** tumour >7cm in greatest dimension, limited to the kidney.
- **T3:** tumour extends into major veins or directly invades adrenal gland or perinephric tissues, but not beyond Gerota's fascia.
- **T3a:** tumour directly invades adrenal gland or perinephric tissues, but not beyond Gerota's fascia.
- **T3b:** tumour grossly extends into renal vein(s) or its segmental branches, or the vena cava below the diaphragm.
- **T3c:** tumour grossly extends into vena cava or its wall above diaphragm.
- **T4:** tumour directly invades beyond Gerota's fascia.

### Regional lymph nodes (N)

- **NX:** regional lymph nodes cannot be assessed.
- **N0:** no regional lymph node metastasis.
- **N1:** metastasis in a single regional lymph node.
- **N2:** metastases in more than 1 regional lymph node.
- **pN0:** lymphadenectomy specimen ordinarily includes 8 or more lymph-nodes. If the lymph nodes are negative, but the number ordinarily examined is not met, classify as pN0.

### Distant metastasis (M)

- **MX:** distant metastasis cannot be assessed.
- **M0:** no distant metastasis.
- **M1:** distant metastasis.

### TNM stage grouping

- **Stage I:** T1, N0, M0.
- **Stage II:** T2, N0, M0.
- **Stage III:** T3, N0, M0; T1, T2, T3, N1, M0.
- **Stage IV:** T4, N0, N1, M0; any T, N2, M0; any T, any N, M1.

### Histological
- Higher Fuhrman grade, presence of sarcomatoid features, microvascular invasion, tumour necrosis, and collecting system invasion.
- Histological subtype. Trend of better prognosis for chromophobe, papillary and conventional (clear cell) RCCs, respectively.

### Clinical
Worse prognosis with patient performance status, localized symptoms, cachexia, anaemia, low platelet count.

### Molecular
Numerous molecular markers being investigated including: carbonic anhydrase IX (CaIX), vascular endothelial growth factor (VEGF), hypoxia inducible factor (HIF), Ki67 (proliferation), p53, PTEN (cell cycle), E-cadherin, and CD44 (cell adhesion).

### Fuhrman nuclear grade
- Most widely used and predictive grading system for RCC.
- Scale of I–IV, where grade I carries the best prognosis and grade IV the worst.
- Nuclear grade means that the system is based on just the appearance of nuclei, rather than appearance or structure of cells as a whole.

#### *Nuclear characteristics used in the Fuhrman system*
- Size/shape of the nucleus as a whole.
- Number/size of nucleoli.
- Chromatin clumping.

# Localized renal cell carcinoma: management

## Radical nephrectomy

Gold standard. In selected cases with lymph node disease limited to the retroperitoneal space, extended lymphadenectomy might improve a patient's clinical prognosis. In general, extended lymphadenectomy is not the therapeutic standard. Adrenalectomy can be spared in the majority of patients, except in the case of large upper pole tumours (>7cm), where direct invasion of the adrenal gland is likely. Palliative embolization in patients unfit for surgery with refractory haematuria or profound local pain.

## Nephron-sparing surgery

Standard indications for nephron-sparing surgery are divided into the following categories:

### Anatomical or functional solitary kidney

- Functioning opposite kidney that is affected by a condition, which might impair renal function in future (include patients with hereditary forms of RCC, who are at high risk of developing a tumour in the contralateral kidney).
- Localized unilateral RCC with a healthy contralateral kidney (<4cm, although can be performed on 4–7cm tumours in expert centres).

### Laparoscopy for radical or nephron-sparing nephrectomy:

Lower morbidity when compared with open surgery. Tumour control rates equivalent for T1–2 and possibly T3a tumours in experienced hands.

### Advantages of laparoscopic surgery

Includes significantly shorter hospital stay, less blood loss, lower analgesic requirement and quicker return to normal activities. Disease-specific survival for T1 disease is about 90–95% for 3–5 years, equivalent to open nephrectomy. No randomized data exist for lap vs. open, but two RCTs comparing lap retroperitoneal vs. lap transperitoneal essentially demonstrated equivalence in terms of complications and other operative parameters.

## Minimally-invasive ablative techniques

Image-guided percutaneous and minimally invasive techniques, e.g. percutaneous radiofrequency (RF) ablation, cryoablation, microwave ablation, laser ablation, and high-intensity focused ultrasound ablation (HIFU) suggested as alternatives to the surgical treatment of RCC, but under evaluation. All these techniques have demonstrated ability to destroy tissue on histological verification, but are still experimental with no long-term data on cancer-specific survival.

# Operative technique: radical nephrectomy

Preparation

- DMSA renogram to assess differential renal function in order to assess for likelihood of renal support of contralateral normal kidney peri-operatively; informed consent; antibiotic prophylaxis at time of induction; DVT prophylaxis (compression stockings and subcutaneous heparin administered until discharge).
- *Patient position:* lateral decubitus with table flexed to elevate flank (patient properly secured) for flank incision. Otherwise supine.
- *Incisions:* flank/loin, thoraco-abdominal, subcostal, midline laparotomy.

Technique

Procedure for 'flank' described since most common.

- 11th or 12th rib incision (dependent on tumour and kidney size, patient habitus) from tip of rib to posterior axillary line to lateral border of rectus abdominis.
- Latissimus dorsi divided. Periosteal elevator used to strip rib without damage to intercostal neurovascular bundle. Rib cutter used to excise rib.
- Alternatively, space between two ribs used by dividing costovertebral ligament.
- Pleura secured superiorly. Anteriorly, external and internal oblique fibres divided with transversus abdominis fibres separated to reveal peritoneum.
- Peritoneum moved medially and retroperitoneal cavity connective tissue divided. Appropriate self-retaining retractor maintains exposure.
- *Left:* lienorenal ligament incised to move spleen cephalad.
- *Right:* hepatic flexure of colon mobilized with duodenum kocherized.
- Ureter identified and can be tied off at this stage for greater mobilization.
- Renal vein identified and isolated.
- Renal artery identified and isolated for 2–3cm. 3 ties placed (2 on aortic side) and artery divided. Renal vein ligated (2 ties on vena caval side) and divided.
- Gerota's gascia mobilized with adrenal gland separated unless adrenalectomy required.
- Specimen removed and haemostasis ensured. Check pleura and close in layers with continuous non-absorbable size no. 1 sutures.

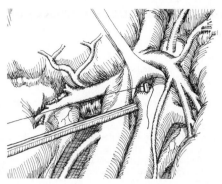

**Fig. 11.1** Line diagram radical nephrectomy. Taken from McLatchie and Leaper (2006). Reproduced with permission of Oxford University Press © 2006.

# Operative technique: laparoscopic nephrectomy

## Transperitoneal

- Pneumoperitonuem created via 12mm incision either 2–3cm medial and cranial to anterior superior iliac spine or transumbilical or mid-clavicular subcostal approaches.
- Increase abdominal pressure to 15mmHg. Two 12mm trocars placed 2cm below costal margin in mid-clavicular line and lateral to rectus abdominis 5–10cm above umbilicus.
- Fourth trocar usually subcostal in posterior axillary line. For right-sided nephrectomies 5th trocar for liver retraction may be needed.
- Line of Toldt incised to expose Gerota's fascia and retroperitoneum. On right side, duodenum kocherized. Secure gonadal vessel, adrenal vein, and ureter.
- Expose renal hilum. Renal vein dissected clean and renal artery exposed. Place five 9 or 11mm vascular clips on renal artery (3 on aortic side) and divide (endo-GIA vascular stapler may be required for broad vessels). Ligate and divide renal vein in a similar fashion.
- Free specimen intact with Gerota's fascia and deliver in a sack through an enlarged incision of the midline 12mm port site.
- Ensure haemostasis and close wound sites appropriately. Fascial closure with no 1 sized suture is necessary for 12mm port sites.

## Retroperitoneal

- Primary port at tip of 12th rib using open technique.
- Blunt finger dissection to open retroperitoneal space. Balloon dilator used to increase space.
- Pneumoperitoneum established and further ports inserted at lower mid-axillary line 2–3cm cephalad to iliac crest (12mm), anterior axillary line at level of primary port (5mm), and upper mid-axillary line port near tip of 11th rib (5mm).
- Dissection along psoas muscle will reveal pulsation of renal artery. Gerota's fascia incised to dissect renal artery free of hilum. Renal artery and vein ligated and divided with technique described above. Cephalad dissection will reveal adrenal vein to secure. Identify ureter and secure.
- Retrieve specimen after completion of dissection from surrounding tissues and deliver through widened primary port site in a sack.
- Ensure haemostasis. Port site closure, but formal fascial closure not required.

# Operative technique: nephron sparing partial nephrectomy

Performed either open or laparoscopic depending on patient status, size, and position of tumour.

- **Access:** as for open or laparoscopic radical nephrectomy, but location and size of tumour will determine whether extra- or transperitoneal approach.
- Small peripheral tumours can be excised without renal arterial occlusion, although most cases warrant this manoeuvre to reduce bleeding and renal tissue turgor.
- **Ischaemia:** 30min of warm ischaemia is sufficient for most procedures, but if longer procedure anticipated, then cold ischaemia time of 3h with ice-slush possible.
- Mannitol administered prior to renal artery occlusion.
- **Partial nephrectomy** performed using segmental nephrectomy, wedge resection, or transverse resection.
- **Segmental nephrectomy** used for tumours confined to upper or lower pole of kidney. Segmental apical or basilar artery can be isolated, and ligated without need for main renal artery occlusion.
- **Wedge resection** used for peripheral tumours on surface of kidney, particularly those not confined to either pole.
- **Transverse resection** is performed to remove larger tumours extensively involving either lower or upper part of the kidney.
- For either technique, 5–10mm margin of normal tissue must surround the resection.
- Hilar tumours can be excised with a 3–4mm margin. The tumours can extend deeply and the collecting system may need to be opened.
- **After resection,** the collecting system should be closed with absorbable 3/0 interrupted sutures.
- Edges of the kidney should be approximated with 3/0 absorbable sutures inserted through the renal capsule and a small amount of parenchyma.
- Surgicel®/Oxycel or perirenal fat can be inserted into the defect for inclusion in the defect closure to ensure sutures are tension-free.
- If the collecting system has been opened, a Robinson/Penrose drain should be inserted. Release renal artery occlusion and ensure meticulous haemostasis.
- Closure as appropriate for type of access.

Complications:
- Wound infection, abscess, haemorrhage +/– emergency laparotomy.
- Conversion to open if laparoscopic.
- Pneumothorax.
- Myocardial ischaemia/infarction, pulmonary embolus [blood clot, tumour thrombus], deep venous thrombus, pneumonia, incisional hernia, renal impairment, neuropathic local pain, recurrence [local, metastatic, contralateral].

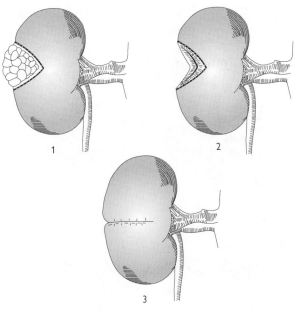

1

2

3

**Fig. 11.2** Partial wedge nephrectomy.

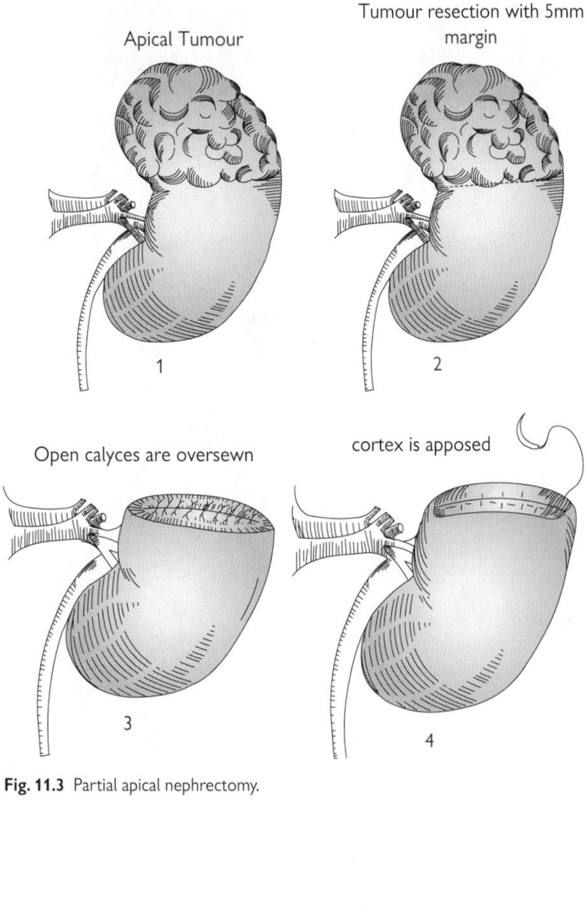
Apical Tumour
Tumour resection with 5mm margin
1
2
Open calyces are oversewn
cortex is apposed
3
4

**Fig. 11.3** Partial apical nephrectomy.

# Surveillance

Surveillance after radical surgery aims to identify post-operative complications, renal function, local recurrence (1.8%), recurrence in the contralateral kidney (1.2%), development of metastases.

Surveillance type and intensity dependent on risk of recurrence. *Mayo scoring system* for risk of recurrence dependent on staging and histological factors.

**Table 11.1** Mayo scoring system

| T-stage | Points |
| --- | --- |
| *Primary tumour* | |
| T1a | 0 |
| pT1b | 2 |
| pT2 | 3 |
| pT3–pT4 | 4 |
| *Tumour size* | |
| <10cm | 0 |
| >10cm | 1 |
| *Regional lymph node status* | |
| pNx/pN0 | 0 |
| pN1–pN2 | 2 |
| *Grade* | |
| Grade 1–2 | 0 |
| Grade 3 | 1 |
| Grade 4 | 3 |
| *Tumour necrosis* | |
| No necrosis | 0 |
| Necrosis | 1 |

**Risk groups stratification**
- *Low-risk:* 0-2.
- *Intermediate risk:* 3–5.
- *High-risk:* >6.

**Table 11.2** Risk of metastases (%) after nephrectomy in patients with clear cell renal cell carcinoma according to Mayo scoring risk groups system

| Risk group | Year 1 | Year 3 | Year 5 | Year 10 |
|---|---|---|---|---|
| Low | 0.5 | 2.1 | 2.9 | 7.5 |
| Intermediate | 9.6 | 20.2 | 26.2 | 35.7 |
| High | | 42.3 | 62.9 | 68.8 |

*Low risk:* Chest radiograph and USS.

*Intermediate-risk:* intensified follow-up including CT scans at regular time intervals.

*High-risk:* routine CT scans.

## Guidelines for surveillance (National Comprehensive Cancer Network)

### Stages I, II, and III

- Can be observed or encouraged to participate in trials of adjuvant agents.
- Chest and abdominal CT at 4–6 months, then as indicated.
- Clinical follow-up with blood tests every 6 months for first 2 years, then annually for 5 years.

# Advanced renal cell carcinoma

- Tumour nephrectomy is recommended for metastatic RCC in patients with good performance status when combined with interferon-alpha as survival is increased.
- Synchronous metastases treated with metastasectomy, where disease is resectable and good performance status.
- Metastasectomy should be performed in patients with residual and resectable metastatic lesions previously responding to immunotherapy, and/or a limited number of metachronous metastases in order to improve prognosis.
- Prognosis worse in patients undergoing surgery for metachronous metastases.

### Adjuvant therapy
Radiotherapy for symptomatic relief, e.g. pain relief from single bony deposit.

### Chemotherapy
- RCCs develop from proximal tubules; therefore, express high levels of multiple-drug resistance protein, P-glycoprotein. Therefore, resistant to most chemotherapeutic agents.
- Chemotherapy effective only if 5-fluorouracil (5-FU) combined with immunotherapeutic agents.

### Immunotherapy
- Interferon-alpha beneficial for metastatic RCC if good performance status, and progression-free survival following initial diagnosis of >1 year with lung metastasis as sole metastatic site.
- Selected metastatic RCC with a good risk profile and clear cell subtype derive benefit from interleukin-2 or interferon-alpha.

### Anti-angiogenesis drugs
Tyrosine kinase inhibitors now considered first- or second-line treatment for metastatic RCC:
- *Sunitinib:* first-line in good-and intermediate-risk patients.
- *Temsirolimus:* considered first-line in poor-risk patients.
- *Sorafenib:* second-line.

# Bladder and upper urinary tract cancer

# Bladder tumours

- 90% transition cell carcinomas.
- 10% squamous cell carcinoma or adenocarcinoma.
- 30% present with muscle-invasive or metastatic disease.
- Of those with non-invasive disease treated with organ-preserving modalities, 30% will represent with muscle-invasive disease.
- *Incidence:* 10 000 (UK); 60 000 (USA).
- *Mortality:* 4700 (UK); 13 000 (USA). 5-year survival in non-invasive disease is 80–90% and <50% for invasive disease (UK).
- *Presentation:* macroscopic haematuria (>75%), lower urinary tract symptoms (urgency, frequency), dysuria, recurrent urinary tract infections.

## Risk factors

- *Smoking:* implicated in half of all cases; risk remains high in ex-smokers for 20 years.
- *Occupational carcinogens:* 5–10% of all cases in Europe; aromatic amines; printing, iron and aluminium processing, industrial painting, gas and tar manufacturing.
- *Pelvic radiotherapy;* cyclophosphamide chemotherapy.
- *Chronic irritation;* recurrent urinary infections and long-term catheters (e.g. paraplegics); chronic urolithiasis, chronic residual urine leads to squamous cell carcinoma or adenocarcinoma.
- *Bilharziosis (schistosomiasis)* usually leads to invasive squamous cell carcinoma, but one-third TCC.

# Investigation and staging

### Urine cytology

High specificity (over 90%), but low sensitivity (below 50%), as it is related to the tumour grade. Therefore, negative cytology cannot rule out a low-grade tumour.

### Tumour markers

Bladder tumour antigen, nuclear matrix protein 22 (NMP 22), fibrin-degradation products (e.g. Quanticyt, Immunocyt). Better sensitivity for bladder cancer, but lower specificity (false positives lead to unnecessary further investigations).

### Imaging

* *Intravenous urography/CT-IVU:* can show filling defect in bladder and ureters. Should be performed routine for tumours close to ureteric orifices and high-grade tumours (7% incidence of synchronous upper tract tumours). CT-IVU increasingly used.
* *Ultrasound:* if combined with abdominal plain radiograph is as accurate in haematuria screen as IVU alone.
* *Cystoscopy.*
* Gold-standard for detection of bladder tumours. Information on location and size, as well as other synchronous tumours or suspicious areas for CIS. If no lesions are seen and cytology positive, but negative upper tract imaging, selected 'cold-cup' bladder biopsies should be taken with biopsy forceps or resection loop. These should be labelled and sent separately from each region. Positive trigonal and bladder neck biopsies will require further biopsies from prostatic urethra.

### New techniques

* *Fluorescence cystoscopy* using blue light and a porphyrin-based photosensitizer, (hexi)-aminolaevulinic acid (HAL or ALA), can demonstrate suspicious areas for *cis-* or papillary tumour not visible with white-light cystoscopy.
* *Cross-sectional imaging:* both CT and MRI have staging error of 30% as they are unable to detect extravesical or extrarenal disease accurately. This may be as a result of inflammatory changes post-endoscopic resection. In large or flat tumours, cross-sectional imaging prior to resection may be useful.
* *N-staging:* both MRI and CT miss microscopic disease in up to 70%.
* *PET-scans currently under evaluation:* lymphadenectomy is gold standard for excluding lymph node disease, but extent of dissection and role for laparoscopic procedure is unknown.
* *M-staging:* a chest radiograph or CT-chest and bone-scan are required in invasive or high grade tumours.

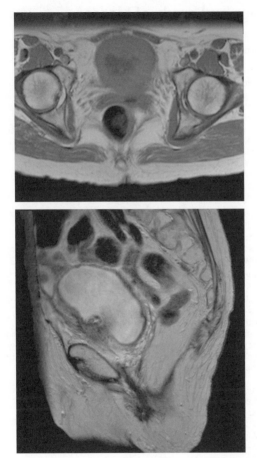

**Fig. 12.1** T4 bladder Ca concentric wall thickening seen on T1 axial and T2 sagittal sequences.

# Stage and grade of bladder tumours

## Histology
Non-invasive and invasive categories.

### Non-invasive tumours
*(Tis, Ta, T1)*
- Usually resected using transurethral procedure. However, CIS and T1 tumours can be highly malignant and invasive, so term 'superficial' is no longer recommended.
- The new WHO/ISUP classification differentiates between papillary urothelial neoplasms of low malignant potential (PUNLMP) and low-grade and high-grade urothelial carcinomas.
- **PUNLMP** are lesions that do not have cytological features of malignancy, but show normal urothelial cells in a papillary configuration. Although they have a negligible risk for progression, they are not completely benign and have a tendency to recur.

### 1973 WHO grading
Urothelial papilloma.
- **Grade 1:** well differentiated.
- **Grade 2:** moderately differentiated.
- **Grade 3:** poorly differentiated.

### 2004 WHO grading
- Urothelial papilloma.
- Papillary urothelial neoplasm of low malignant potential (PUNLMP).
- Low-grade papillary urothelial carcinoma.
- High-grade papillary urothelial carcinoma.
- As most clinical trials have used the 1973 system, it is recommended that all future reports give both grading systems in order to allow for comparison until such time that only the 2004 classification can be adopted.

## Muscle-invasive tumours (T2, T3, T4)

### 1988 grading system
- **GX:** grade of differentiation cannot be assessed.
- **G1:** well differentiated.
- **G2:** moderately differentiated.
- **G3–4:** poorly differentiated/undifferentiated.

## Staging of bladder cancer (2002, UICC TNM)

### Primary tumour (T)
- **TX:** primary tumour cannot be assessed.
- **T0:** no evidence of primary tumour.
- **Ta:** non-invasive papillary carcinoma.
- **Tis:** carcinoma *in situ*: 'flat tumour'.
- **T1:** tumour invades subepithelial connective tissue.
- **T2:** tumour invades muscle.
- **T2a:** tumour invades superficial muscle (inner half).
- **T2b:** tumour invades deep muscle (outer half).
- **T3:** tumour invades perivesical tissue:
  - *T3a* – microscopically;
  - *T3b* – macroscopically (extravesical mass).
- **T4:** tumour invades any of the following: prostate, uterus, vagina, pelvic wall, abdominal wall:
  - *T4a* – tumour invades prostate, uterus or vagina;
  - *T4b* – tumour invades pelvic wall or abdominal wall.

### Lymph nodes (N)
- **NX:** regional lymph nodes cannot be assessed.
- **N0:** no regional lymph node metastasis.
- **N1:** metastasis in a single lymph node 2cm or less in greatest dimension.
- **N2:** metastasis in a single lymph node more than 2cm, but not more than 5cm in greatest dimension, or multiple lymph nodes, none more than 5cm in greatest dimension.
- **N3:** metastasis in a lymph node more than 5cm in greatest dimension.

### Distant metastasis (M)
- **MX:** distant metastasis cannot be assessed.
- **M0:** no distant metastasis.
- **M1:** distant metastasis.

# Upper urinary tract tumours

- Account for 5–10% of renal tumours and 5–6% of all urothelial cancers. Renal pelvis 75%; ureteric 25%. Multiple ipsilateral tumours in 27–36%, but bilateral tumours in 2–8%. 30–75% have primary (at time of diagnosis) or secondary (developed subsequently) bladder tumours. Bladder tumours have primary or secondary ureteric tumours in 0.3–4%.
- *Incidence*: peak age 50–70 years; male:female 3:1.
- *Presentation:* gross or microscopic haematuria (75%), flank pain (30%), other symptoms (see above, 10%).
- *Risk factors:* >40 years age, cigarette smoking, abuse of analgesics, occupational factors, cyclophosphamide, coffee consumption, chronic infections, stones.

Pathology
- Transitional cell carcinoma accounts >90%.
- Squamous cell carcinoma 0.7–7%.
- Adenocarcinoma <1%.
- Inverted papilloma.
- Non-urothelial tumours (sarcomas).

## Staging (UICC 2002 TNM)

- *T:* primary tumour.
- *TX:* primary tumour cannot be assessed.
- *T0:* no evidence of primary tumour.
- *Ta:* non-invasive papillary carcinoma.
- *Tis:* carcinoma *in situ* (CIS).
- *T1:* tumour invades subepithelial connective tissue.
- *T2:* tumour invades muscularis.
- *T3:* (renal pelvis) tumour invades beyond muscularis into peripelvic fat or renal parenchyma; (ureter) tumour invades beyond muscularis into peri-ureteric fat.
- *T4:* tumour invades adjacent organs or through the kidney into perinephric fat.
- *N:* regional lymph nodes.
- *NX:* regional lymph nodes cannot be assessed.
- *N0:* no regional lymph node metastasis.
- *N1:* metastasis in a single lymph node 2cm or less in greatest dimension.
- *N2:* metastasis in a single lymph node (more than 2cm, but not more than 5cm) in greatest dimension, or multiple lymph nodes, none more than 5cm in greatest dimension.
- *N3:* metastasis in lymph node more than 5cm in greatest dimension.
- *M:* distant metastasis.
- *MX:* distant metastasis cannot be assessed.
- *M0:* no distant metastasis.
- *M1:* distant metastasis.

# Treatment of non-invasive bladder cancer (TURBT)

Intravesical instillations: reduce risk of recurrence and progression

### Intravesical chemotherapy

- Meta-analysis of 7 RCTs (1476 patients with a median follow-up of 3.4 years) demonstrated one immediate instillation of chemotherapy after TURBT decreases relative risk of recurrence by 40% for both single and multiple tumours.
- **Mechanism:** destruction of circulating tumour cells or ablative effect (chemoresection) of residual tumour cells at site of resection.
- All studies demonstrated instillation within 24h. If first instillation not given within 24h, risk of recurrence increased 2-fold.
- Agents include mitomycin-C, epirubicin, and doxorubicin.
- Immediate instillation can lead to severe pain as extravasation occurs due to unsuspected bladder perforation. Therefore, this is not recommended. Approximate 8 or 9 patients need to have intravesical therapy to prevent one recurrence requiring further TURBT.

### Intravesical immunotherapy (Bacillus Calmette–Guerin, BCG)

- BCG is superior to chemotherapy for preventing recurrences.
- Patients with intermediate-risk and high-risk tumours are suitable for BCG therapy.
- BCG delays or prevents progression to muscle-invasive bladder cancer.
- Maintenance therapy is necessary for optimal efficacy, but the optimal schedule and dose have not yet been defined.
- At least 1 year of maintenance therapy is advised.

### Indications for intravesical BCG

- High-risk tumours and cystectomy not carried out (unfit; i.e. multiple T1G2 tumours.
- Ta–T1G3 tumours with or without CIS, and CIS alone (15% or more will progress).
- Intermediate-risk tumours (multifocal T1G1, TaG2, and single T1G2): either intravesical BCG or chemotherapy. This group have a 1.8% risk of progression and 45% risk of recurrence, so intravesical BCG indication less clear.

### Summary of intravesical therapy for bladder cancer

- Low to moderate risk of recurrence and very low risk of progression, single post-operative dose of intravesical chemotherapy.
- Low to moderate risk of progression, regardless of risk of recurrence, single post-operative dose of intravesical chemotherapy followed by either more chemotherapeutic instillations for 6–12 months (maintenance) or intravesical BCG instillations for minimum 1 year (maintenance).
- High risk of progression, intravesical BCG (at least 1 year of maintenance) or immediate radical surgery.

# Surveillance of non-invasive bladder tumours

- Follow-up for life is not recommended.
- **Low-risk** (TaG1, 50%): cystoscopy at 3 months. If negative, next cystoscopy at 9 months, then annual cystoscopies for 5 years.
- **High-risk** (15%): cystoscopy at 3 months. If negative, cystoscopies every 3 months for 2 years, every 4 months in third year, every 6 months thereafter until 5 years, and annually thereafter. Annual IVU.
- **Intermediate-risk** (1/3rd): adapt above regimens according to personal and subjective factors.

# Operative technique: transurethral resection of bladder tumour (TURBT)

## Preparation

Informed consent, prophylactic antibiotics, thrombo-embolism prophylaxis.

## Technique

- Bi-manual examination (and vaginal in women) is required prior to and after resection to ascertain clinical T-stage.
- Cystoscopy and resectoscope inserted.
- Resection should be as complete as possible going deep to muscle.
- Care must be taken around anterior dome of bladder as perforation here would be intraperitoneal.
- Selected biopsies of deep muscularis propria should be sent as separate sample.
- If more than one tumour, attempt should be made to send as separate samples.
- If ureteric tumours are visible or tumour around ureteric orifices, then carry out retrograde studies at the same time to demonstrate extent of invasion and limits, as well as synchronous tumours in ipsilateral and contralateral ureters.
- After adequate haemostasis, if large resection then 3-way irrigation catheter is required.

## Second resection

- Second TURBT leads to lower recurrence rate and improved prognosis.
- Timing between 2 and 6 weeks.

### Indications

- Inadequate initial resection (large or multiple tumours requiring time or risking haemorrhage or perforation).
- Inadequate muscle tissue in high-grade or large tumour.
- Ta/T1 high grade tumour requires further resection of tumour base (for correct staging – 10% incorrectly staged at initial TURBT).

### Complications

Infection; bleeding (uncommonly requires emergency cystoscopy and diathermy); dysuria; failed trial without catheter +/– prolonged catheterization; bladder perforation +/– prolonged catheterization (extraperitoneal) +/– laparotomy (intraperitoneal); recurrence, deep venous thrombosis/pulmonary embolus, pneumonia, and myocardial infarction.

# Treatment of invasive bladder cancer

Radical cystectomy remains treatment of choice, but bladder sparing may be requested by patient or patient may not be fit for surgery.

- Involves removal of the bladder and neighbouring organs (e.g. prostate and seminal vesicals in men, uterus and adnexa in women).
- Urethrectomy if the tumour involves bladder neck in women and prostatic urethra in men.
- Mortality of radical cystectomy 1.2–3.7%.
- No direct comparison between radical radiotherapy and cystectomy.

## Indications for radical cystectomy

- T2–T4a, N0–NX, M0; recurrent T1G3 and Tis (BCG resistant); extensive papillary disease impossible to resect adequately.
- Pre-operative radiotherapy has shown no benefit.
- Neoadjuvant chemotherapy prior to radiotherapy and cystectomy has shown some benefit from randomized study data.
- Limited lymph node dissection should be carried out.
- Preservation of the urethra if margins are negative.
- 10% of specimens are T0 reflecting a prior radical TURBT.
- *Survival (5 year):* pT1 – 75%; pT2 – 63%; pT3 – 31%; pT4 – 21%.

## Radical radiotherapy

- Modern 3D-radiotherapy, with or without chemotherapy or radiosensitizers (carbogen or carbogen nicotinamide), is a treatment option in patients who wish to preserve their bladder.
- Requires multi-disciplinary approach from surgical, oncology, radiology, and pathology specialists.
- Regular follow-up to detect recurrent disease for possible salvage cystectomy.
- Candidates for total cystectomy, but wish bladder preservation, with salvage cystectomy in case of persistent disease.
- No modern trial has compared this strategy with primary total cystectomy.

Total cystectomy is not therapeutic option in locally advanced disease (T4b, eventually T3B) or high age, major co-morbidity, and/or decreased performance status.

# Surveillance protocol

**Table 12.1** Surveillance protocol

| | |
|---|---|
| Cystectomy | *3 months post-operatively:* physical examination to exclude surgical complications; serum creatinine; urine analysis; ultrasound/CT (kidney, liver, and retroperitoneum); chest radiograph. If clear, then regular follow-up every 4 months.<br>*If pN+:* regular CT scans and bone-scan.<br>*If pTis:* regular assessment of upper urinary tract.<br>*If urethra intact:* regular urethroscopy and barbotage cytology |
| Radiotherapy | *3 months post-radiotherapy:* serum creatinine; urine analysis; ultrasound/CT (kidney, liver, retroperitoneum); CT pelvis; cystoscopy and urine cytology; chest radiograph |

# Treatment of upper urinary tract tumours

**Nephro-uretectomy:**
- Gold standard curative treatment.
- Whole ureter removed due to high recurrence rate in any remaining distal ureteric segment (16–58%) and multicentricity on ipsilateral side (15–44%).

**Conservative surgery**
- If distal third ureteric tumours then partial uretectomy with surveillance of the remaining ureter and pelvis has some early encouraging results. Long-term results are awaited.
- Low-grade, non-invasive tumours, which do not occlude the lumen can be resected using laser ablative modalities using rigid or flexible ureteroscopy.

**Local chemotherapy (mitomycin-C) or immunotherapy (BCG)**
- Early results suggest similar efficacy for prevention of recurrence and progression as with non-invasive bladder TCC.
- Intra-ureteral therapy can be given via a nephrostomy, ureteral catheter or bladder instillation using double JJ stents into the ureters in order to make them reflux.

**Advanced cases**
- Locally advanced cases may benefit from palliative radiotherapy.
- Systemic chemotherapy has similar indications to advanced bladder TCC.

**Surveillance**
- Intravenous urography or CT-urography at 3 months, then yearly.
- Cystoscopy at 3 months and then yearly.
- Cytology at every visit. CT scans are required yearly to exclude metastases.

**Table 12.2** Follow-up schedules for nephro-ureterectomy and for a conservative approach

| | |
|---|---|
| Follow-up schedule for nephro-ureterectomy | ≥T2 tumours: cystoscopy at 3 months, then annually for 5 years. |
| | Chest radiograph and CT-abdomen/pelvis every 6 months for 2 years and annually thereafter. |
| | Ta–T1 tumours: cystoscopy at 3 months, then once a year. |
| | Chest radiograph, CT scan, and bone scan if symptomatic. |
| Follow-up schedule for conservative approach | IVU and urine cytology at 1–3 months. Repeated at 9 months and then annually for 5 years. |
| | Cystoscopy, ureteroscopy, urine cytology, and upper tract cytology at 3 months and 9 months, then annually for 5 years. |
| | Carcinoma *in situ*: cystoscopy, ureteroscopy, bladder, and upper tract cytology every 3 months for 2 years, then every 6 months for 5 years. |
| | Chest radiograph, CT- abdomen/pelvis, and bone scan in symptomatic patients. |

# Operative technique: radical cystectomy

## Preparation
- Informed consent; bowel preparation (low residue diet and enemas); thromboembolic prophylaxis; IV fluids; prophylactic antibiotics at induction and continued for 2–3 days post-operatively.
- ***Position and pre-cystectomy check:*** assess bladder tumour mobility and adherence to surrounding structures.

## Incision
Either midline, paramedian, or transverse.

## Technique
Palpate pelvic and para-aortic lymph nodes. Frozen section of suspicious lymph nodes may be asked for prior to proceeding to cystectomy. Peritoneal cavity should be inspected thoroughly.

## Lymphadenectomy
- The exact role of lymphadenectomy is controversial.
- Limited lymph node dissection consists of removing the tissue in the obturator fossa.
- Extended lymphadenectomy with removal of the obturator, internal, external and common iliac nodes, the presacral nodes, and lymph nodes at aortic bifurcation.

## Cystectomy
- Urachal remnant dissected off umbilicus. Peritoneal incision extended either side along lateral border of external iliac and common iliac vessels up to aortic bifurcation.
- Vas deferens identified and ligated. Iliopsoas fascia incised and reflected medially.
- Obturator nerve identified and preserved. Internal iliac artery dissected free and anterior division divided and ligated.
- Ureters identified at crossing with common iliac bifurcation, dissected free for 3–4cm and ligated. Using ureter stump, the posteromedial border opens up Denonvillier's space.
- Endopelvic fascia opened on either side of prostate. Blunt dissection to develop posterior space using already created space posteromedial to ureters. Denonvilliers fascia opened between prostate and rectum: care taken to protect rectum.
- Puboprostatic ligaments anteriorly divided and prostatic plexus controlled with 1–2 sutures of 2/0 vicryl or PDS placed near prostate apex.
- Division distal to prostate apex made and specimen with bladder, prostate and seminal vesicals removed.
- Urethral remnant over sewn and haemostasis achieved. 2 tube drains placed in pelvic cavity and wound closed in layers.

### Women
- The fallopian tubes, ovaries, uterus, cervix, and anterior vagina are usually removed.
- In a woman keen to preserve sexual function with a tumour away from the trigone, the anterior vaginal wall and urethra are preserved.

- The reproductive organs should be spared if future fertility is a consideration in the younger patient.
- Urethrectomy must be avoided in women considering bladder substitution if tumour is away from bladder neck.
- To allow for ureteral mobilization and ligation, the uterine and vaginal arteries branching from hypogastric artery are ligated.
- To mobilize anterior pelvic organs, incision in posterior peritoneum is made to rectovaginal space.
- Posterior vaginal wall mobilized to facilitate reconstruction of anterior wall later in the procedure.
- Dissection is carried down to bladder neck and if urethrectomy performed perineal dissection to mobilize the urethra is carried out and a total urethrectomy performed.
- From the perineal side, the anterior vaginal wall is incised on either side to allow the specimen to be removed *en bloc*.
- The vagina is reconstructed using the apex of the posterior wall rotated anteriorly in order to preserve vaginal width.

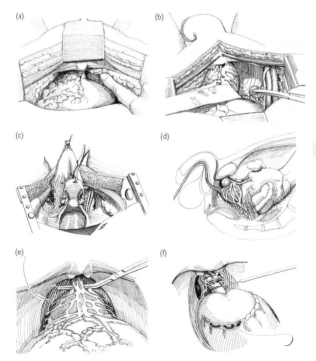

**Fig. 12.2** Radical cystoprostatectomy. Taken from McLatchie and Leaper (2006). Reproduced with permission of Oxford University Press ©2006.

# Operative technique: ileal conduit formation

- After completion of the cystectomy, healthy terminal ileum is identified with area between ileocolic artery and right colic artery selected as distal mesenteric incision (15–20cm from ileocaecal valve; this ensures maintenance of bile salt and vitamin B12 absorption).
- Proximal ileal incision depends on length of ureter and patient body habitus, but must ensure tension-free anastomosis and stoma formation.
- Small bowel anastomosis carried out as per surgeon's preference. Conduit and mesentery placed caudal to rejoined bowel and its mesentery.
- Either stoma or ureteroileal anastomosis can be performed first.
- Either end-side (Bricker) or conjoined end-to-end (Wallace) techniques used for ureteroileal anastomosis (both refluxing).
- Stents placed into both ureters and fed through ileal conduit into stoma bag to facilitate easy removal later.

## Complications

- Infection, bleeding, pelvic haematoma/abscess, bowel anastomotic leak, ileal conduit urine leak, ureteroileal anastomotic stenosis
- Stoma complications (parastomal hernia, prolapse, retraction, stenosis, necrosis).
- Sexual dysfunction.
- Cancer recurrence.
- Mortality rate <5%, deep venous thrombosis/pulmonary embolus, pneumonia, myocardial infarction.

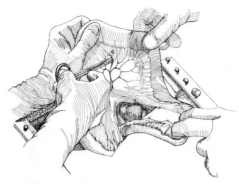

**Fig. 12.3** Preparation of Ileal conduit. Taken from McLatchie and Leaper (2006). Reproduced with permission of Oxford University Press ©2006.

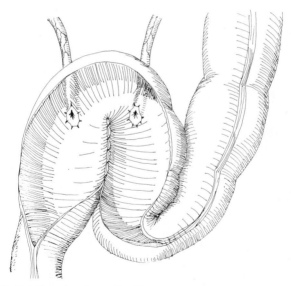

**Fig. 12.4** Alternative technique: Mainz II Sigma rectum. Taken from McLatchie and Leaper (2006). Reproduced with permission of Oxford University Press ©2006.

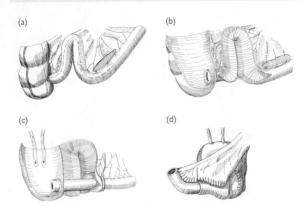

(a)

(b)

(c)

(d)

**Fig. 12.5** The Mainz pouch. Taken from McLatchie and Leaper (2006). Reproduced with permission of Oxford University Press ©2006.

# Operative technique: orthotopic bladder substitution

- A number of techniques have been described for constructing a neobladder from segments of bowel.
- Key to a successful neobladder follow the principles of LaPlace's law, i.e. good capacity, low-pressure, minimal outlet resistance, as well as preserved sphincter function.
- Studer pouch involves taking a U-shaped 54cm segment of ileum, which is opened along its antimesenteric border.
- Medial borders of the opened U-shaped ileal segment are over sewn together, and the same is carried out for the lateral borders creating a roughly spherical reservoir to which the ureters are anastomosed end-side with *in situ* stents.
- Caudal part of the reservoir has a hole cut out and anastomosed to the membranous urethral remnant.
- Cystostomy tube is placed into the reservoir and then through the skin to allow a 'pouchogram' to be performed 10 days later to ensure the reservoir is watertight before catheter removal.
- Other types of pouch include using 70cm of ileum with a W-shape reservoir formation in order to get a larger capacity.
- Others have described using colonic orthotopic bladder substitution.

## Complications

- As above for cystectomy
- Pouch leak.
- Pouch necrosis.
- Ureteral strictures.
- Ureteral necrosis.
- Intestinal obstruction.
- Metabolic (salt-loss syndrome, metabolic acidosis).
- Incontinence.
- Spontaneous pouch rupture (rare).
- Substitute bladder to intestine or cutaneous fistulae (rare).

# Nephro-uretectomy

## Preparation

Preparation and initial approach as for radical nephrectomy.

## Two-incision approach

- Ureter is ligated distal to bifurcation of iliac vessels.
- Distal cut end is securely ligated to prevent tumour spillage.
- If flank approach is used, once renal dissection is complete and specimen removed, an inguinal or midline approach in the supine position is made in the lower abdomen to remove the distal ureter segment with a cuff of bladder.

## Intravesical endoscopic excision of ureter

This approach can be used to remove the distal ureter segment without a lower incision.

## Treatment of metastatic transitional cell carcinoma

- 50% after cystectomy develop metastatic disease (70% distant metastases; 30% pelvic metastases).
- MVAC (methotrexate, vinblastine, doxorubicin (Adriamycin®), and cisplatin) and GC (gemcitabine) are both used as up-front chemotherapy for metastatic disease (median survival 12–14 months).

## Palliation of transition cell carcinoma

Uncontrollable symptoms due to large bladder tumours (haematuria, urgency, pain) can be palliated by radiotherapy of short duration (7Gy × 3; 3–3.5Gy × 10).

# Prostate carcinoma

# Clinical presentation and evaluation

### Incidence
There are 35 000/year in the UK and 250 000/year in the USA. 24% of all new cancers in men (most common) (UK). Increasing year on year due to formal and informal screening practices in Western world.

### Risk factors
Age >50, Black ethnic origin (3× increased risk), lowest rates in Asian men, family history, alcohol consumption, dietary fat, and dairy products.

### Mortality
10 000/year. 3% lifetime risk of death. Mortality rate has shown little increase.

### Screening
Autopsy studies have demonstrated that men over the age of 50 have >30% incidence of prostate cancer. This indolent or insignificant disease did not manifest clinically during their lifetime. Screening has not been definitively proven to reduce mortality, and would certainly lead to a large proportion of men with indolent disease detected and treated (with the subsequent genitourinary and rectal morbidity associated with treatment). Trials in USA, UK, and Europe are currently evaluating role of screening and treatment.

### Prostate specific antigen
PSA (kallikrein-like serine protease) produced almost exclusively by prostatic epithelial cells. Organ-specific not cancer-specific: elevated levels in benign prostatic hypertrophy, prostatitis, urinary tract infection. No accepted lower cut-off value, although >4ng/mL often used. In younger men, aged 50–66 years, prostate cancer detection rate about 13% in PSA interval 3–4ng/mL; majority of these cancers deemed clinically significant. Even lower cut-off levels have been proposed. It is estimated that if USA took 2.5ng/ml as cut-off value, number of cases per year would rise to 750 000 (Table 13.1).

**Table 13.1** Risk of PCa in relation to low PSA values PSA level

| PSA values (ng/mL) | Risk of PCa |
| --- | --- |
| 0–0.5 | 6.6% |
| 0.6–1 | 10.1% |
| 1.1–2 | 17.0% |
| 2.1–3 | 23.9% |
| 3.1–4 | 26.9% |

### Other PSA parameters
Some use. Free:total ratio <20% and PSA velocity >0.75ng/ml/year have a better detection rate.

# Transrectal ultrasound and biopsy

If clinical suspicion of prostate cancer, transrectal ultrasound (TRUS) guided biopsy required.

## Procedure

- Informed consent, antibiotic prophylaxis, left lateral position, and peri-prostatic anaesthetic block usually required.
- Biplanar or end-firing USS probe used with attachment for allowing biopsy needle to traverse probe.
- Volume measurements taken and gland, fully assessed for hypoechoic areas and calcification. Biopsies taken in systematic fashion.
- Although 6-core biopsies were the standard recent evidence shows 12-core systematic biopsies with targeting of the lateral peripheral zone raises detection rates.
- TRUS biopsies miss 10–20% of disease or undergrade/overgrade cancer due to sampling error and undersampling of areas, such as the apex and anterior transition zone.
- Targeted biopsies using USS Doppler signal, tissue characterization, elastography, and new MRI techniques, significantly increase detection, but are not yet in widespread use.
- Transperineal biopsies with systematic 5mm sampling of the prostate under general/spinal anaesthetic in lithotomy position: accuracy of 95% without increased morbidity, but have cost implications.
- ***Complications:*** infection (1–2%), sepsis rare, but life-threatening, haematuria (most cases), prostate bleed (most cases), dysuria (most), retention (0–5%).

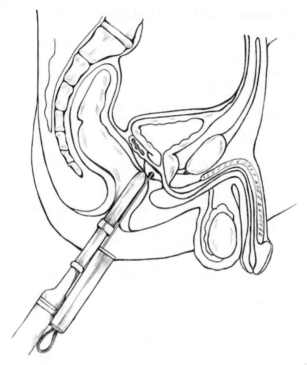

**Fig. 13.1** Trans-rectal ultrasound biopsy of the prostate

# Gleason grading and staging

## The 2002 TNM (tumour node metastasis) classification for prostate cancer

### Primary tumour (T)
- **TX:** primary tumour cannot be assessed.
- **T0:** no evidence of primary tumour.
- **T1:** clinically not apparent tumour, not palpable or visible by imaging.
- **T1a:** tumour incidental histological finding in 5% or less of tissue resected.
- **T1b:** tumour incidental histological finding in more than 5% of tissue resected.
- **T1c:** tumour identified by needle biopsy [e.g. because of elevated prostate-specific antigen (PSA) level].
- **T2:** tumour confined within the prostate.[1]
- **T2a:** tumour involves half of one lobe or less.
- **T2b:** tumour involves more than half of one lobe, but not both lobes.
- **T2c:** tumour involves both lobes.
- **T3:** tumour extends through the prostatic capsule.[2]
- **T3a:** extracapsular extension (unilateral or bilateral).
- **T3b:** tumour invades seminal vesicle(s).
- **T4:** tumour is fixed or invades adjacent structures other than seminal vesicles: bladder neck, external sphincter, rectum, levator muscles, or pelvic wall.

### Regional lymph nodes (N)[3]
- **NX:** regional lymph nodes cannot be assessed.
- **N0:** no regional lymph node metastasis.
- **N1:** regional lymph node metastasis.

### Distant metastasis (M)[4]
- **MX:** distant metastasis cannot be assessed.
- **M0:** no distant metastasis.
- **M1:** distant metastasis.
- **M1a:** non-regional lymph node(s).
- **M1b:** bone(s).

M1c Other site(s)

1 Tumour found in one or both lobes by needle biopsy, but not palpable or visible by imaging, is classified as T1c.

2 Invasion into the prostatic apex or into (but not beyond) the prostate capsule, is not classified as T3, but as T2.

3 Metastasis no larger than 0.2cm can be designated pN1mi.

4 When more than one site of metastasis is present, the most advanced category should be used.

## Guidelines for staging

### Local staging (T-staging)
- Based on findings from DRE, TRUS, and possibly CT or MRI.
- Further information is provided by the number and sites of positive prostate biopsies, tumour grade, and level of serum PSA

### Lymph node status (N-staging)
- Only important when potentially curative treatment is planned for.
- Patients with stage T2 or less, PSA <20ng/mL and Gleason score <6 have less than a 10% likelihood of having node metastases and may be spared nodal evaluation.
- Accurate lymph node staging can only be determined by operative lymphadenectomy

### Skeletal metastasis (M-staging)
- Best assessed by bone scan.
- This may not be indicated in asymptomatic patients if the serum PSA level is less than 20ng/mL in the presence of well or moderately differentiated tumours

# Management 1

- RCT published in 2005 (Bill Axelson et al.) demonstrated that the absolute difference in cancer-related mortality between watchful waiting and radical prostatectomy was 5% (14 *vs.* 9%).
- Although significant, this small difference is probably smaller in the current PSA-screen detected population.
- RCT-recruited men clinically diagnosed with palpable disease on digital rectal examination and therefore recruited men with high risk disease.
- PSA-screening leads to over diagnosis of indolent disease and introduces lead time bias.
- It is estimated that this 5% difference will not become apparent in the current population of men until after 15 years or more.
- In a subset of low-risk men, the effect may not be seen within their lifetimes.
- ***Problem:*** treatment carries >50% risk of impotence, 10–20% risk of incontinence and bowel toxicity in 5–20% (for radiotherapy).
  The options for men diagnosed with prostate cancer therefore include:
- ***Watchful waiting*** (if progression, then palliative care is instituted): usually reserved for those unfit for surgery or radiotherapy or if patient's wish.
- ***Active surveillance*** with selective delayed intervention: radical therapy is instituted when progression is detected. PSA 3-monthly, repeat biopsy after 1 year and then every 2–3 years. Progression judged as PSA rise, increased disease burden on biopsy or increased Gleason grade.
- ***Radical prostatectomy*** (open, laparoscopic, robotic assisted): operative morbidity (haemorrhage +/− transfusion, collection, anastomotic leak, DVT/PE, chest infection), anastomotic stricture (10–20%), incontinence (5–20% +/− requirement for pads/artificial sphincter), impotence (30–50%). Positive margins ~20% requiring radiotherapy.
- ***Radical radiotherapy:*** rectal toxicity (10%, diarrhoea, proctitis/rectal pain, prostate bleed, incontinence (10%), impotence (50–100%). Biochemical recurrence 20–30% within 5–10 years.
- ***Brachytherapy:*** low dose brachytherapy involves radioactive seed implants (e.g., $^{125}$I) – prostate bleed, haematuria, perineal ecchymoses, obstructive urinary symptoms +/− retention, seed migration +/− embolism, rectal toxicity.
- ***Minimally-invasive therapies*** cryosurgery, high intensity focused ultrasound (HIFU). Generally fewer operative complications. Incontinence 5–10%, but impotence varies between 30 and 90% (higher figures in cryosurgery). Rectal fistula <0.5% (more common in early experience and if used as salvage procedures). Long-term cancer control not known, but early to medium term good.

## Comparison of modalities

- Different toxicity profile.
- Differing follow-up periods with different cancer control rates.
- **_Long lead time in prostate cancer:_** cancer survival is not always possible to measure in any evaluation of treatment for PCa.
- Surrogate indicators of efficacy, mainly biochemical PSA endpoints used.
- Each modality and different studies have used slightly different PSA criteria (e.g. <0.2ng/ml, <0.5ng/ml, 3 consecutive PSA rises indicates failure, PSA nadir +2 indicates failure).
- Comparison across studies extremely difficult.
- New research fields are evaluating the role of focal therapy – destruction of tumour foci only in a similar fashion to wide-local excision in breast cancer.

## Risk categories and nomograms (Table 13.2)

- Partin or Kattan nomograms used to stratify men who need treatment against those who probably don't.
- D'amico risk categories into low, intermediate, and high:

**Table 13.2** Risk categories and nomograms

| | |
|---|---|
| Low risk | PSA <=10 and Gleason <=6 and Stage <=T2a<br>For low risk, all these parameters must be met. |
| Intermediate risk | PSA 10.1-20 or Gleason <= 7 or Stage T2b<br>For intermediate, any one of these or a combination of all of these equals intermediate, provided no high risk parameters are present. |
| High risk | PSA >20 or Gleason 8–10 or Stage T2c or greater<br>For high risk, the presence of any of these parameters equals high risk. |

Parameters such as disease burden, as measured by number of biopsies positive and percentage of each positive core involved, and PSA velocity have also been shown to have prognostic value for failure.

## Further reading

Bill-Axelson A, Holmberg L, Ruutu M, Haggman M, Andersson SO, Bratell S, et al. Radical prostatectomy versus watchful waiting in early prostate cancer. N Engl J Med 2005; **352(19)**:1977–84.

# Management 2

## Radical prostatectomy

### Indications
- Patients with stage T1b–T2, Nx–N0, M0 disease, and a life expectancy >10 years.
- Patients with a long life expectancy and stage T1a disease.
- Patients with stage T3a disease, a Gleason score of >8 and a PSA of <20ng/mL.
- Short-term (3 months) neoadjuvant therapy with gonadotropin releasing-hormone analogues is not recommended in the treatment of stage T1-T2 disease.
- Nerve-sparing surgery may be attempted in pre-operatively potent patients with low risk for extracapsular disease (T1c, Gleason score <7, and PSA <10ng/mL or Partin tables/nomograms).
- Unilateral nerve-sparing procedure is an option in stage T2a disease.
- The role of radical prostatectomy in patients with high-risk features, lymph node involvement (stage N1 disease) or as a part of a planned multimodality treatment (with long-term hormonal and/or adjuvant radiation therapy), has not been evaluated.

## Neoadjuvant and adjuvant hormonal treatment and radical prostatectomy
- Neoadjuvant hormonal therapy before radical prostatectomy *vs.* radical prostatectomy alone. No benefit in overall survival or disease free survival.
- However, *does* substantially improve local pathological variables such as organ-confined rates, pathological down-staging, positive surgical margins, and rate of lymph node involvement.
- Adjuvant hormonal therapy following radical prostatectomy shows no survival advantage at 10 years.
- Adjuvant hormonal therapy following radical prostatectomy: the overall survival estimate was highly statistically significant ($p < 0.00001$) in favour of hormonal therapy.

## Radiotherapy

### Indication
- Localized PCa T1c–T2c N0 M0, 3D-conformal radiotherapy, is recommended, even for young patients who refuse surgical intervention.
- Intermediate-risk patients benefit from dose escalation.
- High-risk group, short-term androgen deprivation therapy prior to and during radiotherapy may result in increased cancer control.

### Transperineal interstitial brachytherapy with permanent implants
May be proposed to patients cT1–T2a, Gleason score <7 (or 3 + 4), PSA <10ng/mL, prostate volume <50mL, without a previous TURP and with a good IPSS.

*Immediate external irradiation after radical prostatectomy*
- *For pathological tumour stage T3, N0, M0:* prolongs biochemical and clinical disease-free survival.
- Alternative is radiation at time of biochemical failure but before PSA reaches greater than 1–1.5ng/mL.

*New radiotherapy techniques*
Include intensity modulated (IMRT) and conformal radiotherapy that attempt to boost the local dose to the prostate without deposition of energy in the surrounding tissue.

## Locally advanced prostate cancer

Overall survival improved by concomitant and adjuvant hormonal therapy (total duration 2–3 years) with external irradiation.

## Minimally-invasive techniques

- *High intensity focused ultrasound:* HIFU involves focusing of ultrasound energy to one point, thus raising the temperature to ~80–90°C causing coagulative necrosis. Other mechanical effect includes cavitation. Transrectal probe (combined imaging and therapeutic probe) inserted under general anaesthetic. Planning axial images of the prostate taken and treatment area defined by operator. Pulses fired with specific 'on' and 'off' times to allow cooling. Built-in cooling of probe to prevent rectal heating.
- *Cryotherapy:* temperatures of −20°C over two cycles. Transperineal needles inserted under transrectal ultrasound guidance. Temperature sensors inserted near rectal wall and at posterolateral aspects of the prostate to minimize damage to neurovascular bundles. Some operators insert normal saline into denonvilliers fascia to prevent iceball damaging rectal wall.

# Operative technique: radical prostatectomy

## Preparation

Informed consent, prophylactic antibiotics, thrombo-embolism prophylaxis, Foley catheter placed into bladder, cystoscopy to identify ureteric orifices, and stents placed if close to bladder neck.

## Technique

- Lower midline incision just short of umbilicus. Anterior rectus sheath incised, rectus muscles retracted laterally. Peritoneal cavity mobilized superiorly. Care around epigastric vessels. Self-retaining retractor used (e.g. Bookwater).
- If clinically indicated, bilateral pelvic lymphadenectomy is performed at this stage: boundaries for dissection are external iliac artery laterally, common iliac artery bifurcation superiorly, bladder wall medially, and point of superficial epigastric artery crossing over external iliac artery, distally with dissection carried into obturator fossa.
- Levator ani muscle separated laterally from lateral margin of prostate on both sides (endopelvic fascia).
- Superficial dorsal vein exposed overlying prostate, cauterize, and divided.
- Puboprostatic ligaments identified. Deep dorsal venous complex ligated and divided with size 1 absorbable suture along with puboprostatic ligaments.
- For nerve-sparing, lateral fascia overlying prostate, which carries neurovascular bundle posterolaterally gently lifted.
- Urethra divided at apex, Foley catheter cut and proximal end of catheter brought out through cut urethra. Posterior portion of urethra divided under vision.
- Plane between prostate and rectum developed with mainly sharp dissection as blunt dissection can risk rectal injury.
- Denonvilliers fascia incised to expose seminal vesicles and ampulla of vas deferens.
- Lateral to seminal vesicles is vascular pedicle which is ligated and divided.
- Ampulla of vas ligated and divided medial to seminal vesicles. The seminal vesicles are then dissected free.
- Bladder neck is cleared and incised circumferentially, and specimen removed.
- Care must be taken to avoid ureteric orifices (stents placed in orifices will facilitate this if distance to bladder neck is short or prominent median lobe of prostate).
- Interrupted, absorbable, anastomotic sutures placed (a grooved urethral sound can aid this). Long-term Foley catheter placed through urethra and into bladder.
- Anastomotic sutures tied. Bladder instillation will identify leaks requiring further sutures. Drain placed over anastomosis. Mass closure of abdomen.

## Post-operative

- Sips of water until the following morning at which point a light diet can be started.
- Drain removed after 2–3 days.
- Foley catheter removed after 7–10 days (some surgeons carry out cystogram to check for leaks prior to this).

## Other approaches

- Laparoscopic and robotic-assisted techniques are now increasingly popular, and have shown fewer operative morbidity (pain, bleeding, hospital stay), but long-term genitor-urinary morbidity, and cancer control has not shown superior results for either technique over open surgery.
- Once access has been achieved via appropriate ports, the technique is essentially similar to that described above.

## Complications

Infection, bleeding +/– emergency laparotomy (uncommon), anastomotic leak +/– prolonged catheter, anastomotic stricture, incontinence (urge, stress, insensory) +/– bladder neck bulking procedure, or sling, or artificial urinary sphincter), impotence, rectal injury (rare) +/– defunctioning colostomy, positive margins +/– adjuvant radiotherapy, recurrence, deep venous thrombosis/pulmonary embolus, pneumonia, myocardial infarction.

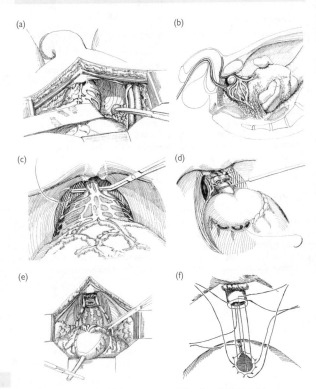

**Fig. 13.2** Line diagram radical prostatectomy. Taken from McLatchie & Leaper. Reproduced with permission of Oxford University Press ©2006.

# Hormonal therapy strategies

- *Prostate cells* physiologically dependent on androgens to stimulate growth, function, and proliferation.
- *Testosterone*, essential for growth of tumour cells. Testes main source of androgens, with 5–10% (androstenedione, dihydroepiandrosterone, and dihydroepiandrosterone sulphate) from adrenals.
- *Testosterone secretion* regulated by hypothalamic-pituitary-gonadal axis. The hypothalamic luteinizing hormone-releasing hormone (LHRH) stimulates anterior pituitary gland to release luteinizing hormone (LH) and follicle-stimulating hormone (FSH).
- *Luteinizing hormone* stimulates Leydig cells of testes to secrete testosterone. In prostate cells, testosterone converted by 5-alphareductase into more active form, 5-alpha-dihydrotestosterone (DHT).
- *Circulating testosterone* peripherally aromatized and converted into oestrogens, which, alongside circulating androgens, have negative feedback control on hypothalamic LH secretion.
- *Apoptosis of prostate cells* if deprived of androgenic stimulation.
- Treatment resulting in suppression of androgen activity referred to as **androgen deprivation therapy** (ADT).

# Testosterone-lowering therapy (castration)

## Bilateral orchidectomy (gold standard)

### Oestrogens (e.g. diethylstilboestrol)

**Mechanism of action is multi-fold:** down-regulation of LHRH secretion, androgen inactivation, direct suppression of Leydig cell function and direct cytotoxicity to prostate epithelium (only *in vitro* evidence).

### Luteinizing hormone-releasing hormone (LHRH) agonists (standard of care for hormonal therapy; e.g. buserelin, goserelin, leuprorelin, and triptorelin)

Long-acting depot injection. Initially stimulate pituitary LHRH receptors, inducing transient rise in LH and FSH release, and consequently elevate testosterone production (known as 'testosterone surge' or 'flare' phenomenon), which begins approximately 2–3 days after first injection lasting approximately first week of therapy. Anti-androgens should be started on same day as the depot injection and treatment continued for 2 weeks. Chronic exposure to LHRH agonists eventually results in down-regulation of LHRH-receptors, with subsequent suppression of pituitary LH and FSH secretion, and testosterone production. Level of testosterone decreases to castration levels usually within 2–4 weeks. However, approximately 10% of patients treated with LHRH agonist fail to achieve castration levels.

### Anti-androgen

Compete with testosterone and DHT for binding sites on receptors in prostate cell nucleus, promoting apoptosis, and inhibiting growth. Orally administered. Two types (chemical structure).

- **Steroidal** (e.g. CPA, megestrol acetate, and medroxyprogesterone acetate): act as competitors of androgens at receptor level; steroidal anti-androgens have additional progestational properties (inhibition of pituitary gland).
- **Non-steroidal or pure (e.g. nilutamide, flutamide, and bicalutamide):** sole action of non-steroidal anti-androgens to compete for androgen receptors; do not lower testosterone levels (testosterone normal or slightly elevated).

### Maximal androgen blockade (MAB)

Serum testosterone levels reduced by 95% after castration, but intraprostatic androgen stimulus is sustained by conversion of circulating androgens from adrenals into DHT within prostate cells. Action of adrenal androgens blocked by anti-androgen in addition to surgical or pharmacological castration.

### *Intermittent vs. continuous androgen deprivation therapy (ADT)*

Long-term maximal androgen blockade stimulates prostate cell apoptosis, but fails to eliminate the entire malignant cell population. After variable periods (averaging 24 months) tumour inevitably relapses. Characterized by androgen-independent growth. Giving ADT intermittently encourages androgen sensitive cell clones to accumulate during periods of no androgen deprivation, whilst at the same time reducing toxicity of treatment. This strategy has been shown to prolong the time to androgen independence and also reduce progression rates.

# Side effects of hormonal approaches (Table 13.3)

**Table 13.3** Side effects of hormonal treatment

| Treatment/prophylaxis | Side effects |
| --- | --- |
| *Castration* | |
| Loss of libido | None |
| Erectile dysfunction | Phosphodiesterase-5 (PDE5)-inhibitors, intracavernosal injection (ICI), vacuum device |
| 'Hot flushes' (55–80%) | Venlafaxine, clonidine |
| Gynaecomastia and breast pain (49–80% DES; 50% complete androgen blockade (CAB), (10–20% castration) | Prophylactic radiotherapy, mammectomy, tamoxifen, aromatase inhibitors |
| Increase in body fat | Exercise |
| Muscle wasting | Exercise |
| Anaemia (severe in 13% CAB) | Erythropoietin (EPO) |
| Decrease in bone mineral density (not DES) | Exercise, calcium+ vitamin D, bisphosphonates |
| *Oestrogens* | |
| Cardiovascular toxicity (acute myocardial infarction, congestive heart failure, cerebrovascular accident, deep vein thrombosis, pulmonary embolism) | Parenteral administration, anticoagulants |
| *Anti-androgens* | |
| *Steroidal:* pharmacological side-effects: loss of libido, erectile dysfunction, rarely gynaecomastia | |
| *Non-steroidal:* Pharmacological side-effects: gynaecomastia (49–66%), breast pain (40–72%), 'hot flashes' (9–13%) | Prophylactic radiotherapy, mammectomy, tamoxifen, Aromatase inhibitors |

# Follow-up after treatment with curative intent

- **In asymptomatic patients**, a disease-specific history and a serum PSA measurement supplemented by DRE are the recommended tests for routine follow-up. These should be performed at 3, 6, 9, and 12 months after treatment, then every 6 months until 3 years, and then annually.
- **After radical prostatectomy**, a serum PSA level of more than 0.2ng/mL can be associated with residual or recurrent disease.
- **After radiation therapy**, a rising PSA level over 2ng/mL above the nadir PSA, rather than a specific threshold value, is the most reliable sign of persistent or recurrent disease.
- Both a palpable nodule and a rising serum PSA level can be signs of local disease recurrence.
- Detection of local recurrence by TRUS and biopsy is only recommended if it will affect the treatment plan. In most cases, TRUS and biopsy are not necessary before second-line therapy.
- Metastasis may be detected by pelvic CT and MRI or bone scan.
- In asymptomatic patients, these examinations may be omitted if the serum PSA level is less than 30ng/mL, but data on this topic is sparse.
- Routine bone scans and other imaging studies are not recommended in asymptomatic patients.
- If a patient has bone pain, a bone scan should be considered, irrespective of the serum PSA level.

# Management of PSA relapse after radical prostatectomy

- Local recurrences are best treated by salvage radiation therapy with 64–66Gy at a PSA serum level <1.5ng/mL.
- Expectant management is an option for patients with presumed local recurrence unfit for, or unwilling to undergo, radiation therapy.
- PSA recurrence indicative of systemic relapse is best treated by early ADT resulting in decreased frequency of clinical metastases.

# Management of PSA relapse after radiation therapy

- Local recurrences may be treated by salvage radical prostatectomy in carefully selected patients.
- Cryosurgery, interstitial brachytherapy, and high intensity focused ultrasound are alternative experimental procedures in patients not suitable for surgery.
- ADT is an option in patients with presumed systemic relapse.

# Chemotherapy

Hormone-refractory prostate cancer (HRPC) requires a number of criteria to be fulfilled. Androgen independence without secondary hormonal manipulations does not automatically equate to HRPC.

- Serum castration levels of testosterone.
- Three consecutive rises of PSA 2 weeks apart resulting in two 50% increases over the nadir.
- Anti-androgen withdrawal for at least 4 weeks*.
- PSA progression despite secondary hormonal manipulations.
- Progression of osseous or soft tissue lesions.

The treatment of these patients may involve chemotherapy. In patients with metastatic HRPC, who are candidates for cytotoxic therapy, docetaxel at 75mg/m$^2$ every 3 weeks has shown a significant survival benefit.

In patients with symptomatic osseous metastases due to HRPC, either docetaxel or mitoxantrone with prednisolone or hydrocortisone are options.

# Testicular cancer

# Clinical presentation and evaluation

## Incidence

3–6 per 100 000 males/year. 1–1.5% of male neoplasms. >1900 cases/year (UK). Double peaks of incidence (young and middle-age groups). Peak at age 25–34 years. 50% occur at age <35years, 90% in age <55 years.

## Risk factors

- Age.
- Race (Caucasian).
- Cryptorchidism (2–4× increased risk; 10% of testicular tumour patients have history of this), correction of cryptorchidism before age of 4 (ideal), or at latest puberty required, but risk is still higher.
- Previous testicular tumour.
- Inguinal hernia .
- Subfertility.
- Microlithiasis of testes; hypotrophic (<12mL) or atrophic testicle.
- Klinefelter syndrome.
- Familial history of testicular tumours among first-grade relatives (brothers, father).

## Mortality

70 deaths/year (UK). 98% 5- and 10-year overall survival due to introduction of platinum-based chemotherapy. Prior to 1970 only ~5% with metastatic testicular cancer survived, but approximately 80% survive now.

## Presentation

Usually present as a painless lump, although occasionally present as painful lump, which may have been noticed after direct trauma to the area. Rarely, present with symptoms of advanced disease (breast tenderness, back pain, shortness of breath, and haemoptysis). Ultrasound with high resolution 7.5MHz probe has 100% sensitivity for testicular tumours.

# Testicular cancer histology

Testicular tumours
- 95% germ-cell tumours (GCTs).
- 4% lymphomas.
- 1% various rare histologies.

Lymphomas are almost always in men aged >50 (generally treated as different disease entity from GCTs).

GCTs can be divided into two main groups:
- 40–45% are seminomas.
- 55–60% non-seminomas.
- 10–15% mixed seminoma and non-seminoma (classified and treated as non-seminomas).

*Non-seminoma*
- Malignant teratoma differentiated (MTD).
- Malignant teratoma intermediate (MTI).
- Malignant teratoma undifferentiated (MTU).

GCTs probably develop from non-invasive lesion – carcinoma *in situ* (CIS) of testis [≡ intratubular germ-cell neoplasia unclassified (IGCNU) or testicular intra-epithelial neoplasia (TIN)], whose malignant transformation is likely to be influenced by hormones at or after puberty.

# Staging

Ultrasound

Diagnostic, but also evaluates whether intratesticular or extratesticular.

Tumour markers
- *Alpha-foetoprotein* (AFP): produced by yolk sac cells.
- *Human chorionic gonadotropin* (hCG): expression of trophoblasts.
- *Lactate dehydrogenase* (LDH): marker of tissue destruction.

Mean serum half-life of AFP is 5–7 days; hCG approximately 2–3 days. Markers should be measured before orchidectomy and weekly intervals until normalization. Overall, increase in markers in 51% of cases of testicular cancer.

*Negative marker levels do not exclude the diagnosis of a germ cell tumour.*

AFP increases in 50–70% non-seminomatous germ cell tumour (NSGCT).

hCG increases in 40–60% of patients with NSGCT.
- ~90% NSGCTs present with rise in either AFP and/or hCG markers.
- Up to 30% of seminomas can present or develop elevated hCG level
- Lactate dehydrogenase is less specific (concentration is proportional to tumour volume; may be elevated in 80% advanced testicular cancer).

CT scan

Assessment of pulmonary and abdominal lymph node status (70–80% sensitivity) and liver metastases. Supraclavicular nodes can be assessed using physical examination and if suspicious, CT-neck.

*Clinical stage classifications according to the American Joint Committee on Cancer (1997)*
- *Stage I*: no regional lymph node metastases are present.
- *Stage IIA*: lymph nodes are smaller than 2cm.
- *Stage IIB*: lymph nodes are larger than 2cm, but smaller than 5cm.
- *Stage IIC:* lymph nodes are larger than 5cm.
- *Stage III*: supradiaphragmatic lymph nodes, visceral involvement, or persistently elevated marker values are present.

## TNM classification for testicular cancer

### Primary tumour (pT)

- **pTX:** primary tumour cannot be assessed.
- **pT0:** no evidence of primary tumour (e.g. histological scar in testis).
- **pTis:** intratubular germ cell neoplasia (carcinoma in situ).
- **pT1:** tumour limited to testis/epididymis without vascular/lymphatic invasion – tumour may invade tunica albuginea, but not tunica vaginalis.
- **pT2:** tumour limited to testis/epididymis with vascular/lymphatic invasion, or tumour extending into tunica albuginea tunica vaginalis.
- **pT3:** tumour invades spermatic cord +/– vascular/lymphatic invasion.
- **pT4:** tumour invades scrotum +/– vascular/lymphatic invasion.

### Regional lymph nodes clinical (N)

- **NX:** regional lymph nodes cannot be assessed.
- **N0:** no regional lymph node metastasis.
- **N1:** metastasis with a lymph node mass ≤2cm in greatest dimension or multiple lymph nodes, none >2cm.
- **N2:** metastasis with a lymph node mass >2cm, but ≤5cm in greatest dimension, or multiple lymph nodes, any one mass >2cm, but ≤5cm.
- **N3:** metastasis with a lymph node mass >5cm.

### Pathological (pN)

- **pNX:** regional lymph nodes cannot be assessed.
- **pN0:** no regional lymph node metastasis.
- **pN1:** metastasis with a lymph node mass ≤2cm and 5 or fewer positive nodes, none >2cm.
- **pN2:** metastasis with a lymph node mass >2cm, but ≤5cm; or more than 5 nodes positive, ≤5cm; or evidence or extranodal extension of tumour.
- **pN3:** metastasis with a lymph node mass >5cm.

### Distant metastasis (M)

- **MX:** distant metastasis cannot be assessed.
- **M0:** no distant metastasis.
- **M1:** distant metastasis.
- **M1a:** non-regional lymph node(s) or lung.
- **M1b:** other sites.

### Serum tumour markers (S)

- **Sx:** serum marker studies not available or not performed.
- **S0:** serum marker study levels within normal limits.

|    | LDH (U/L)       | hCG (mIU/mL)     | AFP (ng/mL)      |
|----|-----------------|------------------|------------------|
| S1 | <1.5 × N        | and <5000        | and <1000        |
| S2 | 1.5–10 × N      | or 5000–50 000   | or 1000–10 000   |
| S3 | >10 × N         | or >50 000       | or >10 000       |

N indicates the upper limit of normal for LDH assay.

# Prognostic groups

Metastatic disease (TNM stage > 2) has to be classified additionally according to the International Germ Cell Cancer Collaborative Group (IGCCCG) staging system: prognostic-factor based staging system for metastatic testicular tumour. Uses histology, location of the primary tumour, location of metastases and serum marker levels as prognostic factors to categorize patients into 'good', 'intermediate', or 'poor' prognostic groups.

## Good prognosis group

| *Non-seminoma (56% of cases, all criteria)* | |
|---|---|
| 5-year PFS 89%<br>5-year survival 92% | Testis/retroperitoneal primary<br>No non-pulmonary visceral metastases<br>AFP <1000ng/mL<br>hCG <5000IU/L (1000 ng/mL)<br>LDH <1.5 × ULN |
| *Seminoma (90% of cases; all criteria)* | |
| 5-year PFS 82%<br>5-year survival 86% | Any primary site<br>No non-pulmonary visceral metastases<br>Normal AFP<br>Any hCG<br>Any LDH |

## Intermediate-prognosis group

| *Non-seminoma (28% of cases) (any criteria)* | |
|---|---|
| 5-year PFS 75%<br>5-year survival 80% | Testis/retroperitoneal primary<br>No non-pulmonary visceral metastases<br>AFP >1000 and <10 000 ng/mL or<br>hCG >5000 and <50 000 IU/L or<br>LDH >1.5 and <10 × ULN |
| *Seminoma (10% of cases) (any criteria)* | |
| 5-year PFS 67%<br>5-year survival 72% | Any primary site<br>Non-pulmonary visceral metastases<br>Normal AFP<br>Any hCG<br>Any LDH |

## Poor-prognosis group

| *Non-seminoma* (16% of cases) (any criteria) | |
|---|---|
| 5-year PFS 41%<br>5-year survival 48% | Mediastinal primary<br>Non-pulmonary visceral metastases<br>AFP >10 000ng/mL or<br>hCG >50 000 IU/L (10 000ng/mL) or<br>LDH >10 × ULN |
| *Seminoma* | |
| No patients classified as poor prognosis | |

PFS: progression-free survival; ULN: upper limit of normal range.

# Treatment: seminomas

## Stage 1

- 15–20% relapse due to microscopic metastases in retroperitoneum. Therefore, following radical inguinal orchidectomy, adjuvant radiotherapy to retroperitoneum (20Gy) recommended (relapse rate drops to 1–3%).
- Alternative is surveillance: avoids need for radiotherapy toxicity, but requires more intensive follow-up.
- Survival 97–100% for surveillance. 70% relapse within 2 years after orchidectomy, 7% occur >6 years.
- *Adjuvant chemotherapy:* carboplatin can be used as alternative to radiotherapy, but efficacy seems to be similar.
- *Radical retroperitoneal lymph node dissection:* no benefit.

## Metastatic

### Stage 2A/2B

- Radiotherapy to retroperitoneum ('hockey stick' field including para-aortic and inguinal regions).
- 6-year relapse-free survival for stages 2A and B is 95 and 89%, respectively.
- Overall, survival is 100%.
- Chemotherapy good alternative (BEP; bleomycin-etoposide-cisplatin) for stage 2B disease.

## Advanced disease

- 3–4 cycles of BEP chemotherapy.
- Side-effects of BEP predominantly reflect decreased bone-marrow turnover: bruising/bleeding (decreased production of platelets), anaemia (decreased red blood cell production), immunosuppression (decreased white blood cell count); nausea/vomiting/diarrhoea, lethargy, alopecia (hair loss), mouth ulcers, peripheral neuropathy (caused by platinum), skin changes (darker, pruritus), renal impairment (cisplatin), tinnitus (cisplatin), infertility.

# Treatment non-seminomatous germ cell tumours

### Stage 1

- 30% have subclinical metastases and, therefore, relapse if surveillance only after inguinal orchidectomy (pathological vascular invasion is the main predictor for this).
- One-third on surveillance have normal serum markers.
- 30% relapse, 60% in retroperitoneum. 11% have large volume disease. 80% relapse in year 1, 12% in year 2 and 6% in year 3, decreasing to 1% in years 4–5.

### CS1A (pT1, no vascular invasion), low risk

- Long-term (at least 5 years), close follow-up if the patient is willing and able to comply.
- Adjuvant chemotherapy or nerve-sparing RPLND in low-risk patients if not willing to undergo surveillance.
- chemotherapy with two courses of cisplatin, etoposide, and bleomycin (PEB), if RPLND reveals PN+ (nodal involvement).

### CS1B (pT2–pT4), high risk

- Primary chemotherapy with two courses of PEB should be recommended.
- Surveillance or nerve-sparing RPLND in high-risk patients remain options for those not willing to undergo adjuvant chemotherapy.
- If pathological stage II is revealed at RPLND, further chemotherapy should be considered

# Treatment of metastatic germ cell tumours

- *Low-volume NSGCT stage IIA/B with elevated markers* should be treated like 'good' or 'intermediate prognosis' advanced NSGCT with three and four cycles of PEB, respectively.
- *Stage II without marker* elevation (in suspicion of differentiated teratoma) can be treated either by RPLND or close surveillance with delayed surgery.
- *Metastatic NSGCT* (> stage IIC) with a good prognosis, three courses of PEB is the primary treatment of choice.
- *Metastatic NSGCT with an intermediate or poor prognosis*, the primary treatment of choice is four courses of standard PEB.
- *Surgical resection of residual masses after chemotherapy* in NSGCT is indicated in the case of a residual mass >1cm and when serum levels of tumour markers are normal or normalizing.
- *Metastatic seminoma with less than N3M1 disease* can be treated initially with radiotherapy. When necessary, chemotherapy can be used as a salvage treatment with the same schedule as for the corresponding prognostic groups of NSGCT.
- *Advanced seminoma (N3 or M1)* should be treated with primary chemotherapy according to the same principles used for NSGC.

# Operative technique: radical orchidectomy

## Preparation

Informed consent, determine whether prosthesis is required, sperm freezing may need to be organized, prophylactic antibiotics at induction.

## Incision

Inguinal incision as per inguinal herniorrhaphy (in order to avoid scrotal skin violation leading to inguinal lymphadenopathic spread).

## Technique

- Scarpa's fascia and external oblique divided.
- Cord freed and soft clamp applied to cord near deep inguinal ring in order to prevent malignant cells spreading during manipulation.
- Testis gently pushed into incision from scrotal end and freed from gubernaculum.
- Cord divided and transfixed with non-absorbable sutures so as to allow for subsequent identification of proximal end of cord if RPLND is required.
- Haemostasis. Closure in layers.

## Complications

Infection, bleeding, scrotal haematoma/abscess, inguinal paraesthesia, chronic pain, recurrence +/– RPLND.

# Operative technique: retroperitoneal lymph node dissection

## Preparation

Informed consent, antibiotic prophylaxis, thromboembolic prophylaxis.

## Incision

Midline laparotomy incision.

## Technique

Assess abdominal contents and retroperitoneum. Posterior peritoneum incised along right colic gutter to caecum. Small bowel mesentery incised superiorly to ligament of Treitz. Inferior mesenteric vein divided to allow pancreas to be rotated superiorly. Small bowel removed outside the abdomen and hepatic flexure of colon may need mobilizing in some cases. Care should be taken to preserve ureters and sympathetic chain.

### Right side tumours

Left para-aortic nodes (lateral to ureter from upper border of renal vein to inferior mesenteric artery level); all interaortocaval nodes; precaval and paracaval nodes; right common iliac nodes (with right ureter as lateral limit).

### Left-sided tumours

- Left para-aortic nodes (from renal vein to bifurcation of common iliac lateral to left ureter); nodes in front of aorta; interaortocaval region (inferior to renal vein to inferior mesenteric artery).
- If gross disease is palpated, consideration must be given to specific removal or even bilateral RPLND.

### Complications

Renal/great vessel vascular damage, lymphocoele, ureteric damage, small bowel damage, recurrence +/− re-exploration, deep venous thrombosis, pulmonary embolus, pneumonia

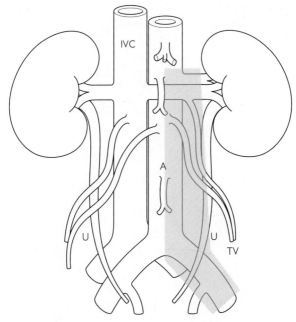

**Fig. 14.1** Retroperitoneal lymph node dissection extent of resection—left sided tumours.

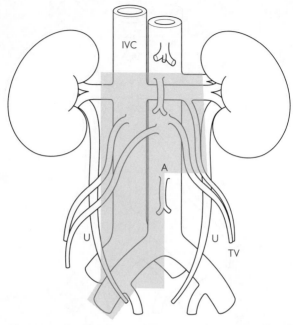

**Fig. 14.2** Retroperitoneal lymph node dissection extent of resection—right sided tumours.

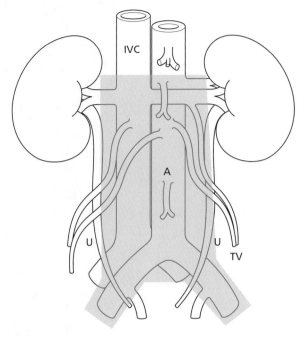

**Fig. 14.3** TV, testicular vessels; U, ureter; A, aorta; IVC, inferior vena cava. Bilateral RPLND.

# Soft tissue sarcoma

# Introduction

Soft tissue sarcomas are a heterogeneous group of rare malignancies that arise in cells of mesenchymal origin. There are approximately 1400 new soft tissue sarcomas diagnosed every year in UK.

They commonly present as an asymptomatic mass, with the timing of presentation and the size at presentation are largely dependent on the site of the tumour, i.e. patients are more likely to present earlier with small distal extremity tumours than they are to present with small retroperi-toneal or proximal extremity tumour as they tend to reach a larger size before they become noticeable to the patient.

Soft tissue sarcoma sites include limbs (50%), gastrointestinal tract (25%), retroperitoneal sarcomas (15–20%), and head and neck tumours (9%).

Treatment is primary surgical excision of the tumour with *en-bloc* resection of any involved structures with the aim of achieving clear margins. Radiotherapy and chemotherapy have a more limited role and are used where margins are threatened, the tumour is high grade, or there is unresectable or metastatic disease.

# Biopsy in sarcoma surgery

Biopsy to obtain a histopathological specimen remains the only definitive means of diagnosis in soft tissue sarcoma. It allows for microscopic and immunohistochemical examination to guide further treatment. It also allows the surgeon to establish the grade of the tumour pre-operatively; however, many tumours are heterogeneous and the grade may be worse than suggested by needle biopsy.

In certain cases biopsy is not recommended due to the risk of haemorrhage and the increased risk of tumour dissemination (e.g. in GIST and retroperitoneal sarcoma). Pre-operative biopsy may therefore not always be appropriate. The need to get pre-operative histology is based on the extent of the disease, the likelihood of complete surgical resection, suspicion of a different tumour type (e.g. lymphoma or germ cell tumour), and the need for neoadjuvant therapy.

Some controversy exists as to the recommended biopsy method. Types of biopsy include:
- *Core needle biopsy:*
  - advantages – quick, cheap, few complications, can be performed in outpatients, reliable;
  - disadvantages – less tissue for diagnosis, sampling error, e.g. underestimate grade.
- *Incision biopsy:*
  - advantages – more tissue for diagnosis;
  - disadvantages – higher complication rate than core biopsy, usually requires day case admission.
- *Excision biopsy:*
  - advantages – large amount of tissue for diagnosis;
  - disadvantages – following excision biopsy the anatomy of the excision site becomes distorted making further treatment more difficult.

# Staging

Several staging systems are recognized in soft tissue sarcoma (Table 15.1).

**Table 15.1** Surgical staging system by Musculoskeletal Tumour Society

| Stage | Grade | Local extent | Metastasis |
|---|---|---|---|
| I–A | Low | Intracompartmental | None |
| I–B | Low | Extracompartmental | None |
| II–A | High | Intracompartmental | None |
| II–B | High | Extracompartmental | None |
| III | Any | Any | Present |

*Intra-compartmental* tumours are confined to the boundaries of well-defined anatomical structures.

*Extra-compartmental* tumours are those that are within or involve secondarily extrafascial spaces or planes that have no natural anatomical barriers to extension.

**Table 15.2** Staging of soft tissue sarcomas (AJCC, 2002)

| Stage | | | | | | |
|---|---|---|---|---|---|---|
| I | T1a, 1b, 2a, 2b | N0 | M0 | G1–2 | G1 | Low |
| II | T1a, 1b, 2a | N0 | M0 | G3–4 | G2–3 | High |
| III | T2b | N0 | M0 | G3–4 | G2–3 | High |
| IV | Any T | N1 | M0 | Any G | Any G | High or low |
| | Any T | N0 | M1 | Any G | Any G | High or low |

## AJCC Cancer Staging

### Primary tumour (T)

- **TX:** primary tumour cannot be assessed.
- **T0:** no evidence of primary tumour.
- **T1:** tumour 5cm or less in greatest dimension.
- **T1a:** superficial tumour.
- **T1b:** deep tumour.
- **T2:** tumour more than 5cm in greatest dimension.
- **T2a:** superficial tumour.
- **T2b:** deep tumour.

### Regional lymph nodes (N)

- **NX:** regional lymph nodes cannot be assessed.
- **N0:** no regional lymph node metastasis.
- **N1:** regional lymph node metastasis.

### Distant metastases (M)

- **MX:** distant metastasis cannot be assessed.
- **M0:** no distant metastasis.
- **M1:** distant metastases.

### Histologic grade (G)

- **GX:** grade cannot be assessed.
- **G1:** well differentiated.
- **G2:** moderately differentiated.
- **G3:** poorly differentiated.
- **G4:** poorly differentiated or undifferentiated (4-tiered systems only).

Superficial tumour is located exclusively above the superficial fascia without invasion of the fascia; deep tumour is located either exclusively beneath the superficial fascia, superficial to the fascia with invasion of or through the fascia, or both superficial to and beneath the fascia.

Retroperitoneal, mediastinal, and pelvic sarcomas, deep tumours.

## The Intergroup Rhabdomyosarcoma Study group staging system

- **Group I:** localized disease with complete surgical resection. No evidence of regional nodal involvement.
- **Group II:**
  - IIA – macroscopically resected disease with microscopic residual disease and no regional involvement;
  - IIB – complete resection with no residual disease, but they also have regional disease with involved nodes;
  - IIC – microscopic residual disease and involved nodes.
- **Group III:** gross residual disease.
- **Group IV:** distant metastasis at the time of diagnosis.

### Further reading

AJCC. *Cancer Staging*, 6th edn. 2002.

# Principles of sarcoma surgery

## NICE recommendations

- All patients with a diagnosis of soft tissue sarcoma should have their care supervised by or in conjunction with a specialist sarcoma MDT.
- Cancer networks should arrange diagnostic services for the investigation of patients with suspected soft tissue sarcomas and all patients with probable bone sarcoma on X-ray should be referred directly to a bone tumour treatment centre for diagnosis and management
- All patients with a provisional diagnosis of sarcoma should have their histology and/or radiology reviewed by a specialist sarcoma histopathologist and/or radiologist who are part of a sarcoma MDT.
- Soft tissue sarcoma MDT should manage at least 100 new cases per year. If the MDT manages bone and soft tissue sarcoma it needs to manage at least 50 new bone sarcoma and at least 100 new soft tissue sarcoma per year.
- All patients managed by the MDT need to be allocated a key worker.
- Patients should undergo definitive resection by a surgeon who is a member of a sarcoma MDT or a surgeon in consultation with the MDT.
- Chemotherapy and radiotherapy should be carried out at designated centres by appropriate specialists as recommended by the MDT.
- Patients should be informed about relevant clinical trials.
- All sarcoma MDTs should participate in national audit, data collection, and training.
- Patients with functional disabilities as a consequence of their sarcoma should have access to support and rehabilitation services.

## Sarcoma surgery

- **Pre-operative biopsy** by a sarcoma specialist, where appropriate, to diagnose and grade sarcomas.
- **Resection margins >1cm:** this should be noted at time of surgery and at histopathological evaluation.
- **Margins <1cm** should be evaluated carefully for post-operative adjuvant therapy or re-resection if possible.

  - R0 resection – no residual microscopic disease;
  - R1 resection – microscopic residual disease;
  - R2 resection – gross residual disease.

- An experienced sarcoma pathologist should review all biopsies and resected specimens.
- Limb salvage surgery is preferred to achieve local tumour control with minimal morbidity.

- Amputation to treat extremity sarcoma should only be considered for patient preference or if one or more of the following tumour characteristics occur:
  - extensive soft tissue mass and/or skin involvement;
  - involvement of a major nerve or blood vessel;
  - extensive bony involvement necessitating whole bone resection;
  - failure of pre-operative chemo/radiation therapy;
  - tumour recurrence after prior adjuvant radiation.

# Gastrointestinal stromal tumours (GIST)

GIST was described as a separate clinico-pathological entity in 1983 by Mazur and Clark. They reviewed the histogenesis of gastric stromal tumours and found a subset that lacked the immunohistochemical features of Schwann cells and the ultrastructural characteristics of smooth muscle cells.

As with other sarcomas, the mainstay of treatment is complete surgical resection. GIST are relatively chemoresistant: prognosis with recurrent or metastatic disease treated with conventional chemotherapy is poor. New therapies selectively inhibit their mutated transmembrane receptor. GIST is a possible model for future targeted cancer therapies.

## Epidemiology

- Rare. <1% of malignant tumours of the GI tract (GIT).
- Incidence 11–14.5 per million. 10% detected at post-mortem.
- 70% symptomatic.
- Median age at diagnosis 66–69. Majority of patients age 40–80 years. <3% age under 21 years.
- Equal sex incidence.
- *Aetiology:* unknown.
- Arise from interstitial cells of Cajal: pacemaker cells of the gut.

## Tumour biology

- KIT proto-oncogene (c-kit) encodes the KIT protein.
- KIT protein is:
  - a transmembrane type III receptor tyrosine kinase;
  - its ligand is stem cell factor;
  - essential for haematopoiesis, proliferation, and migration of germ cells during embryogeneisis;
  - responsible for pacemaker function in interstitial cells of Cajal.
- PDGFRA encodes PDGFRα a similar transmembrane type III receptor tyrosine kinase.
- Mutation lead to constitutive activation of the intracellular tyrosine kinase leading to uncontrolled cell growth and prevention of apoptosis.
- KIT mutation is seen in 85%, PDGFRA mutation is seen in 5%.
- Both mutations do not co-exist, no mutation in 10–15%.

## Presentation

- Can occur anywhere in GIT. 51% stomach, 36% small intestine, 7% colon, 5% rectum, 1% oesophagus.
- Most present as bleeding into peritoneal cavity or GIT (50%).
- Non-specific symptoms (20–50%) pain, nausea, bloating, dysphagia, weight loss.
- Obstruction (10–30%).
- Asymptomatic abdominal mass (20%).
- Metastatic disease (10–25%), peritoneal, omental, mesenteric liver, lymph node metastasis is rare.

### Diagnosis

- Endoscopy may reveal a submucosal tumour.
- Endoscopic USS may aid diagnosis.
- *Biopsy:* not always indicated.
- *Options:* endoscopic biopsy:
  - endoscopic ultrasound-guided biopsy improved accuracy;
  - percutaneous biopsy (CT or USS guidance).

### Imaging

- *Local staging:* endoscopic ultrasound, CT, MRI for rectal GIST.
- *Staging of distant spread:* CT chest/abdomen/pelvis, PET, CT.

### Pathology

- *Macroscopically:* well circumscribed mass surrounded by pseudocapsule.
- *Microscopically:* 70% spindle shaped, 20% epithelioid, 10% pleomorphic. Large tumours often have cystic degeneration or central necrosis.
- *Immunohistochemistry:* 95% KIT (CD117) positive, >70% protein kinase c-θ positive, 95% desmin negative, 95% S-100 negative.

### Chemotherapy and radiotherapy

GIST are chemotherapy resistant. Radiotherapy limited by toxicity to surrounding organs.

### Surgery

- Surgery is standard treatment for non-metastatic GISTs.
- *En-bloc* resection of intact tumour with pseudocapsule and any involved structures (i.e. negative margins).
- Avoid tumour spillage.
- No need for lymphadenectomy.
- Local recurrence may be managed surgically.

### Imatinib (GLIVEC, Novartis)

- Selective tyrosine kinase inhibitor binds to Mutant KIT.
- Acts to block intracellular signal transduction and turns off abnormal cell activation.
- Treatment is for inoperable or recurrent/metastatic disease and should be continued until there is disease progression.
- At 52 months phase 2 trial B2222 showed: 16 % stable disease, 67% partial response, 1% complete response.

### Prognosis

- *Pre Imatinib:* 45–65% 5-year survival, 40–90% chance of recurrence (local or distant), 10–20-month survival after diagnosis of recurrence.
- *Post-Imatinib:* median overall survival 4.8 years.
- All GIST should be managed by a specialist sarcoma MDT.
- Gastro-intestinal stromal tumours (GIST) are managed differently to other intra-abdominal sarcoma.
- Local staging includes CT abdomen and pelvis with contrast +/– MRI, endoscopy and endoscopic ultrasound.
- Distant staging includes chest CT/CXR.

- Biopsy may cause tumour dissemination or haemorrhage.
- Endoscopic ultrasound guided biopsy is preferred over percutaneous.
- If the tumour is easily resectable biopsy may not be indicated.
- Need biopsy for neoadjuvant therapy.
- 85–95% GIST CD117 (KIT) positive immunochemistry.
- Consider using investigational mutational analysis in KIT negative tumours.
- Surgical resection is the primary treatment for GIST.
- Rupture of tumour capsule should be avoided.
- Imatinib mesylate (Glivec®) is a selective tyrosine kinase inhibitor and can improve progression-free survival in unresectable/metastatic KIT positive GIST.
- Sunitinib malate (Sutent®) is a multi-targeted tyrosine kinase inhibitor that can invoke response in imatinib resistant GIST.
- Imatinib may be used in the neo-adjuvant setting to downsize the tumour prior to resection in patients with marginally resectable GIST.
- Imatinib should be continued unless side effects become too severe.
- KIT negative GIST may also respond to imatinib and should be given a therapeutic trial.
- Complete surgical resection is possible in 85% of patients but recurrence rate is 50%.
- Recurrent disease represents loco-regional metastasis/ infiltrative spread and carries the same prognosis as metastatic disease.
- Stopping imatinib in GIST that is refractory may result in a tumour flare and increased rate of progression.
- Radiotherapy is only considered for bone metastasis (rare).
- Patients with limited progressive disease or widespread systemic disease and good performance status dose of imatinib may be increased or sunitinib may be considered.

**Table 15.3** Surgical procedure for GISTs by tumour location

| | |
|---|---|
| Gastric fundus, greater curve | Laparoscopic / open stapled wedge resection or partial gastrectomy |
| Lesser curve | Laparoscopic / open wedge resection or laparoscopic transgastric resection |
| Posterior wall | Laparoscopic/ open anterior gastrotomy + wedge resection intraluminally or lap transgastric resection |
| Pyloric/antral | Laparoscopic/ open resection after Kocher's |
| Duodenal | Local resection or PPPD Whipple's |
| Pancreatic | PPPD, Standard Whipple's , splenic preserving distal pancreatectomy |
| Small or large bowel | Laproscopic or open standard resection |
| Rectum | Trans endoscopic mucosal resection if possible |
| Retroperitoneal | En-bloc resection |

**Further reading**

Mazur MT, Clark HB. Gastric stromal tumors. Reappraisal of histogenesis. *Am J Surg Pathol* 1983; **7**(6):507–19.

# Other intra-abdominal sarcomas

- All intra-abdominal sarcoma should be managed by a specialist sarcoma MDT.
- Imaging with CT chest/abdomen/pelvis.
- Biopsy.
- Primary surgical resection is treatment of choice.
- Patients with solitary metastasis may benefit from resection of the primary and resection/ablation of the metastasis.
- Unresectable primary or metastatic GI sarcomas have a poor prognosis.
- Palliation with chemotherapy, radiotherapy, surgery, supportive care.
- Recurrent disease may be surgically resected.

# Desmoid tumours

Desmoid tumours are a locally aggressive tumour with a high local recurrence rate. Although they are histologically benign they have been included due to their locally aggressive nature. They are commonly found in the rectus abdominis muscle, although they may arise in any skeletal muscle and are thought to arise from myofibroblast cells.

## Epidemiology
- Rare. account for 0.03% neoplasms, 3% soft tissue tumours.
- Associated with familial ademomatous polyposis coli/Gardner syndrome (may develop in 10–25% of patients).
- Most common in ages 10–40 years, but can occur at any age.

## Aetiology
- History of trauma to site.
- Bi-allelic adenomatous polyposis coli (APC) gene mutation in FAP.
- Family history desmoid tumours.
- Oestrogen exposure:
  - tumours are most commonly seen in young women during or after pregnancy;
  - desmoids may regress during the menopause or with tamoxifen treatment;
  - fibroblasts are known to proliferate in response to oestrogen.
- Adults female>male (2:1). Children equal sex incidence.

## Presentation
- Peripheral desmoid tumours:
  - firm, smooth mobile lump;
  - adherant to surrounding structures;
  - overlying skin intact.
- Intra-abdominal desmoid tumours:
  - symptoms due to involvement/ extrinsic pressure on other structures (e.g. intestinal, vascular, ureteric);
  - palpable mass.

## Staging
- CT scan is useful in assessing the primary lesion and is an aid to diagnosis.
- MRI allows for better definition of the tumour and its relationships to surrounding structures.
- Both modalities help plan surgical excision.
- MRI is useful to look for local recurrence after resection.

## Diagnosis
- *Biopsy:* flexible sigmoidoscopy/colonoscopy to exclude FAP.
- **Fundal examination** to look for multifocal pigmented lesion of the fundus (previously known as CHRPE, seen in Gardner syndrome – a variant of FAP).

## Histopathology

- *Macroscopically:*
  - hard fibrous mass/infiltrating and adherant to local tissues;
  - pale tan colour with poor vascularization/infiltration may extend beyond the mass.
- *Microscopically:*
  - bundles of spindle cells surrounded by collagen;
  - regular nuclei, pale cytoplasm;
  - no mitoses or giant cells;
  - immune cells (e.g. macrophages, lymphocytes) present in periphery.

## Treatment

### Surgery

- Primary resection with wide margin is treatment of choice.
- Microscopically involved margins may be accepted if consequences of complete resection too excessive.
- Surgery is the only effective method of cure.
- Reconstruction of abdominal wall, e.g. Marlex mesh.

### Chemotherapy

- Chemotherapy is usually restricted to those tumours that are inoperable.
- Low dose cytotoxic drugs, e.g. methotrexate and vinblastine, or doxorubicin may be considered.
- Imatinib: some activity against unresectable desmoid tumours.
- Cytostatic therapy includes tamoxifen, interferon-alpha, NSAIDS, and sulindac.
- Hormonal therapy, e.g. tamoxifen, prostaglandins.
- Extra-abdominal desmoids: doxorubicin, dacarbazine, carboplatin.
- Intra-abdominal desmoid (in association with Gardner syndrome): doxorubicin and ifosfamide.
- Response rates are approximately 40–50%.

### Radiotherapy

- Radiotherapy considered in patients whose tumours are inoperable or who have recurrent disease.
- Radiotherapy can improve local recurrence rates where margins are involved.

## Prognosis

Local recurrence rates are up to 70%.

## Follow-up

- OPA review and physical examination. 3–6 monthly for first 3 years.
- Monthly for next 2 years, annually thereafter.
- CXR with every outpatient appointment. CT abdomen/pelvis with every outpatient appointment if retroperitoneal primary.
- Consider reimaging primary site if not easily palpable, e.g. proximal limb.

## Retroperitoneal sarcoma

- All patients should be managed by a sarcoma MDT.
- Local staging with CT abdomen/pelvis +/– MRI.
- Distant staging with chest X-ray +/– CT chest.
- Consider differential diagnosis of desmoid, lymphoma, and germ cell tumour.
- Biopsy is necessary when there is doubt regarding diagnosis or if pre-operative therapy is being considered.
- Complete surgical resection is the treatment of choice, but occur in <70%.
- Local recurrence rates are 50%.
- Pre-operative radiotherapy allows for smaller radiation field, but may be associated with more post-operative would problems.
- Unresectable tumours may be treated with chemotherapy +/– radiotherapy, but need biopsy.
- Subsequent resection may be possible if there is a good response.
- Palliative treatment for symptom control in unresectable or metastatic disease.

# Angiosarcomas

Angiosarcomas arise from the endothelial cells lining blood (haemangio-sarcoma) and lymphatic (lymphangiosarcoma) vessels. They can occur any-where in the body, but are most frequently seen in skin and soft tissues. They tend to be aggressive and have a high rate of both lymphatic and systemic metastasis. They tend to recur locally and have a high associated mortality.

## Epidemiology
- Rare.
- Account for 1% of all soft tissue sarcomas.
- In the USA annual incidence is 2–3 cases per 1 000 000.
- Most commonly affected site is in the head and neck (50%).
- Angiosarcoma of the lower extremities is more frequent than that of the upper extremity. Visceral angiosarcoma is the least frequent.
- Can occur at any age. Cutaneous angiosarcoma of the head and neck is more common in the elderly, whereas angiosarcoma of the breast occurs in women in there third and fourth decades.
- Cutaneous angiosarcoma and angiosarcoma of the liver are more frequently seen in males.
- Breast angiosarcoma is more common in females.

## Aetiology
- Exposure to radiation:
  - post-radiotherapy angiosarcomas occur after radiotherapy for carcinoma of cervix, breast, ovary, endometrium, and Hodgkins disease;
  - arises in area of previous irradiation;
  - risk increases with increased dose;
  - approximately 10-year interval between radiotherapy and development of tumour.
- Chronic lymphoedema:
  - Stewart–Treves syndrome is angiosarcoma in post-mastectomy patients with chronic lymphoedema;
  - Kettles syndrome is angiosarcoma in patients who have chronic lymphoedema due to radical inguinal lymphadenopathy;
  - congenital, idiopathic, traumatic, or infectious chronic lymphoedema also predisposes to angiosarcoma.
  - ***Foreign body:*** association with Dacron, steel, plastic graft material, surgical bone wax.
- Exposure to carcinogens:
  - 1% potassium arsenite (Fowler's solution) used to treat psoriasis and by vintners who use it as a crop spray;
  - thorotrast exposure (an intravenous contrast solution used by radiologists in the 1950s);
  - vinyl chloride used in plastic industry.

## Presentation

- Often present late as have an insidious onset.
- Symptoms and signs may be dependant on site.
- Lymphadenopathy (secondary to metastasis), weight loss, haemorrhage.
- Newly appearing or changing skin lesion (commonly an enlarging bruise, area of ulceration, or a black-blue nodule).
- Mass or symptoms associated with compression of adjacent structures.
- Chronic lymphoedema with area of ulceration, nodularity, papules, or bruising.
- Anaemia, thrombocytopenia.
- Hepatic angiosarcoma can present with hepatomegaly, ascites, and hepatic dysfunction.
- Head and neck angiosarcomas of the face often present as nodules with ulceration, plaques, or bruises.
- Breast angiosarcoma presents with a painless rapidly enlarging palpable ill-defined spongy mass without tenderness. Often arise deep causing diffuse enlargement.

## Imaging

- **Local staging:** MRI.
- **Accurate assessment** of local invasion into surrounding structures and is an aid to surgical planning and assess local response to radiotherapy and chemotherapy.
- **Staging of distant spread:** CT chest/abdomen/pelvis. Include CT of head and neck in cutaneous angiosarcoma of head and neck.

## Diagnosis

- Core biopsy.
- Avoid breaching tissue planes and risking direct spread of tumour.
- Biopsy should be planned to allow biopsy tract to be included in any subsequent resection.
- Care with haemostasis after procedure.
- FNA is associated with a high false negative rate.

## Histopathology

- Microscopically.
- Vascular tumours with the vascular spaces lines with atypical cells.
- Low grade lesions may resemble benign haemangiomas.
- High grade lesions may resemble other soft tissue tumours.
- **Immunohistochemistry:** Weible-palade bodies may be seen. Majority express vimentin.
- Focally factor VIII-related antigen positive.
- CD34/CD31 positive in the majority of cases.
- BNH9 positive in 72% cases.
- Cytokeratin positive in 35%.
- Epithelial membrane antigen negative.
- S100 and gp100 negative.

## Chemotherapy

- Neoadjuvant therapy.
- Doxorubicin-based reserved for high grade lesions.
- Improved local control improved disease-free survival.
- No long-term survival advantage.
- Single agent paclitaxel for angiosarcoma of face or scalp.
- Angiosarcoma of breast is relatively chemoresistant.
- Combination chemo- and radiotherapy can be used to achieve local control.
- Adjuvant therapy: high grade tumours. Doxorubicin based.

## Radiotherapy

- Improves local control, but has no impact on survival.
- Pre-operative radiotherapy may be associated with a higher wound complication rate.
- *Adjuvant radiotherapy:* threatened margins with no option for further resection (i.e. limb salvage). Reduces local recurrence with larger high grade soft tissue angiosarcomas. In breast angiosarcoma if tumour is >5cm, margins are positive or nodes or skin involved.

## Surgery

- Complete resection is dependent on the site of the tumour and its anatomical relationships.
- *En-bloc* resection of tumour with at least 2cm margin.
- *Cutaneous angiosarcoma of the scalp:*
  - may spread horizontally and vertically;
  - full thickness scalp excision with 5cm margins.
- *Breast angiosarcoma:*
  - wide local excision an option;
  - mastectomy if large central tumour, multifocal disease, patient preference.
- Hepatic angiosarcoma is associated with a high early recurrence rate after surgical resection.

## Prognosis

### Soft tissue angiosarcomas

- Poor prognosis.
- Up to 50% have metastatic disease on presentation.
- Adverse prognostic indicators are elderly patient, retroperitoneal tumour, high grade, large tumour.
- 2/3 retroperitoneal angiosarcomas recur locally.

### Cutaneous angiosarcoma.

Poor prognosis tumour, grade not a predictor of survival, 5-year survival <33%, median survival 15–24 months.

### Breast angiosarcoma

Poor prognosis, 90% mortality at 2 years for primary breast angiosarcoma

**Follow-up**
- High recurrence rate, 80% recur within 2 years.
- OPA review and physical examination:
  - 3–6 monthly for first 3 years;
  - monthly for next 2 years;
  - annually thereafter.
- CXR with every outpatient appointment.
- CT abdomen/pelvis with every outpatient appointment if retroperitoneal primary.
- Consider reimaging primary site if not easily palpable, e.g. proximal limb.
- Re-image based on clinical suspicion.

# Dermatofibrosarcoma protuberans

Dermatofibrosarcoma protuberans (DFSP) is a locally aggressive soft tissue sarcoma arising from the dermis. It invades deeper structures and rarely metastasizes.

## Epidemiology

Rare. 1% of all soft tissue sarcomas.
- Annual incidence in USA is 4 cases per million per year.
- Metastasis is rare, <4% of cases, but is associated with poor prognosis. Usually occurs in adults age 20–50 years old, but has been reported at any age. Slightly increased incidence in males.

## Aetiology

Unknown. Anecdotal evidence to suggest previous trauma to site (burn/vaccine site).

## Presentation

- Slow growing tumour. Small asymptomatic skin papule.
- As enlarges becomes more nodular, indurated plaque. Firm to touch. Colour varies .May ulcerate as increases in size.
- Imaging.
- No agreed classification system of staging.
- *Local staging:* MRI.
- *Staging of distant spread:* CT chest/abdomen/pelvis (only if suspicion of metastatic disease as metastasis rare).
- *Diagnosis:* biopsy.

## Histopathology

- *Microscopically (plaque type):* slender tumour cells. Large spindle shaped nuclei. Sparse mitotic figures.
- *Microscopically (nodular type):* storiform pattern to tumour cells Cartwheel pattern around hub of fibrous tissue. Cellular atypia. May show focal fibrosarcomatous change.
- *Rare pigmented variant* (Bednar tumour) seen in black patients. Melanin containing dendritic cells are seen between the spindle cells.

## Immunohistochemistry

- Cd34 positive in DFSP.
- CD34 positivity may be lost in areas of fibrosarcomatous change.

## Treatment

### Chemotherapy

- Conventional chemotherapy has a limited role in the treatment of DFSP.
- Imatinib mesylate (Glivec®), a tyrosine kinase inhibitor, is indicated for treatment of adult patients with unresectable, recurrent and/or metastatic DFSP.

### Radiotherapy
- Post-operative radiotherapy for patients with involved resection margins reduces local recurrence.
- May be considered as an adjunct to surgery where a wide local excision would not be feasible.

### Surgery
- Wide local excision (WLE) with margin of at least 3cm, including fascia
- Average recurrence rates for DFSP treated with WLE 18% (range 0–60%).
- Average recurrence rates for DFSP with undefined or conservative margins 43% (range 26–60%).
- Mohs micrographic surgery (MMS) has been reported to give less local recurrence.
- Allows intra-operative mapping of tumour margins with further resection as required.
- Time consuming.
- Average recurrence rate 0.6% (range 0–6.6%) when treated with MMS.

## Prognosis
- Poor prognostic features include:
  - <1mm resection margin;
  - fibrosarcomatous change;
  - 5-year recurrence-free survival 75%;
  - fibrosarcomatous change reduces 5-year recurrence-free survival to 25%.

## Follow-up
- OPA review and physical examination.
- 3–6-monthly for first 3 years.
- Monthly for next 2 years.
- Annually thereafter.
- CXR with every outpatient appointment.
- CT abdomen/pelvis with every outpatient appointment if retroperitoneal primary.
- Consider reimaging primary site if not easily palpable, e.g. proximal limb.
- Re-image based on clinical suspicion.

## Fibrosarcoma

Fibrosarcoma is a rare soft tissue tumour that is comprised of malignant fibroblasts. As with other sarcomas the treatment comprises surgical excision with the aim of clear margins.

### Epidemiology
- Accounts for 10% of all musculoskeletal sarcomas.
- Can occur at any age, but more common in third to fifth decades of life.
- Can be seen in children (infantile fibrosarcoma).

### Aetiology
Associated with neurofibromatosis.

### Presentation
Painless mass. May cause neurovascular deficit (late sign).

### Imaging
- *Local staging:* plain radiography may show bone invasion, MRI.
- *Distant staging:* CT chest.

### Diagnosis
Biopsy taken after radiological investigation.

### Histopathology
Microscopically can range from multiple fibroblasts with deep-staining nuclei to high grade anaplastic pleomorphic lesions.

### Treatment
*Chemotherapy/radiotherapy*
Pre-operative radiotherapy with a boost for close or involved margins.

*Surgery*
- Local resection with wide margins >1cm where anatomically possible.
- Aim for limb salvage as amputation has no survival benefit.
- Surgical reconstruction of tissue deficit with plastic surgeon may be necessary.

### Prognosis
40–60% 5-year survival. Infantile 80% 5-year survival.

**Follow up**
- OPA review and physical examination.
- 3–6-monthly for first 3 years.
- Monthly for next 2 years.
- Annually thereafter.
- CXR with every outpatient appointment.
- CT abdomen/pelvis with every outpatient appointment if retroperitoneal primary. Consider re-imaging primary site if not easily palpable, e.g. proximal limb.
- Re-image based on clinical suspicion.

# Kaposi's sarcoma

Kaposis sarcoma was first described by Hungarian dermatologist Moritz Kaposi in 1872. It is a spindle cell tumour of endothelial cell linage and is most commonly associated with HIV as an AIDS defining illness. It can occur without HIV infection and is seen in those taking immunosuppresants following organ transplant. Other forms of Kaposis sarcoma are classic Kaposis and endemic African Kaposis sarcoma.

## Epidemiology

- Most common HIV associated malignancy.
- Endemic African Kaposis sarcoma occurs in HIV negative men or women in Africa.
- Classic Kaposis Sarcoma occurs in elderly men of Mediterranean or Eastern European background.

## Aetiology

Human Herpes Virus 8 has been identified by PCR in 90% of all types of Kaposis sarcoma.

## Presentation

- *Cutaneous lesions:* pink, purple, red, brown-black nodules, or plaques.
- Mucous membrane involvement common.
- Tumour associated lymphoedema.
- Pain on walking (plantar lesions).
- *GI symptoms due to lesions within GIT:* dysphagia, pain, haematemesis/malena, obstruction.
- *Pulmonary symptoms:* cough, haemoptysis, dyspnoea, pain.

## Diagnosis

Biopsy, bronchoscopy if pulmonary symptoms, endoscopy if GI symptoms.

## Imaging

- *CXR:* variable non-specific radiographic findings.
- *Thallium scans:* can help differentiate from infective causes vs. Kaposi sarcoma in lung (intense thallium uptake in kaposis sarcoma).

## Histopathology

*Microscopy:* proliferation of spindle cells. Prominent slit-like vascular spaces.

## Treatment

*Chemotherapy*
- *Local therapy:* intralesional vinblastine.
- *Systemic therapy:* palliative.
- *Liposomal doxorubicin.*
- *Liposomal daunorubicin.*
- *Paclitaxel.*

*Radiotherapy*
- Radiotherapy improves the probability of disease-free survival.
- Considered for any patient with stage I disease with resection margins <1cm. Stages II and III disease. Palliation.

## Prognosis
- Cutaneous leiomyosarcoma follows an indolent course and carries a low risk of metastasis.
- Uterine 5-year survival 30–48%.
- Limb – 5-year disease free survival 30%.
- Stomach (with curative resection) 68–90%.
- Small bowel (curative resection) 40–50%.

## Follow-up
- OPA review and physical examination: 3–6-monthly for first 3 years.
- Monthly for next 2 years, annually thereafter.
- CXR with every outpatient appointment, CT abdomen/pelvis with every outpatient appointment if retroperitoneal primary.
- Consider reimaging primary site if not easily palpable, e.g. proximal limb.
- Re-image based on clinical suspicion.

# Liposarcomas

Liposarcoma, as the name suggests, is a sarcoma arising from fat cells and is one of the most common adult sarcomas. Several different subtypes exist and can range from a well differentiated liposarcoma with low risk of metastasis to a high grade dedifferentiated aggressive lesion. Most liposarcoma arise from the deep stroma, and not the subcutaneous or submucosal fat and are not thought to arise from a benign lipoma.

There are 5 subgroups of liposarcoma. Well differentiated liposarcoma and dedifferentiated liposarcoma are found mainly in the retroperitoneum, whilst myxoid, round cell, and pleomorphic liposarcoma occur in the extremities.

### Epidemiology
- Rare. Incidence 2.5 per million. 20% of all soft tissue sarcomas.
- Very rare in children. Average age 50 years.
- *Aetiology:* no known causative factors.

### Presentation
- Slow growing mass, non-tender. Diffuse increase in abdominal girth with retroperitoneal disease. Pain. Decreased function due to mass effect. Venous engorgement. Weight loss. Nausea. Vomiting.
- *Diagnosis:* biopsy.

### Imaging
- *Local staging/diagnostic imaging:* CT, MRI, USS.
- *Staging for distant metastasis:* CT chest/abdomen/pelvis, PET, CT.

### Histopathology
- Microscopy.
- *Lipoblasts:* cells with non-membrane bound intracytoplasmic lipid that shifts and causes indentations (scalloping) of the nuclear membrane.
- Well differentiated liposarcoma has widely scattered lipoblasts within a background of mature fat cells.
- Myxoid liposarcoma has a plexiform capillary network with both primitive mesenchymal cells and lipoblasts.
- Round cell liposarcoma has lipoblasts within sheets of poorly differentiated round cells.
- Dedifferentiated/pleomorphic liposarcoma has atypical stromal cells and multivacuolated lipoblasts. Haemorrhage and necrosis are common.

### Treatment
#### Chemotherapy
- Doxorubicin +/− ifosfamide.
- Trabectedin undergoing phase II trials.

### Radiotherapy

- Radiotherapy can reduce local recurrence rates, but has no effect on overall survival.
- Radiotherapy should be considered for any sarcoma that has <1cm resection margin.
- AJCC Stages II and III sarcomas.
- Palliation.

### Surgery

Wide excision of the tumour with >1cm margin.

## Prognosis

**5-year survival:** well differentiated liposarcoma – 100%; myxoid liposarcomas – 88%; round cell – 50%; dedifferentiated – 50%.

## Follow-up

- **OPA review and physical examination:** 3–6-monthly for first 3 years.
- Monthly for next 2 years, annually thereafter.
- CXR with every outpatient appointment.
- CT abdomen/pelvis with every outpatient appointment if retroperitoneal primary. Consider reimaging primary site if not easily palpable eg proximal limb. Re-image based on clinical suspicion.

# Malignant peripheral nerve sheath tumours

Malignant schwannoma, neurofibrosarcoma.

Malignant peripheral nerve sheath tumours (MPNST) are sarcomas that arise from the mesenchymal cells of the neural crest. They can arise in a peripheral nerve with or without the presence of neurofibroma however the development of MPNST is associated with neurofibromatosis type 1 (von Recklinghausen's disease).

MPNST are highly malignant sarcoma with a high risk of local recurrence and metastasis. Common sites of primary tumour are the limbs (especially the sciatic nerve), head and neck and the retroperitoneum, but they can occur anywhere.

## Epidemiology
- 50% of all cases associated with neurofibromatosis type 1.
- Incidence approximately 4%.
- Accounts for 5–10% soft tissue sarcomas.
- Slight male>female incidence in some studies.
- Can occur at any age (median age 30–40 years).
- **Aetiology:** unknown.
- **Presentation:** mass, pain, paraesthesia, weakness.
- **Diagnosis:** biopsy.

## Imaging
- **Local staging/diagnosis:** CT – able to detect bone invasion.
  MRI – allows definition of surrounding structures.
- **Staging for distant metastasis:** CT chest (abdomen/pelvis).

## Histopathology
- **Macroscopically** fusiform enlargement of nerve or a mass within the nerve.
- **Microscopically:** spindle cells. Mitoses with bizarre nuclear shapes
- **Immunohistochemistry:** S-100 positive.

## Treatment
### Chemotherapy
Doxorubicin +/– ifosfamide.

### Radiotherapy
- Radiotherapy can reduce local recurrence rates, but has no effect on overall survival.
- Radiotherapy should be considered for any sarcoma that has <1cm resection margin.
- **Stage II and III sarcomas:** palliation.

### Surgery
Wide excision of the tumour with >1cm margin.

## Prognosis
- *Stage I:* 80% 5-year survival.
- *Stage III:* <20% 5-year survival.

## Follow-up
- OPA review and physical examination: 3–6-monthly for first 3 years. monthly for next 2 years, annually thereafter.
- CXR with every outpatient appointment. CT abdomen/pelvis with every outpatient appointment if retroperitoneal primary.
- Consider reimaging primary site if not easily palpable, e.g. proximal limb. Re-image based on clinical suspicion.

# Malignant fibrous histiocytomas/ myxofibrosarcomas

Malignant Fibrous histiocytoma was the most common soft tissue sarcoma. No definable criteria for diagnosis other than a lack of differentiation. Advances in cytogenetics and immunohistochemistry have questioned the existence of MFH as a separate entity.

## Epidemiology

- Accounts for 10–25% of all soft tissue sarcoma. More common in elderly. Male:female 2:1. Angiomatoid MFH seen in children.
- *Aetiology:* unknown.

## Presentation

- Painless enlarging soft tissue mass. Symptoms associated with mass effect.
- Diagnosis biopsy.

## Imaging

- *Local staging:* CT/MRI.
- *Staging of distant metastasis:* CT chest+/– abdomen/pelvis.

## Treatment

### Chemotherapy

Doxorubicin +/– ifosfamide.

### Radiotherapy

- Radiotherapy can reduce local recurrence rates, but has no effect on overall survival.
- Radiotherapy should be considered for any sarcoma that has <1cm resection margin.

### Surgery

- Complete surgical resection with negative margins (>1cm).
- Re-resection for positive margins if anatomically possible.

## Prognosis

- Poor prognosis associated with:
  - retroperitoneal primary, head and neck primary;
  - high grade tumour;
  - high staging (AJCC), overall 5-year survival 15–60%.

## Follow-up

- OPA review and physical examination. 3–6-monthly for first 3 years, monthly for next 2 years, annually thereafter. CXR with every outpatient appointment. CT abdomen/pelvis with every outpatient appointment if retroperitoneal primary. Consider reimaging primary site if not easily palpable, e.g. proximal limb.
- Re-image based on clinical suspicion.

# Rhabdomyosarcoma

- Rhabdomyosarcoma is the commonest paediatric soft tissue tumour. It is rare in adults. The name is derived from the Greek words 'rhabdo' – rod shaped – and 'myo' – muscle.
- The most commonly affected sites are the head and neck, limbs, genitourinary tract, trunk, orbit, and retroperitoneum. Like other sarcomas it can arise in any part of the body.
- Rhabdomyosarcoma metastasizes to lung, bone marrow, bone, lymph nodes, breast and brain.

## Epidemiology

- Incidence 6 per million. 85% are aged <15 years.
- Males:females 2:1 for genitourinary tract primary. Rare in adults.
- Young children <6 years tend to head and neck, or genitourinary primary. Adolescents tend to have extremity/truncal/paratesticular primary.
- Several congenital syndromes are associated with an increased risk of rhabdomyosarcoma.
- Neurofibromatosis Type 1.
- *Li–Fraumeni syndrome:* inherited mutation in TP53 tumour suppressor gene.
- *Rubinstein–Taybi syndrome:* chromosome 16 abnormality leading to short stature, mental retardation, distinctive facial features, broad thumbs.
- *Gorlin basal cell nevus syndrome:* autosomal dominant condition – mutation in tumour supressor gene located on chromosome 9.
- *Beckwith–Wiedemann syndrome:* 80% associated with defect in chromosome 11.
- *Costello syndrome:* mutation in *HRAS* gene.

## Aetiology

Parental cocaine use. Intrauterine exposure to radiation. Alkylating agents.

## Presentation

Mass. Pain. Proptosis in orbital disease. Urinary outflow problems with prostatic. Anaemia. Metastatic disease.

## Diagnosis

- Biopsy. Cytogenetics – fluorescent *in situ* hybridization.
- Looking for translocations t(1;13) or t(2;13), which are associated with the alveolar subtype.
- Reverse-transcriptase polymerase chain reaction test.
- Screening for translocations associated with soft tissue sarcoma.
- Bone marrow aspirate.

## Imaging

- Local staging/diagnosis.
- **CT:** able to detect bone invasion.
- **MRI:** allows definition of surrounding structures.
- Staging for distant metastasis.
- **CT chest** (+abdomen/pelvis for lower extremity or genitourinary primary). USS liver. Bone scan.

## Histopathology

- **Microscopically:** small round blue-cell tumour with variable differentiation.
- **Immunohistochemistry:** stain for myoglobin, actin, desmin.
- Four histological subtypes:
  - embryonal – 60–70% of cases, more common in head and neck;
  - botryoid and spindle cell – 5–10% of cases, loose tumour cells just below epithelial surface;
  - alveolar – 20% of cases, resembles lung alveoli on microscopy;
  - pleomorphic/anaplastic – 20% of cases. subtype associated with adult rhabdomyosarcoma.

## Treatment

### Chemotherapy

- Vincristine and dactinomycin (actinomycin D) +/– cyclophosphamide.
- Other chemotherapeutic regimens have been trailed with no survival advantage (e.g. ifosfamide/doxorubicin).
- High dose chemotherapy (myeloablative) and stem cell rescue have been investigated with no evidence to suggest definite benefit.

### Radiotherapy

- Completely resected tumours of embryonal subtype may not require adjuvant radiotherapy, but other subtypes may benefit.
- Radiotherapy indicated for microscopic residual/ gross residual disease.

### Surgery

- Wide excision of primary tumour with >2cm margin, where possible, +/– nodal sampling of regional lymph node drainage basin dependant on primary site.
- Paratesticular rhabdomyosarcoma treated with radical inguinal orchidectomy.
- Bladder conservation where possible, using neoadjuvant chemoradiotherapy to reduce tumour bulk.
- Conservative surgery for vaginal/vulval/uterine rhabdomyosarcoma with adjuvant chemotherapy.
- Second look surgery for residual tumour.

*Prognosis*
- **Localized disease:** 80% 5-year survival.
- **Metastatic disease:** <30% 5-year survival.
- **Poor prognostic factors:**
  - age <1 or >10 years;
  - multiple metastatic sites;
  - bone marrow involvement;
  - primary parameningeal or extremity tumour.
- Favourable prognosis with orbital and genitourinary (non-bladder, non-prostate) primary.

Follow-up
- OPA review and physical examination.
- 3–6 monthly for first 3 years.
- Monthly for next 2 years.
- Annually thereafter.
- CXR with every outpatient appointment.
- CT abdomen/pelvis with every outpatient appointment if retroperitoneal primary.
- Consider reimaging primary site if not easily palpable, e.g. proximal limb.
- Re-image based on clinical suspicion.

# Synovial sarcomas

- Synovial sarcoma was originally named as it resembled synovial cells at histology, but is actually unrelated to the synovium. It arises from multipotent stem cells that differentiate into mesenchymal and/or epithelial structures.
- Three subtypes of synovial sarcoma exist: monophasis, biphasic, and poorly differentiated.
- They typically occur within 5cm of a joint, but are rarely intra-articular. Commonest site are lower limb (70%), upper limb (25%) with other regions being less common.

## Epidemiology

- Accounts for 8% soft tissue sarcomas.
- 30% occur before age 20.
- Most common in age 30–50 years.
- 0.7 cases per million.
- Equal sex incidence.
- *Aetiology:* unknown.

## Presentation

- Painless slow growing mass (often noticed after trauma).
- Pain (in up to 50%) and tenderness with no mass.
- Contracture.
- 25% present
- *Diagnosis:* biopsy.

## Imaging

- Local staging.
- *CT:* calcification common. Also able to show bony invasion (occurs in 11–20% cases).
- *MRI:* can be misdiagnosed as benign as tumour is often well defined and cystic.
- Staging of distant metastasis.
- CT chest.
- Bone scan if suspicious of bone involvement.

## Histopathology

- *Microscopically:* monophasic – spindle cells.
- *Biphasic:* both spindle cell and epitheloid morphology.
- *Poorly differentiated:* high cellularity, pleomorphism, and polygonal or small-round cell morphology.
- Immunohistochemistry.
- Negative desmin/smooth muscle actin.
- Negative S-100.
- *Monophasic:* positive keratin and EMA.
- *Poorly differentiated:* CD56 and CD99 expression.
- *Cytogenetics:* 90% have characteristic t(X;18) translocation (p11.2;q11.2).

## Treatment

### Chemotherapy
- Doxorubicin +/− Ifosfamide.
- Paediatric Oncology Group Trial of adjuvant chemotherapy with vincristine, dactinomycin, cyclophosphamide, and doxorubicin showed no survival advantage in completely resected tumours.
- For high risk paediatric/adults tumours (Grade 3 and >5cm tumours) adjuvant chemotherapy may confer a survival benefit.

### Radiotherapy
Improves local control where surgical resection margins are compromised.

### Surgery
- Complete surgical resection with the aim of microscopically clear margins (>1cm).
- Re-resection where possible if margins close or involved.

## Prognosis
- Approx 85–89% 5-year survival for completely resected tumour.
- ***Poor prognostic features:*** metastatic disease. Tumour size >5cm. High grade tumour. Positive resection margin.

## Follow-up
- OPA review and physical examination. 3–6-monthly for first 3 years, monthly for next 2 years, annually thereafter.
- CXR with every outpatient appointment. CT abdomen/pelvis with every outpatient appointment if retroperitoneal primary.
- Consider reimaging primary site if not easily palpable, e.g. proximal limb. Re-image based on clinical suspicion.

# Extremity sarcoma

- All patients should be managed by a sarcoma MDT.
- Pre-operative imaging to provide information on local staging, tumour size and relationship to other anatomical structures (MRI +/− CT) and distant metastasis (CT chest +/− abdomen/pelvis).
- FDG-PET CT may have a role in prognostication and assessment of response to chemotherapy.
- Diagnosis and grade should be confirmed where appropriate by biopsy.
- Pre-operatively tumours are placed into groups. Low grade (stage I), high grade (stage II and III), unresectable, or recurrent/metastatic disease. This guides their management.

## Low grade tumours (Stage I)

- Surgery is the primary treatment.
- Radiotherapy may not be needed in small <5cm tumours as they are associated with less local recurrence.
- ***Stage I (T1a-b, N0, M0) low grade tumours:***
  - surgical margin >1cm or fascial plane intact no further treatment;
  - surgical margin <1cm post-operative radiotherapy.
- ***Stage I (T2a-b, N0, M0) low grade tumours:***
  - surgical resection +/− radiotherapy.

## High grade tumours (Stage II and III)

- High grade tumours >10cm are at high risk of local recurrence and metastasis.
- Pre-operative chemo/chemoradiotherapy can downstage prior to resection.
- Local control rates are improved with concurrent chemoradiation.
- Doxorubicin based chemotherapy prolongs disease-free survival in adults with localized resectable disease and decreases recurrence rates.
- No benefit to overall survival with adjuvant chemotherapy.
- Surgery followed by radiotherapy +/− chemotherapy is the primary treatment for resectable high grade sarcomas.

## Recurrent disease/metastatic disease

- Patients with local recurrence can be managed as though this were a new primary lesion.
- Isolated or limited metastasis may be suitable for lymph node dissection or keratectomy.
- Isolated limb perfusion with tumour necrosis factor α and Memphian is used to treat unresectable limb sarcoma.
- Palliation of symptoms.

# Index